Drug Carriers

Edited by Luis Jesús Villarreal-Gómez

Published in London, United Kingdom

Drug Carriers
http://dx.doi.org/10.5772/intechopen.98117
Edited by Luis Jesús Villarreal-Gómez

Contributors
Sudarshan Kumar Singh, Tanvi R Dodiya, Rajesh Dodiya, Yogesh V. Ushir, Slamet Widodo, Fikadu Ejeta, Ramakant Joshi, Wasim Akram, Rajendra Chauhan, Navneet Garud, Pankaj Sharma, Mukul Tailang, Vinay Jain, Melika Masoudi, Davood Mansury, Amirhosein Tashakor, Sona Gandhi, Ashi Mittal, Indrajit Roy, Itziar Vélaz Rivas, Sarai Rochin-Wong, Lourdes Rodriguez-Fragoso, Juan Pablo González-Castillo, Esdras Alfredo Zamora-Morán, Luis Jesús Villarreal-Gómez, Graciela Lizeth Pérez-González

First published in London, United Kingdom, 2022 by IntechOpen
IntechOpen is the global imprint of INTECHOPEN LIMITED, registered in England and Wales, registration number: 11086078, 5 Princes Gate Court, London, SW7 2QJ, United Kingdom

British Library Cataloguing-in-Publication Data
A catalogue record for this book is available from the British Library

Additional hard and PDF copies can be obtained from orders@intechopen.com

Drug Carriers
Edited by Luis Jesús Villarreal-Gómez
p. cm.
Print ISBN 978-1-80355-831-8
Online ISBN 978-1-80355-832-5
eBook (PDF) ISBN 978-1-80355-833-2

For EU product safety concerns:
IN TECH d.o.o., Prolaz Marije Krucifikse Kozulić 3, 51000 Rijeka, Croatia, info@intechopen.com or visit our website at intechopen.com.

Meet the editor

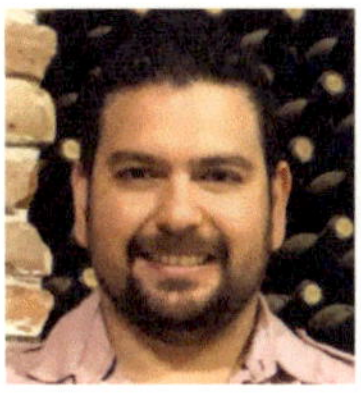

Dr. Luis Jesús Villarreal-Gómez is a research professor from the Facultad de Ciencias de la Ingeniería y Tecnología, Universidad Autónoma de Baja California, México. Dr. Villarreal is the editor-in-chief and founder of the *Revista de Ciencias Tecnológicas* (RECIT) and is a member of several editorial and reviewer boards for numerous international journals. He has published more than 35 international papers and reviewed more than 142 manuscripts. His research interests include biomaterials, nanomaterials, bioengineering, biosensors, drug delivery systems, and tissue engineering.

Contents

Preface

Traditional drug administration faces numerous challenges, such as full dosage absorption and efficient targeting, undesirable secondary effects and damage to the liver and kidneys, and inflammation and immune response. Drug carriers can combat these challenges by promoting drug absorption, enhancing targeting, and avoiding or decreasing secondary effects. Some drug carriers can even camouflage the drug from the immune system. Moreover, carriers can permit controlled release, which provides prolonged delivery of a drug while maintaining its blood concentration within therapeutic limits. This book discusses different novel and traditional strategies to create and characterize drug carrier systems using nanotechnology, microfluidics devices, and more.

This book is divided into two sections. The first section describes several drug carrier systems, and the second section focuses on nanotechnology. The book includes nine chapters.

Chapter 1 presents, describes, and discusses some examples of drug carriers such as electrospun nanofibers, aptamers, micelles, and liposomes, unfolding the properties and polymers used in each system. It is observed that fast dissolving administration is the most recommended strategy for a drug carrier system. Drug carriers have numerous advantageous properties such as biocompatibility, biodegradability, good mechanical properties, and high surface area, among others. Drug carriers are becoming crucial to avoid or diminish secondary effects and improve the targeting of administered drugs to enhance their effectiveness.

Chapter 2 discusses the selection and role of polymers in designing a drug carrier. It describes the main characteristics and properties of polymers in order of their importance in a drug carrier approach. Depending on the polymer's characteristics, the drug carrier system will regulate the delivery of bioactive molecules in reproducible dosages in a certain period of time. The nature of the polymer governs the kind of drug-loaded and the strategy of delivery. The hydrophobicity and hydrophilicity of the polymer surface determines the bioactive molecule that will be selected for each drug carrier. It is intended that polymers became inert systems with their only function being to carry the drug to the target in the best way.

Chapter 3 discusses thin films and their potential properties as drug carriers. Thin films have attracted interest due to their capacity to safely load bioactive molecules and deliver them in a regulated manner thus improving their efficiency. The chapter proposes oral, buccal, sublingual, ocular, and transdermal administrations of thin films for local and systemic effects.

Chapter 4 explains metal-organic frameworks (MOFs) as drug carriers and their physicochemical properties. These systems offer a high drug loading capacity and controlled release at the target site.

Graphene is an allotrope of carbon consisting of a single layer of atoms arranged in a two-dimensional honeycomb lattice nanostructure. Its specific and unique properties make it an ideal cancer drug carrier. Chapter 5 discusses examines how graphene quantum dots (GQDs) are used for cancer drug delivery due to their unique surface, which allows a diverse set of molecules to interact. In addition, their photothermal properties can be used to improve the efficiency of the drug-releasing activity by enhancing their specificity to the target zone. Another important application of GQDs permit is the monitoring of cellular responses thanks to the high-quality images that can be obtained using this drug carrier's platforms. This chapter addresses the advances in the use of GQD platforms for drug delivery and the biocompatibility studies reported so far.

Chapter 6 discusses microfluidics technology as drug carriers. Microfluidics use nano- and micro-scale manufacturing technologies to develop controlled and reproducible liquid microenvironments. Lead compounds with controlled physicochemical properties can be obtained using microfluidics characterized by high productivity and evaluated by biomimetic methods. Microfluidics produce nanoparticles in a well-controlled, reproducible, and high-throughput manner and create three-dimensional environments to mimic physiological and/or pathological processes.

Nanotechnology has been widely used for more effective drug carriers. Because of their size, they can reach difficult areas that pharmaceutical drugs or other drug carriers cannot. Chapter 7 reviews a lipid nanoparticle drug carrier, discussing the use of hybrid lipid polymers that provides a platform for the encapsulation and delivery of lipophilic biomolecules. These lipophilic systems are proposed for dermal, transdermal, mucosal, intramuscular, and ocular administration. They have also proved useful for cancer therapy, delivery of nucleic acids such as DNA and RNA, and as diagnostic imaging agents. The chapter explains that the nanostructure lipidic carriers can decrease the undesired secondary effects of certain drugs. As such, the chapter presents a general discussion of synthetic and natural lipid polymers with the use of surfactants.

Chapter 8 also discusses the potential characteristics of lipid and polymeric nanoparticles. These drug carriers promote stability and are disponible and provide sustained delivery. The chapter describes systems based on natural macromolecules, lipids, or polymeric/polyelectrolyte nanocapsules and their principal chemical and functional characteristics. Special focus is given to nano-vesicular systems that possess core-shell structures in which bioactive molecules can be loaded into the inner area of the particle. Moreover, the chapter examines diverse methodologies in the preparation of these nanosystems and reviews applications of lipid and polymeric nanocapsules, focusing on the encapsulation of drugs.

Chapter 9 discusses plant gum-based drug carriers. These carriers have a diverse set of advantages over chemical drug carriers including being biodegradable, biocompatible, nontoxic, more tolerable to the patient with few side effects, nonallergenic, and non-irritable to the skin or eyes. They have low production costs as well. Despite these favorable characteristics, the use of plant gums as drug carriers is limited due to a series of disadvantages such as microbial contamination because of the moisture in their content. In addition, their viscosity decreases in storage due to contact with water. In the case of green nanoparticle synthesis of these plant gums as drug carriers, the disadvantages can be limited. There are several studies showing that plant gum drug carriers can have a great combination with various drugs and nanoparticles, thus they could be extremely effective against multi-resistant bacteria and even systemic illnesses like cancer. Today, the green synthesis of drug carriers has been gaining importance because of emerging antibiotic-resistant bacteria and climate change.

Dr. Luis Jesús Villarreal-Gómez
Facultad de Ciencias de la Ingeniería y Tecnología,
Universidad Autónoma de Baja California,
Tijuana, Baja California, México

Section 1

Drug Delivery

Chapter 1

Novel Drug Carries: Properties and Applications

Luis Jesús Villarreal-Gómez and Graciela Lizeth Pérez-González

Abstract

Conventional drug administration has several issues and challenges such as full doses absorption and efficient targeting, some generate undesirable secondary effects and promote damage to organs and tissues such as the liver and kidneys, and others trigger inflammation and immune responses. Hence, drug carriers help to promote drug absorption, enhance targeting, avoid or decrease secondary effects, possess the ability to camouflage drugs from immune cells and proteins, and permit controlled release to provide prolonged drug delivery to maintain its blood concentration within therapeutic limits. Drug carriers have gained importance thanks to their various properties such as biocompatibility, biodegradability, mechanical properties, and high surface area, among others. Drug carriers are getting crucial to avoid or diminish secondary effects and improve the targeting of the administered drugs incrementing their effectiveness. Hence, this book chapter aims to introduce some drug carriers (electrospun nanofibers, aptamers, micelles, and liposomes), describing the properties and polymers used. It is observed that fast dissolving administration is the most recommended strategy for the use of drug carriers, where more evident therapeutics benefits can be appreciated.

Keywords: aptamers, drug delivery, drug carriers, nanofibers, micelles, electrospinning, nanogels, liposomes

1. Introduction

Presently, drug carriers can be incorporated in several systems that are available in the market in different presentations such as tablets, syrups, and shots that the patients swallow, chew, or are inoculated administering specific doses of the medical compound. However, children, geriatrics, and patients with specific conditions have still difficulty obtaining the recommended doses through these administration routes and medical presentations [1–4]. Until now, oral administration has been the preferred administration route for its easiness of administration [5–7].

Innovative drug carriers can include several micro and nanostructures such as micelles, nanoparticles, liposomes, emulsions, and nanofibers, among others [8]. The most important technical advantages of drug carriers can be reported as the high stability, high carrying capacity, the feasibility of several administration routes, and the capacity to be used with hydrophilic and hydrophobic molecules. The intention to use drug carriers is to control the drug release using these polymeric matrices and reduce or avoid secondary effects [9].

One of the main properties needed for a drug carrier is biocompatibility, which is the absence or decrease of adverse tissue reactions against the implanted or administered biomaterials avoiding immune response. Biomaterials can include natural and synthetic polymers, ceramics, metals, and a combination of them [10]. However, biomaterials that are applied as a drug carrier need to develop a bioactive role in the tissue such as to respond to chemical, physical, or external stimuli and possess a therapeutic effect [11].

Drug carriers can include nanogels, micelles, mucoadhesives, bacteriophages, magnetic nanoparticles, graphene, dendrimers, carbon-based materials, viral-based nanoparticles, nanofibers, liposomes, films, bacterial vesicles, metal-organic frameworks, and carbon nanotubes, among others [12]. **Figure 1** shows some examples of nanocarriers.

For all the above, this chapter discusses the electrospun nanofibers' properties applied as drug delivery systems, some characteristics of the main polymers used, describing their advantages and disadvantages. Some electrospinning strategies are also compared.

2. Electrospun nanofibers

Electrospun nanofibers (**Figure 2**) are polymeric-based structures that possess diverse customary properties that make them interesting to be used as drug carriers [13], these characteristics include biocompatibility [14, 15], biodegradability [16, 17],

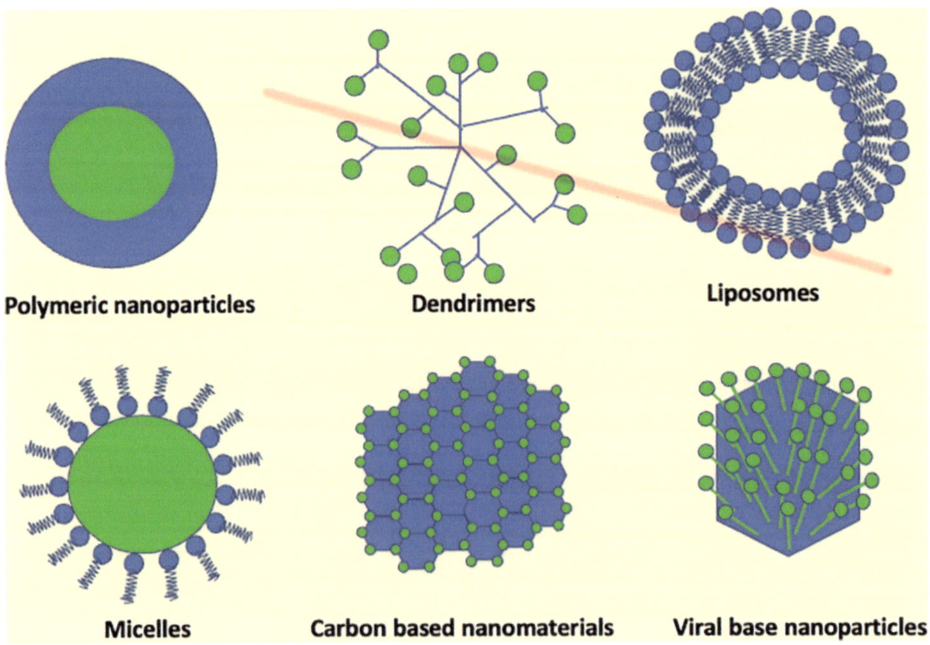

Figure 1.
Some examples of drug carriers.

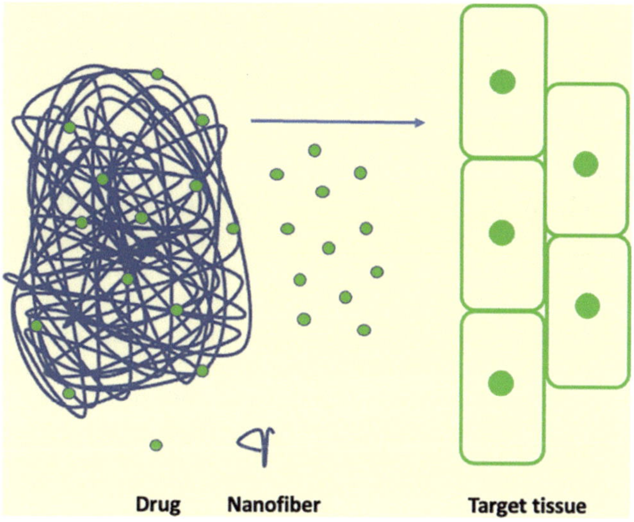

Figure 2.
Electrospun nanofibers as drug carriers.

high surface area [18, 19], adequate mechanical properties [20, 21], highly customizable fiber diameter and structure [22, 23], excellent porosity connectivity [24, 25], ease of handling [26, 27], functionalization [28, 29], and the ability to encapsulation of a diversity of bioactive molecules [30, 31].

Electrospinning is a versatile technique that has expanded through time, where the objective of this technique is to fabricate fibers or particles in the nanoscale range [32] creating a tridimensional scaffold that has wanted characteristics with potential use as drug carriers such as the large surface area, where this property permits a high drug loading capacity in a reduced volume range [33], low cost [10], and adaptability [33]. The electrospinning technique uses a high-voltage electrical field that charges a polymer solution breaking its surface tension when is injected with a specific rate, this polymeric solution is attracted to a conductive collector creating a liquid jet yielding nanofibers (~10–1000 nm) where the solvent evaporates in the air [18, 34].

There are different types of electrospinning techniques that help to incorporate bioactive molecules or drugs into the fibers or over their surface [35, 36]. The objective is to release the loaded drug at the target zone through the polymeric degradation of the fibers controlling its delivery rate depending on the polymer used [37]. Among the reported electrospinning techniques can be listed the blending, coaxial, emulsion, and surface modification electrospinning, each of them has a different strategy for drug incorporation. The advantage of this strategy is that improves the equilibrium between the mechanical and physicochemical characteristics of the functionalized resulting fibers. Moreover, it permits the adjusting of the proportion used of the bioactive component by altering the concentration added to the final solution [38].

One of the advantages of electrospinning is that is a one-step method because the loaded biomolecules or drug solution is dissolved or dispersed directly into the polymeric solution. In this method, it is important to choose correctly the polymeric matrix because its characteristics will determine the efficiency in the drug encapsulation, dispersion in/on the fibers, and delivery rate. It is reported that the equilibrium between hydrophilic and hydrophobic functional groups in all components of the system (drug, polymer, solvent) will improve the optimal functionalization of the resulting fibers [39]. It's important to note that due to the hydrophobic properties of some polymers, lipophilic drugs are easier to dissolve and create a homogeneous solution and vice versa. Such is the case of the polyester's polymers, which are hydrophobic and interact very well with the hydrophobic drug rifampicin and paclitaxel, and gelatin, poly (ethylene glycol), and poly (vinyl alcohol), which are hydrophilic polymers, can dissolve hydrophilic drugs such as doxorubicin [40].

The disadvantage of this method is that some metallic bioactive molecules tend to aggregate in the polymer solution and in the resulting fibers [34]. Moreover, with this process, pharmaceutical drugs that are insoluble in water cannot be encapsulated using hydrophilic polymers [41]. To avoid this issue, cyclodextrins are used to improve the solubility of the insoluble drugs in the polymeric solution [42]. The main advantage of fibrous scaffolds proposed for drug delivery systems is that they possess a high surface area to volume ratio, which can permit high dose load and promote the solubility of the drug in an aqueous environment improving the drug efficiency [43].

3. Aptamers

Aptamers are also used as interesting drug carriers; these molecules are composed of short nucleic acid oligomers. Many pieces of literature have reported the use of aptamers as drug carriers and diagnostic's approaches [44–47]. Aptamers are important because they can be designed and predicted to become a drug carrier for even general drugs and theragnostic drugs for specific pathologies such as Alzheimer's disease and cancer, among others. Since they can be designed, they are able to bind to various important targets such as lipids, nucleic acids, proteins, small organic compounds, or entire organisms. Thanks to their binding specificity, these specific drug carriers have shown less toxicity [44].

Kanwar, et al., 2011, discussed that aptamers can bind to a wide range of targets, which are called epitopes, which possess a high affinity and specificity. Aptamers can be used in chemical biology, therapeutic delivery, diagnosis, research, and monitoring therapy in real-time imaging. As mentioned before, aptamers are interesting for their low immunogenic reaction and also can mimic monoclonal antibodies that are proposed for research, diagnostic, and therapeutic [48].

Ganji et al., 2016, mentioned that aptamers can be generated from libraries of single-stranded nucleic acids against different molecules. The authors discussed that aptamers can be used for dendritic cell targeting, in order to improve immunotherapy in the treatment of allergies and cancers. In this scenario, dendritic cells use several receptors to stimulate the adaptive immune response through the antigen presentation route in naïve T cells [49].

Aptamers are single-stranded oligonucleotides that fold into defined architectures and bind to targets such as proteins. In binding proteins, they often inhibit protein-protein interactions and thereby may produce therapeutic effects (**Figure 3**) [50].

4. Micelles

Micelles have been importantly positioned as a drug carrier [51]. Micelles, which are commonly synthesized from polymers, have been proposed in preclinical studies

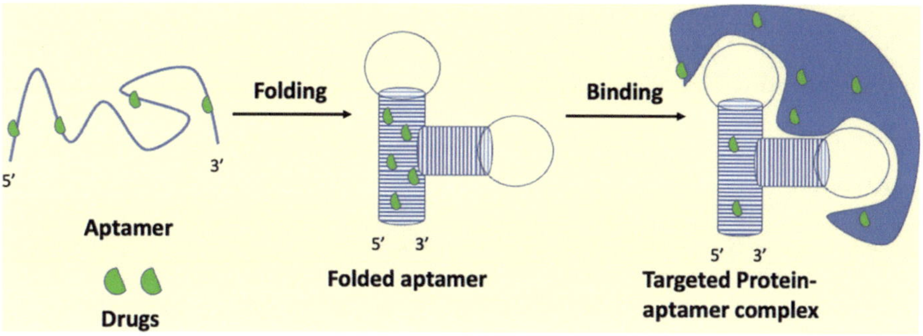

Figure 3.
Aptamers as drug carrier.

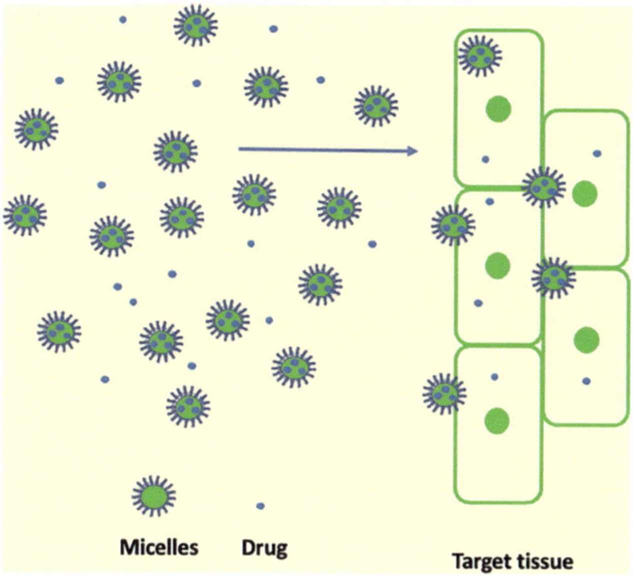

Figure 4.
Micelles as drug carrier.

for the drug release of poorly soluble chemotherapeutic agents in cancer. Polymeric micelles are created via the self-assembly of amphiphilic polymers [52].

Many polymers have been proposed to produce micelles including poly(lactide) (PLA), poly(caprolactone) (PCL), poly(lactide-co-glycolide) (PLGA), polyesters, poly (amino acids), lipids, poly (ethylene glycol), poly(oxazolines), chitosan, dextran, and hyaluronic acids, among others. Micelles can be prepared on a nanoscale enabling the enhanced permeability and retention (EPR) effect (**Figure 4**). Moreover, the stimuli (pH, hypoxia, enzymes) sensitive breakdown offers the micelles an efficient drug release. These micelles can be degraded using light, ultrasound, and temperature among other external stimuli to perform a controlled release of the drug [52].

Soleymani Abyaneh et al., 2015, prepared a block copolymer micelle containing methoxy poly (ethylene oxide) (PEO) as a shell layer, poly (lactic acid) (PLA) of different stereo-chemistries as the outer core, and poly (α-benzylcarboxylate-ε-caprolactone)

(PBCL) or poly(ε-caprolactone) (PCL) as the inner core. The micelles were used as drug carriers of the hydrophobic drug nimodipine, which is a drug used to treat symptoms from a ruptured blood vessel in the brain [53].

5. Liposomes

Liposomes can be defined as spherical vesicles, which involve one or more layers of phospholipids. These drug carriers can be used to load hydrophilic drugs in the inner core and/or lipophilic drugs in the double layer of phospholipids [54].

The main advantages of liposomes are their augmented stability and decreased toxicity of the encapsulated drug, capacity to be fused directly with the target cell membranes (**Figure** 5), biologically inert, non-antigenic, and non-pyrogenic, increased efficacy and therapeutic index of several drugs (actinomycin-D, amphotericin B, Taxol, Daunorubicin), improved stability via encapsulation, nontoxic, flexible, biocompatible, completely biodegradable, and non-immunogenic for systemic and non-systemic administrations, reduce the toxicity of the encapsulated agent, help reduce the exposure of sensitive tissues to toxic drugs, site avoidance effect, flexibility to couple with site-specific ligands to achieve active targeting [55].

On the contrary, the main issues of liposomes are linked to their production; several methods have been developed, but industries prefer to use batch-mode methods, which are characterized by low repeatability. Moreover, raw materials employed are particularly non-economic, low-solubility, with short half-life, sometimes phospholipid undergoes oxidation and hydrolysis-like reaction, leakage and fusion of encapsulated drug/molecules, the production cost is high, and fewer stables [54].

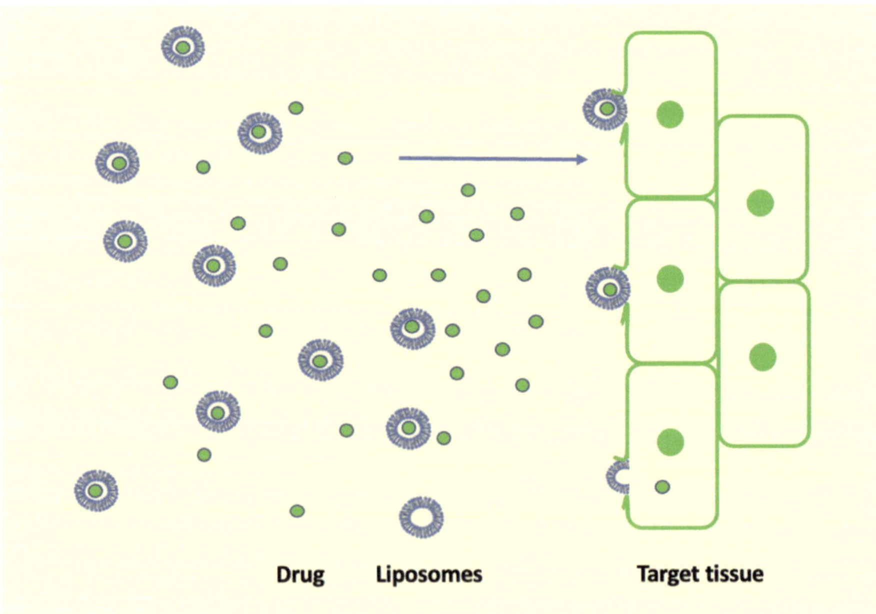

Figure 5.
Liposomes as drug carriers.

6. Carbon-based nanomaterials

Carbon-based nanomaterials (CNBs) possess a singular structural dimension, which gives them special physicochemical properties interesting for several applications including as drug carriers [56]. CNBs can be classified as graphene, carbon nanotubes, mesoporous carbon, nanodiamonds, and fullerenes. All these structures differ in their excellent optical activities and multifunctional surface area, but all of them have demonstrated a high capacity for drug loading, biocompatibility, and low immunogenicity [57].

One of the principal areas of application of CNBs as drug carriers is in the treatment of several kinds of cancer, due to their excellent supramolecular π-π stacking, high absorption ability, and photothermal conversion capacity, among others [58]. Unfortunately, the use of CNBs in cancer therapy comes with undesirable secondary effects related to the cytotoxicity of healthy tissues [59].

Respecting their role as drug carriers, single-walled carbon nanotubes (SWCNTs) have been loaded with paclitaxel, doxorubicin, and isoniazid increasing the capacity of drug delivery, incrementing drug action, improved bioactivity in the destruction of bacterial cells [60–62]. Another example of CNBs such as fullerenes can be loaded with hydroxyurea, ibuprofen, chloroquine, doxorubicin, and N-desmethyl tamoxifen, giving them a better delivery efficiency of these pharmaceutical drugs [63–65].

7. Viral-based nanoparticles

In the case, the viral-based nanoparticles are reported to be useful for photodynamic therapy due to their simple manufacturing and good safety profile [66], also they have interesting characteristics such as to possess great diversity in their structural uniformity, functionalization, expression, and self-assembly. Viral-based nanoparticles are mostly seen as therapeutics adjuvants or excipients that promote, improve, start, and attenuate or avoid the toxicity of the loaded pharmaceutical drug or bioactive compound [67].

Alemzadeh E et al., 2018, discussed that viral-based nanoparticles possess several advantages over other drug carriers, which include biodegradability, biocompatibility, known structure in atomic level, capacity to attach to ligand with high control on structure, accessibility for genetic and chemical alteration and malleable methods of preparation [68].

Several RNA viruses have been used as drug carriers such as *Brome mosaic virus* (BMV), *Red clover necrotic mosaic virus* (RCNMV), *Cowpea mosaic virus* (CPMV), *Cucumber mosaic virus* (CMV), *Hibiscus chlorotic ringspot virus* (HCRSV), *Tobacco mosaic virus* (TMV), *Potato virus X* (PVX), which have icosahedral and helical symmetries, from the pharmaceutical drugs loaded in these particles can be included doxorubicin, proflavine, DAPI, propidium iodide, acridine orange, polystyrene sulfonic acid, polyacrylic acid, phenanthriplatin, Herceptin, among others [68, 69].

7.1 Types of polymers used as drug carriers

Not all polymers can be used for drug carriers, these polymers have to possess specific characteristics such as biocompatibility, biodegradability, permit drug loading, permit mass transfer, and respond to certain stimuli, among other characteristics [70]. Some examples of these polymers and their properties can be listed in **Table 1**:

Polymers	Advantages	Disadvantages	Ref.
PCL	Biodegradable, biocompatible, compatible with a range of other materials, FDA approved	Low melting point, hydrophobic, long degradation rate, inadequate mechanical properties, and soft cell adhesion	[71]
PVA	Bioadhesive, biodegradable, biocompatible, low tendency for protein adhesion, and low toxicity	Humidity reduces the polymer's tensile strength; slow biodegradation	[72]
PVP	Binder, FDA approved, excellent wetting properties, biocompatibility, low toxicity, adhesive characteristics, complexing stability, relatively inert behavior, and is resistant to thermal degradation	Certain allergic reactions, storage disease, subcutaneous granulomas, pulmonary vascularization, and reticuloendothelial system (RES) deposition, high hygroscopic nature which made it tough to store and handle, non-biodegradability in parenteral administration	[36, 73]
PNIPAM	Mechanical strength, biocompatibility, biodegradability, multi-stimuli responsibility, higher drug loading	Low mechanical strength, limited drug loading capacity, and low biodegradability	[74]
PAA	Low toxicity, super hydrophilicity properties, biocompatibility, biodegradability characteristics	Poor mechanical properties, and high solubility in water	[75]

PCL: Poly (caprolactone); PVA: Poly (vinyl alcohol); PVP: Poly (vinyl pyrrolidone); PNIPAM: Poly (N-isopropyl acrylamide); PAA: Poly (acrylic acid).

Table 1.
Most of the reported polymers are used for drug carriers' fabrication in drug delivery systems.

Depending on their polymeric functional groups, antibiotics, anticancer agents, and biomolecules such as nucleic acids and proteins can be loaded [1], where surface morphology and structure of the polymeric nanofibers are key features for regulating the delivery rate and quantity of the drug. Also, the surface of the polymers can protect the bioactive loaded molecules from corrosion or degradation of the enzyme, water, or gastric acid, prolonging the effectivity of the pharmaceutical drug [43].

8. Conclusions

Necessary human equivalent doses still need to be tuned to generate drug carriers with adequate chemical, mechanical, and biological properties that are loaded with the specific doses of the pharmaceutical drug for a certain therapy. Another opportunity for the study is the proposed different taste masking in order to avoid the bad taste of some drugs or polymers. In all these studies, still, biocompatibility, biodegradability, mechanical testing, *in vivo* efficacy, and pharmacokinetics, must be studied. Future work must be focused on the biological response of the tissue and clinical phases must be performed [33].

For all discussed, the use of drug carriers is a promising technology that can be applied in most administration routes such as oral, vaginal, transdermal, ocular, rectal, and nasal tissues. The unique qualities of these drug delivery systems include a large surface area, nanoporosity, high drug encapsulation, and fast disintegration and dissolution properties. The advantages and limitations of various synthetic polymers and natural polymers nanofibers are discussed in the context of producing target drug delivery systems. Also, the bioavailability can be enhanced by exploiting the hydrophilic nature of polymers and their ability to form hydrogen bonds with encapsulated drugs, resulting in uniform distribution of encapsulated molecules throughout the matrices and providing the formulation with rapid dissolution abilities. Despite much literature being found, most of them still test these systems just for *in vitro* approaches. But *in vivo* and clinical trials are still poor.

Conflict of interest

"The authors declare no conflict of interest."

Nomenclature

EPR	Enhanced permeability and retention effect
PAA	Poly (acrylic acid)
PBCL	Poly (α-benzylcarboxylate-ε-caprolactone) (PBCL)
PCL	Poly (caprolactone)
PEO	Poly (ethylene oxide)
pH	Potential hydrogen
PLA	Poly (lactic acid)
PNIPAM	Poly (N-isopropyl acrylamide)
PVA	Poly (vinyl alcohol)
PVP	Poly (vinyl pyrrolidone)

Author details

Luis Jesús Villarreal-Gómez* and Graciela Lizeth Pérez-González
Facultad de Ciencias de la Ingeniería y Tecnología, Universidad Autónoma de Baja California, Unidad Valle de las Palmas, Tijuana, Baja California, México

*Address all correspondence to: luis.villarreal@uabc.edu.mx

References

[1] Dahmash EZ, Iyire A, Alyami HS. Development of orally dissolving films for pediatric-centric administration of anti-epileptic drug topiramate–a design of experiments (DoE) study. Saudi Pharmaceutical Journal. 2021;**29**(7): 635-647. DOI: 10.1016/j.jsps.2021.04.025

[2] He M, Zhu L, Yang N, Li H, Yang Q. Recent advances of oral film as platform for drug delivery. International Journal of Pharmaceutics. 2021;**604**:120759. DOI: 10.1016/j.ijpharm.2021.120759

[3] Özakar RS, Özakar E. Current overview of oral thin films. Turkish Journal of Pharmaceutical Sciences. 2021;**18**(1):111-121. DOI: 10.4274/tjps.galenos.2020.76390

[4] Mehdi M, Hussain S, Gao BB, Shah KA, Mahar FK, Yousif M, et al. Fabrication and characterization of rizatriptan loaded pullulan nanofibers as oral fast-dissolving drug system. Materials Research Express. 2021;**8**(5):055404. DOI: 10.1088/2053-1591/abff0b

[5] Gao S, Li X, Yang G, Feng W, Zong L, Zhao L, et al. Antibacterial perillaldehyde/hydroxypropyl-γ-cyclodextrin inclusion complex electrospun polymer-free nanofiber: Improved water solubility, thermostability, and antioxidant activity. Industrial Crops and Products. 2022;**176**:114300. DOI: 10.1016/j.indcrop.2021.114300

[6] Wang Y, Deng Z, Wang X, Shi Y, Lu Y, Fang S, et al. Formononetin/methyl-β-cyclodextrin inclusion complex incorporated into electrospun polyvinyl-alcohol nanofibers: Enhanced water solubility and oral fast-dissolving property. International Journal of Pharmaceutics. 2021;**603**:120696. DOI: 10.1016/j.ijpharm.2021.120696

[7] Xu C, Ma J, Wang W, Liu Z, Gu L, Qian L, et al. Preparation of pectin-based nanofibers encapsulating *lactobacillus rhamnosus* 1.0320 by electrospinning. Food Hydrocolloids. 2022;**124**:107216. DOI: 10.1016/j.foodhyd.2021.107216

[8] Li Y, Yang L. Driving forces for drug loading in drug carriers. Journal of Microencapsulation. 2015;*32*(3):255-272. DOI: 10.3109/02652048.2015.1010459

[9] Gelperina, S, Kisich, K, Iseman, M. D, and Heifets, L 2005. The potential advantages of nanoparticle drug delivery systems in chemotherapy of tuberculosis. American Journal of Respiratory and Critical Care Medicine, *172*(12), 1487-1490. doi:10.1164/rccm.200504-613PP

[10] Velasco-Barraza RD, Álvarez-Suárez AS, Villarreal-Gómez LJ, Páz-González JA, Iglesias AL, Vera-Graziano R. Designing a low-cost electrospinning device for practical learning in a bioengineering biomaterials course. Revista mexicana de ingeniería biomédica. 2016;**37**(1):7-16. DOI: 10.17488/RMIB.37.1.1

[11] Yeo Y, Kim BK. Drug carriers: Not an innocent delivery man. The AAPS Journal. 2015;**17**(5):1096-1104. DOI: 10.1208/s12248-015-9789-6

[12] Du AW, Stenzel MH. Drug carriers for the delivery of therapeutic peptides. Biomacromolecules. 2014;**15**(4):1097-1114. DOI: 10.1021/bm500169p

[13] Torres-Martínez EJ, Cornejo-Bravo JM, Serrano-Medina A, Pérez-González GL, Villarreal-Gómez LJ. A summary of electrospun nanofibers

as drug delivery system: Drugs loaded and biopolymers used as matrices. Current Drug Delivery. 2018;**15**:1360-1374. DOI: 10.2174/1567201815666180723114326

[14] Vass P, Szabó E, Domokos A, Hirsch E, Galata D, Farkas B, et al. Scale-up of electrospinning technology: Applications in the pharmaceutical industry. Wiley Interdisciplinary Reviews Nanomedicine and Nanobiotechnology. 2020;**12**(4):e1611. DOI: 10.1002/wnan.1611

[15] Villarreal-Gómez LJ, Vera-Graziano R, Vega-Rios MR, Pineda-Camacho JL, Mier-Maldonado PA, Almanza-Reyes H, et al. Biocompatibility evaluation of electrospun scaffolds of poly(L-lactide) with pure and grafted hydroxyapatite. Journal of the Mexican Chemical Society. 2014;**58**:435-443 http://www.scielo.org.mx/scielo.php?script=sci_arttext&pid=S1870-249X2014000400010&lng=es&tlng=en

[16] Birer M, Acartürk F. Electrospun orally disintegrating film formulation of telmisartan. Pharmaceutical Development and Technology. 2021;**26**(6):661-672. DOI: 10.1080/10837450.2021.1916031

[17] Pacheco MS, Barbieri D, da Silva CF, de Moraes MA. A review on orally disintegrating films (ODFs) made from natural polymers such as pullulan, maltodextrin, starch, and others. International Journal of Biological Macromolecules. 2021;**178**:504-513. DOI: 10.1016/j.ijbiomac.2021.02.180

[18] Badgar K, Prokisch J. Elemental selenium enriched nanofiber production. Molecules. 2021;**26**(21):6457. DOI: 10.3390/molecules26216457

[19] Zhang X, Xie L, Wang X, Shao Z, Kong B. Electrospinning super-assembly of ultrathin fibers from single- to multi-Taylor cone sites. Applied Materials Today. 2021;**26**:101272. DOI: 10.1016/j.apmt.2021.101272

[20] Kopp A, Smeets R, Gosau M, Kröger N, Fuest S, Köpf M, et al. Effect of process parameters on additive-free electrospinning of regenerated silk fibroin nonwovens. Bioactive Materials. 2020;**5**(2):241-252. DOI: 10.1016/j.bioactmat.2020.01.010

[21] Huang A, Liu F, Cui Z, Wang H, Song X, Geng L, et al. Novel PTFE/CNT composite nanofiber membranes with enhanced mechanical, crystalline, conductive, and dielectric properties fabricated by emulsion electrospinning and sintering. Composites Science and Technology. 2021;**214**:108980. DOI: 10.1016/j.compscitech.2021.108980

[22] Pérez-González GL, Villarreal-Gómez LJ, Serrano-Medina A, Torres-Martínez EJ, Cornejo-Bravo JM. Mucoadhesive electrospun nanofibers for drug delivery systems: Applications of polymers and the parameters' roles. International Journal of Nanomedicine. 2019;**14**:5271-5285. DOI: 10.2147/IJN.S193328

[23] Mohammadinejad R, Madamsetty VS, Kumar A, Verzandeh M, Dehshahri A, Zarrabi A, et al. Electrospun nanocarriers for delivering natural products for cancer therapy. Trends in Food Science and Technology. 2021;**118**:887-904. DOI: 10.1016/j.tifs.2021.10.007

[24] Rampichová M, Košťáková Kuželová E, Filová E, Chvojka J, Šafka J, Pelcl M, et al. Composite 3D printed scaffold with structured electrospun nanofibers promotes chondrocyte adhesion and infiltration. Cell Adhesion and Migration. 2018;**12**(3):271-285. DOI: 10.1080/19336918.2017.1385713

[25] Yan W, Miao D, Babar AA, Zhao J, Jia Y, Ding B, et al. Multi-scaled interconnected inter- and intra-fiber porous janus membranes for enhanced directional moisture transport. Journal of Colloidal Interface Sciences. 2020;**565**:426-435. DOI: 10.1016/j.jcis.2020.01.063

[26] Sóti PL, Weiser D, Vigh T, Nagy ZK, Poppe L, Marosi G. Electrospun polylactic acid and polyvinyl alcohol fibers as efficient and stable nanomaterials for immobilization of lipases. Bioprocess and Biosystems Engineering. 2016;**39**(3):449-459. DOI: 10.1007/s00449-015-1528-y

[27] Liu H, Zhou Z, Lin H, Wu J, Ginn B, Choi JS, et al. Synthetic nanofiber-reinforced amniotic membrane via interfacial bonding. ACS Applied Materials and Interfaces. 2018;**10**(17):14559-14569. DOI: 10.1021/acsami.8b03087

[28] Niemczyk-Soczynska B, Gradys A, Sajkiewicz P. Hydrophilic surface functionalization of electrospun Nanofibrous scaffolds in tissue engineering. Polymers (Basel). 2020;**12**(11):2636. DOI: 10.3390/polym12112636

[29] Chen W, Zheng D, Chen Y, Ruan H, Zhang Y, Chen X, et al. Electrospun fibers improving cellular respiration via mitochondrial protection. Small. 2021;**17**(46):e2104012. DOI: 10.1002/smll.202104012

[30] Dumitriu RP, Stoleru E, Mitchell GR, Vasile C, Brebu M. Bioactive electrospun fibers of poly (ε-caprolactone) incorporating α-tocopherol for food packaging applications. Molecules. 2021;**26**(18):5498. DOI: 10.3390/molecules26185498

[31] Toprak Ö, Topuz B, Monsef YA, Oto Ç, Orhan K, Karakeçili A. BMP-6 carrying metal organic framework-embedded in bioresorbable electrospun fibers for enhanced bone regeneration. Materials Science and Engineering C: Materials for Biological Applications. 2021;**120**:111738. DOI: 10.1016/j.msec.2020.111738

[32] Villarreal-Gómez LJ, Cornejo-Bravo JM, Vera-Graziano R, Grande D. Electrospinning as a powerful technique for biomedical applications: A critically selected survey. Journal of Biomaterial Sciences Polymer Edition. 2016;**27**(2):157-176. DOI: 10.1080/09205063.2015.1116885

[33] Luraghi A, Peri F, Moroni L. Electrospinning for drug delivery applications: A review. Journal of Controlled Release. 2021;**334**:463-484. DOI: 10.1016/j.jconrel.2021.03.033

[34] Villarreal-Gómez LJ, Pérez-González GL, Bogdanchikova N, Pestryakov A, Nimaev V, Soloveva A, et al. Antimicrobial effect of electrospun nanofibersloadedwithsilvernanoparticles: Influence of Ag incorporation method. Journal of Nanomaterials. 2021;**2021**:e9920755. DOI: 10.1155/2021/9920755

[35] Torres-MartínezEJ,Pérez-GonzálezGL, Serrano-Medina A, Grande D, Vera-Graziano R, Cornejo-Bravo JM, et al. Drugs loaded into electrospun polymeric nanofibers for delivery. Journal of Pharmacy and Pharmaceutical Sciences. 2019;**22**(1):313-331. DOI: 10.18433/jpps29674

[36] Torres-Martínez EJ, Vera-Graziano R, Cervantes-Uc J, Bogdanchikova N, Olivas-Sarabia A, Valdez-Castro R, et al. Preparation and characterization of electrospun fibrous scaffolds of either PVA or PVP for fast release of sildenafil citrate. E-Polymers. 2020;**20**(1):746-758. DOI: 10.1515/epoly-2020-0070

[37] Uhljar LÉ, Kan SY, Radecsi N, Koutsos V, Szabó-Révész P, Ambrus R. In vitro drug release, permeability, and structural test of ciprofloxacin-loaded nanofibers. Pharmaceutics. 2021;**13**(4):556. DOI: 10.3390/pharmaceutics13040556

[38] Tipduangta P, Belton P, Fábián L, Wang LY, Tang H, Eddleston M, et al. Electrospun polymer blend nanofibers for tunable drug delivery: The role of transformative phase separation on controlling the release rate. Molecular Pharmaceutics. 2016;**13**(1):25-39. DOI: 10.1021/acs.molpharmaceut.5b00359

[39] Moreira A, Lawson D, Onyekuru L, Dziemidowicz K, Angkawinitwong U, Costa PF, et al. Protein encapsulation by electrospinning and electrospraying. Journal of Controlled Release. 2021;**329**:1172-1197. DOI: 10.1016/j.jconrel.2020.10.046

[40] Nguyen J, Stwodah RM, Vasey CL, Rabatin BE, Atherton B, D'Angelo PA, et al. Thermochromic fibers via electrospinning. Polymers (Basel). 2020;**12**(4):842. DOI: 10.3390/polym12040842

[41] Balusamy B, Celebioglu A, Senthamizhan A, Uyar T. Progress in the design and development of "fast-dissolving" electrospun nanofibers-based drug delivery systems-a systematic review. Journal of Controlled Release. 2020;**326**:482-509. DOI: 10.1016/j.jconrel.2020.07.038

[42] Costoya A, Concheiro A, Alvarez-Lorenzo C. Electrospun fibers of Cyclodextrins and poly(cyclodextrins). Molecules. 2017;**22**(2):230. DOI: 10.3390/molecules22020230

[43] Meng ZX, Xu XX, Zheng W, Zhou HM, Li L, Zheng YF, et al. Preparation and characterization of electrospun PLGA gelatin nanofibers as a potential drug delivery system. Colloids and Surfaces B: Biointerfaces. 2011;**84**(1):97-102. DOI: 10.1016/j.colsurfb.2010.12.022

[44] Ashrafuzzaman M. Aptamers as both drugs and drug-carriers. BioMed Research International. 2014;**2014**(2014):697923. DOI: 10.1155/2014/697923

[45] Dadwal A, Baldi A, Kumar Narang R. Nanoparticles as carriers for drug delivery in cancer. Artificial Cells Nanomedicine Biotechnology. 2018;**46**(sup2):295-305. DOI: 10.1080/21691401.2018.1457039

[46] Mattice CM. DeRosa MC 2015 status and prospects of aptamers as drug components. BioDrugs. 2015;**29**(3):151-165. DOI: 10.1007/s40259-015-0126-5

[47] Gopinath SC, Lakshmipriya T, Chen Y, et al. 2016. Cell-targeting aptamers act as intracellular delivery vehicles. Applied Microbiology and Biotechnology. 2016;**100**(16):6955-6969. DOI: 10.1007/s00253-016-7686-2

[48] Kanwar JR, Roy K. Kanwar RK 2011 chimeric aptamers in cancer cell-targeted drug delivery. Critical Reviews in Biochemistry and Molecular Biology. 2011;**46**(6):459-477. DOI: 10.3109/10409238.2011.614592

[49] Ganji A, Varasteh A, Sankian M. 2016. Aptamers: New arrows to target dendritic cells. Journal of Drug Targeting. 2016;**24**(1):1-12. DOI: 10.3109/1061186X.2015.1041962

[50] Nimjee SM, White RR, Becker RC, Sullenger BA. Aptamers as therapeutics. Annual Review of Pharmacology and Toxicology. 2017;**2017**(57):61-79. DOI: 10.1146/annurev-pharmtox-010716-104558

[51] Yokoyama M. 2014. Polymeric micelles as drug carriers: Their lights and shadows. Journal of Drug Targeting. 2014;**22**(7):576-583. DOI: 10.3109/1061186X.2014.934688

[52] Ghosh B, Biswas S. Polymeric micelles in cancer therapy: State of the art. Journal of Controlled Release. 2021;**2021**(332):127-147. DOI: 10.1016/j.jconrel.2021.02.016

[53] Soleymani Abyaneh H, Vakili MR, Zhang F, Choi P, Lavasanifar A. Rational design of block copolymer micelles to control burst drug release at a nanoscale dimension. Acta Biomaterialia. 2015;**2015**(24):127-139. DOI: 10.1016/j.actbio.2015.06.017

[54] Trucillo P. Drug carriers: Classification, administration, release profiles, and industrial approach. PRO. 2021;**9**(3):470. DOI: 10.3390/pr9030470

[55] Akbarzadeh A, Rezaei-Sadabady R, Davaran S, Joo SW, Zarghami N, Hanifehpour Y, et al. Liposome: Classification, preparation, and applications. Nanoscale Research Letters. 2013;**8**(1):102. DOI: 10.1186/1556-276X-8-102

[56] Rauti R, Musto M, Bosi S, Prato M, Ballerini L. Properties and behavior of carbon nanomaterials when interfacing neuronal cells: How far have we come? Carbon. 2019;**143**:430-446. DOI: 10.1016/j.carbon.2018.11.026

[57] Mohajeri M, Behnam B, Sahebkar A. Biomedical applications of carbon nanomaterials: Drug and gene delivery potentials. Journal of Cell Physiology. 2018;**234**:298-319. DOI: 10.1002/jcp.26899

[58] Wang SY, Hu HZ, Qing XC, Zhang ZC, Shao ZW. Recent advances of drug delivery nanocarriers in osteosarcoma treatment. Journal of Cancer. 2020;**11**:69-82. DOI: 10.7150/jca.36588

[59] Shannahan J. The biocorona: A challenge for the biomedical application of nanoparticles. Nanotechnology Reviews. 2017;**6**:345-353. DOI: 10.1515/ntrev-2016-0098

[60] Al Garalleh H, Algarni A. Modelling of paclitaxel conjugated with carbon nanotubes as an antitumor agent for cancer therapy. Journal of Biomedical Nanotechnology. 2020;**16**:224-234. DOI: 10.1166/jbn.2020.2886

[61] Jagusiak A, Chłopaś K, Zemanek G, Jemioła-Rzemińska M, Piekarska B, Stopa B, et al. Self-assembled supramolecular ribbon-like structures complexed to single walled carbon nanotubes as possible anticancer drug delivery systems. International Journal of Molecular Sciences. 2019;**20**:2064. DOI: 10.3390/ijms20092064

[62] Zomorodbakhsh S, Abbasian Y, Naghinejad M, Sheikhpour M. The effects study of isoniazid conjugated multi-wall carbon nanotubes nanofluid on mycobacterium tuberculosis. International Journal of Nanomedicine. 2020;**15**:5901-5909. DOI: 10.2147/IJN.S251524

[63] Wang P, Yan G, Zhu X, Du Y, Chen D, Zhang J. Heterofullerene MC59 (M = B, Si, Al) as potential carriers for hydroxyurea drug delivery. Nanomaterials. 2021;**11**:115. DOI: 10.3390/nano11010115

[64] Alipour E, Alimohammady F, Yumashev A, Maseleno A. Fullerene C60 containing porphyrin-like metal center as drug delivery system for ibuprofen drug. Journal of Molecular Modeling. 2020;**26**:7. DOI: 10.1007/s00894-019-4267-1

[65] Bagheri NS, Aram MR. Quantum mechanical simulation of chloroquine drug interaction with C60 fullerene for treatment of COVID-19. Chemical Physics Letters. 2020;**757**:137869. DOI: 10.1016/j.cplett.2020.137869

[66] Lin S, Liu C, Han X, Zhong H, Cheng C. Viral nanoparticle system: An effective platform for photodynamic therapy. International Journal of Molecular Sciences. 2021;**22**(4):1728. DOI: 10.3390/ijms22041728

[67] Nkanga CI, Steinmetz NF. The pharmacology of plant virus nanoparticles. Virology. 2021;**556**:39-61. DOI: 10.1016/j.virol.2021.01.012

[68] Alemzadeh E, Dehshahri A, Izadpanah K, Ahmadi F. Plant virus nanoparticles: Novel and robust nanocarriers for drug delivery and imaging. Colloids and Surfaces. B, Biointerfaces. 2018;**167**:20-27. DOI: 10.1016/j.colsurfb.2018.03.026

[69] Cao J, Guenther RH, Sit TL, Opperman CH, Lommel AS, Willoughby JA. Loading and release mechanism of red clover necrotic mosaic virus derived plant viral nanoparticles for drug delivery of doxorubicin. Small. 2014;**10**:5126-5136. DOI: 10.1002/smll.201400558

[70] Cornejo-Bravo JM, Villarreal-Gómez LJ, Serrano A. Electrospinning for drug delivery systems: Drug incorporation techniques. In: Haider S, Haider A, editors. Electrospinning - Material, Techniques, and Biomedical Applications. London: IntechOpen; 2016. DOI: 10.5772/65939

[71] Aguirre-Chagala YE, Altuzar V, León-Sarabia E, Tinoco-Magaña JC, Yañez-Limón JM, Mendoza-Barrera C. Physicochemical properties of polycaprolactone/collagen/elastin nanofibers fabricated by electrospinning. Materials Science and Engineering. C, Materials for Biological Applications. 2017;**76**:897-907. DOI: 10.1016/j.msec.2017.03.118

[72] Pérez-González GL, Cornejo-Bravo JM, Vera-Graciano R, Adan-López ES, Villarreal-Gómez LJ. Development, characterization, and in vitro evaluation of adhesive fibrous mat for mucosal propranolol delivery. E-Polymers. 2022;**22**(1):58-68. DOI: 10.1515/epoly-2022-0002

[73] Kurakula M, Rao G. Pharmaceutical assessment of polyvinylpyrrolidone (PVP): As excipient from conventional to controlled delivery systems with a spotlight on COVID-19 inhibition. Journal of Drug Delivery Science and Technology. 2020;**60**:102046. DOI: 10.1016/j.jddst.2020.102046

[74] Xu X, Liu Y, Fu W, Yao M, Ding Z, Xuan J, et al. Poly(N-isopropylacrylamide)-based Thermoresponsive composite hydrogels for biomedical applications. Polymers. 2020;**12**(3):580. DOI: 10.3390/polym12030580

[75] Alhalawani AMF, Curran DJ. Boyd, D and Towler, mark R 2016 the role of poly (acrylic acid) in conventional glass polyalkenoate cements. Journal of Polymer Engineering. 2016;**36**(3):221-237. DOI: 10.1515/polyeng-2015-0079

Chapter 2

Selection and Role of Polymers for Designing of a Drug Carrier

Pankaj Sharma, Vinay Jain and Mukul Tailang

Abstract

Polymers have helped to develop drug carrier technologies by allowing for the regulated release of bioactive molecules in consistent dosages over extended periods of time, cyclic dosing, and adjustable delivery of both hydrophobic and hydrophilic medicines. Formulations are released in a coordinated and consistent fashion over long periods of time. Polymers going to act as just an inert carrier whereby a substance can be conjugated having significant advantages. For instance, the polymer enhances the pharmacodynamic and pharmacokinetic characteristics of biopharmaceuticals in a variety of ways, such as plasma half-life, reduces immunogenicity, increases biopharmaceutical consistency, enhances the solubilization of low-molecular-weight substances, and has the prospects for targeted delivery. Smart polymeric delivery systems, in instance, have been investigated as "smart" delivery methods capable of releasing encapsulated pharmaceuticals at the right time and place of activity with respect to certain physiological stimuli. The development of novel polymeric materials and cross-linkers that are more biocompatible and biodegradable would expand and improve present uses. Polymer sensitivity to a particular stimulus may be tuned within a limited range because of the diversity of polymer substrates and their sequential production. The methods through which polymer frameworks are formed *in situ* to construct implanted systems for continuous release of medicinal macromolecules are discussed in this chapter, as well as numerous applicability of enhanced drug delivery.

Keywords: polymeric material, drug delivery, thermally responsive, smart polymer, glucose, enzyme, oxidation-reduction

1. Introduction

Since the 1980s, researchers have been working on polymeric drug delivery systems [1–4]. Several of the frontier scientific fields are the hunt for novel medication delivery mechanisms and novel action mechanisms. These include multidisciplinary research techniques that aim to make significant improvements in therapeutic efficacy and bioavailability just at point of medication administration [5, 6]. One or more traditional medication delivery mechanisms are combined with engineering technologies in a drug delivery system. The technologies allow for precise targeting of the place in the body where a medicine has been delivered and/or the pace at which it has been released.

Short half-lives, low bioavailability, and physicochemical instability are all common limitations of biopharmaceutical therapies. Physiological instability is characterized by changes in the highly organized structure of proteins, which can result in undesired events including denaturation, aggregation, and precipitation. The chemical instability of pharmaceuticals is exacerbated by processes including such oxidation, deamidation, hydrolysis, and racemization. Stimulus-responsive polymers provide a pharmaceutical delivery mechanism for delivering pharmaceuticals at a regulated pace and in a durable and physiologically functional state. Research in stimuli-responsive polymers has grown over the years, and a lot of effort has gone into designing eco-friendly macromolecules that may be molded into novel smart polymers [7]. A composition or platform that allows the administration of a medicinal chemical into the body is known as just polymeric drug carriers. By regulating the pace, duration, and location of medication distribution in the system, it increases its effectiveness and safety. There in previous two decades, delivery of drugs has progressed significantly, but regulating medication entrance into the system, particularly the brain, has remained a tough challenge. Recent development in investigations of nano-drug delivery system distribution across the blood-brain membrane via carrier-mediated carriage is starting to give a reasonable basis for directing medication delivery to the brain. Natural materials such as amino acids, hexose, peptides, monocarboxylate, and stem cells are transported over the blood-brain membrane via ingestion transporters [8–10]. In the type of biomaterials with liposomes, polymers in reservoir-containing drug delivery applications have made tremendous development. Additional applications of the polymers include diffusion-based drug delivery systems and solvent-triggered/activated drug delivery systems. Drugs are dissolved in a non-swellable solution or a completely inflated matrix that does not breakdown throughout their engagement period in diffusion-based drug delivery applications. Whenever subjected to an aquatic media, solvent triggered materials such as hydrogels expand and release the medication. They are naturally hydrophilic. Because of their well-engineered polymeric by the changes in the underlying reasons of the biological function, biocompatible polymers provide a safe pathway for medication transport. Biodegradable polymers disintegrate owing to the breakage of covalent bonds among them, whereas bioerodible polymers cause degradation of the polymer owing to the dissolving of connecting strands without causing any changes in the molecule's chemical properties. Aqueous soluble, safe, as well as non-immunogenic polymers are being used as therapeutic carriers. They act in the background to reduce medication breakdown and increase circulation time. Another crucial consideration is the drug's appropriate elimination. If indeed the polymer is non-degradable, it really should be avoided accumulating in the body, and if it is biodegradable, the fragmented elements should be safe and not cause an immune reaction. Polymers that resemble important biological respond to environmental stimuli such as changes in pH or thermal by altering features such as solubility, hydrophobic/hydrophilic equilibrium, biomolecule (pharmaceutical component) releases, as well as configuration [11, 12].

The polymeric medicinal delivery compositions are classified into several classes, such as, biodegradable (chemically-controlled), diffusion-controlled, externally-responsive systems (e.g., temperature pH,) [13], solvent-actuated [14] and nanosized polymeic delivery platform that accomplish in three prime technologies [15]: (i) PEGylation [16, 17], (ii) active targeting of certain cells and organs [18–20] and (iii) Increased permeability and retaining allows for passive targeting effect [20, 21]. The more sophisticated polymeric therapeutic delivery technologies are indeed being anticipated as multidimensional fully – featured systems that will enable instantly improved pharmacokinetics, decreased toxicity, faster targeting, as well as a programmable drug release pattern. Furthermore, greater appropriate therapy might be provided by combination treatment, which involves the simultaneous administration of 2 or more medicaments/diagnostics substances [22–24]. In reaction to a modest external/internal stimulation, a stimuli-reactive or smart polymer changes its physical characteristics abruptly. Although minor changes take place in subjected to external/internal stimuli stimulus until a crucial limit is found, and they have the potential to revert to their original form when the stimulus is withdrawn, those polymers are indeed known as smart polymers [25–27]. The uniqueness of these polymers resides in their unpredictable reaction, which is initiated by a really tiny stimulus and results in enormous structural changes. Different triggers responsible for modulating the release of the drug using innovative polymeric drug delivery compositions are depicted in **Figure 1**. Modifications in physical state, structure, solubility, solvent interactions, aqueous soluble and lipid soluble equilibrium, and conductance are all reversible transitions. The introduction of oppositely charged polymers or a pH change to neutralize charged groups, as well as variations in the water-loving/lipid-loving balance or hydrogen bonding owing to temperature differences, are the driving factors underlying such transitions. Fewer dosage periodicities, simplicity of preparation, preservation of optimal therapeutic level at a single dose, longer delivery of integrated medication, decreased adverse effects, and increased stability are all advantages of innovative polymer-based medicaments delivery systems [28–30].

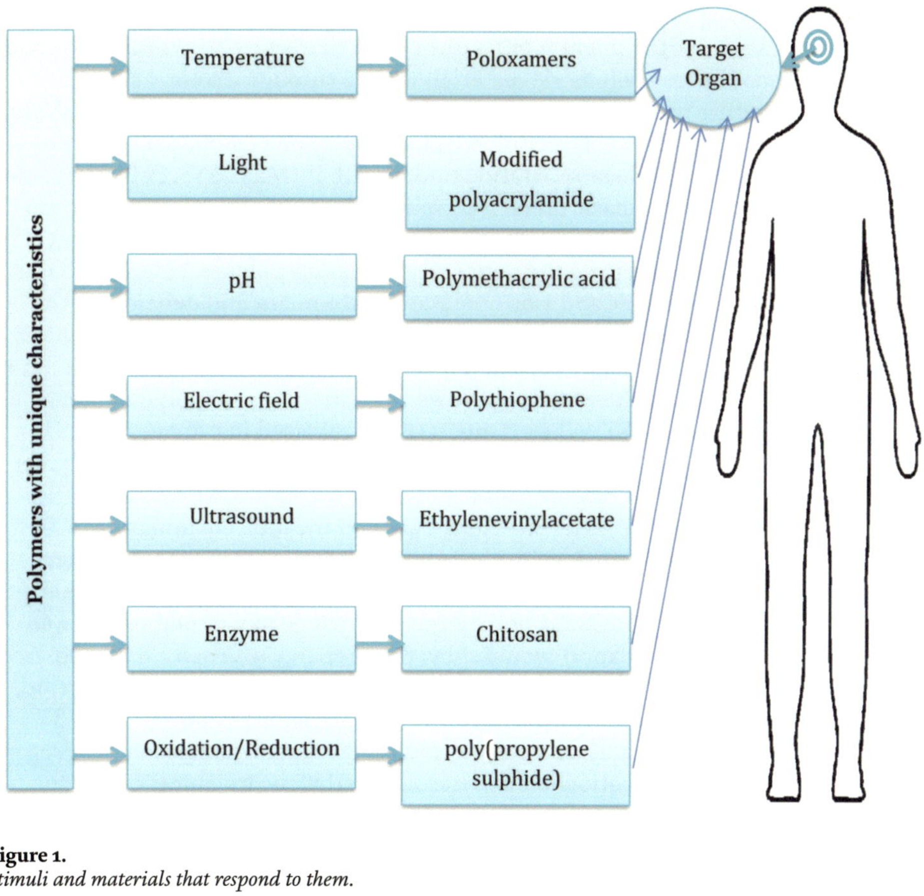

Figure 1.
Stimuli and materials that respond to them.

A dynamic polymeric material can respond in a variety of ways. The breakdown and development of numerous secondary interactions such as hydrogen bonding, van der Waals forces, hydrophobic forces, and electrostatic interaction [31, 32] restrict the responsiveness of such a polymeric solution induced by physicochemical stimuli. Fundamental processes including acid-base reaction, reduction, oxidation, and hydrolysis of components linked to the polymer chain are examples of chemical processes. Destruction of a polymeric structure owing to irreversible bond breaking in response to external stimuli is one example of the significant conformational shift in the polymer backbone. Biodegradability and biocompatibility; sustained-release characteristics; drug-loading potential; the dearth of deleterious characteristics including systemic toxicity, carcinogenic effects, immunogenicity, and reproductive toxicity; as well as outstanding stability characteristics are all important characteristics of a smart polymer.

2. Criteria for choosing a polymeric system

2.1 Polymers with temperature sensitivity

These are polymeric frameworks that are susceptible to thermal fluctuations. These polymers exhibit a gel-to-gel shift as temperature dependent, and can be used to deliver medicinal compounds in vivo. This sort of system seems to have a crucial temperature of the solution (usually in aqua) where the polymer and solution phases shift according to respective content. The solubility of several polymers varies dramatically as a result of ambient temperature. This characteristic was used to create aqueous solutions of these polymeric materials that go through a sol-gel changeover when the temperature varies. A maximum crucial solution temperature (MaxCST) exists for thermally sensitive polymer blends that display one component above a specific temperature with phase separation underneath it (MaxCST). Polymeric solutions that seem to be monophasic under a certain temperature but biphasic beyond that temperature are said to have a minimum crucial solution temperature (MinCST) [33, 34]. The MinCST seems to be the temperature where a polymer solution divides into two portions (anisotropic and isotropic states), abundant and deficient in the polymer. Such solution also is monophasic under a certain temperature but biphasic beyond that degree. The enthalpy parameter, which is connected to hydrogen bonding here between polymer and the water molecules, is accountable for polymer breakdown underneath the MinCST. When temperatures are raised just above MinCST, the entropy component (lipophilic contacts) takes precedence, resulting in polymer deposition. Among the most biocompatible polymers with MinCST characteristics includes poly (ethylene oxide). Nevertheless, based on the molecular mass, the MinCST transition of poly (ethylene oxide) aqueous solutions happens at ambient temperature, spanning between 100° C to 150° C. At minimum temperatures than just the poly (ethylene oxide) MinCST, a polymer with ethylene oxide components and hydrophilic sections (e.g. ethanol) would show phase changes. When a linear polymer with small sufficient Ethylene oxide sections is utilized to avoid micelle production, the precipitating from the aqueous phase can be thought about as a rapid MinCST changeover. Furthermore, in the lack of intermolecular and intramolecular hydrogen bonding, a continuous alternation of ethylene oxide-ethylene monomer copolymer pattern throughout the polymer would result in a MinCST defined either by lipophilic/hydrophilic equilibrium.

Poly(N-alkylacrylamide)s, Poloxamers, Poly(N-vinylcaprolactam)s, Chitosan, poly (ethylene oxide)- poly (propyleneoxide)- poly (ethylene oxide), Cellulose, xyloglucan, etc. are instances of thermally sensitive polymers (lactic acid) – tri blocks of poly (ethylene glycol). Poly (N-isopropyl acrylamide) and Poly (N-alkyl substituted acrylamides) with an annealing temperature of 32° C as well as poly (Nvinylalkylamides) like poly (N-vinyliso-butyramide) with just an annealing temperature of 39° C are perhaps the most extensively utilized thermally sensitive polymers [7, 35].

2.1.1 Thermally responsive smart polymers' mechanisms of action

The occurrence of a minimum crucial solution temperature (MinCST) above which the polymer turns aqueous insoluble is generally the source of thermally-responsive smart polymeric solubility. This is characteristic of polymers that create hydrogen bonds with aqua, and it also has a wide spectrum of biological possibilities, including cell mapping, smart medication delivery, DNA sequencing, and so on. The chemical makeup of the monomers is varied throughout this strategy to regulate the polymer thermal sensitivity in aqua. To accomplish this, a variety of polymers centered on ethyleneoxide/ethylene monomer were developed and produced via multiple condensation processes of polyfunctional ethyleneoxide/ethylene monomer oligomers. The cloud point reflects the hydrophobicity/hydrophobicity balance continuously and may be customized in the spectrum of 7–70°C by adjusting the composition and polymer type.

The lack of organic solvents is an important benefit of such compositions. The shrinking in the volume that emits a considerable quantity of an encapsulating medication has been linked to the strong initial bursting impact of such approaches. The solubility behavior of polymer grafted onto the silicon surface is identical. The solubility cloud levels of grafting polymers are similar to those of bulk polymer solutions, according to binding energy studies.

Thermally responsive smart polymers' dynamic solubility is generated by variations in the lipophilic/hydrophilic balance of the electron-deficient polymer, which are triggered by rising temperature or ionic intensity. Because of hydrogen bonds between aqueous molecules, electron-deficient polymers are soluble in aqua. The efficacy of hydrogen bonding decreases even as the temperature goes up. Whenever the effectiveness of hydrogen bonding is inadequate for macromolecule immersion, a polymer phase transition occurs. A phase transition occurs whenever the temperature of the water solution of innovative polymers is raised beyond a particularly critical point. There is a formation of an aqueous phase with almost minimal polymer and a polymer richer phase. The temperature at which a phase transformation occurs is determined by the amount of polymer present as well as the molecular mass of a polymer [35, 36].

2.2 Polymers with pH sensitivity

pH-Adaptive polymers are a class of stimuli-sensitive polymers that may alter their structural and physical properties in reaction to variations in solution pH, including surface properties, chain conformation, solubility, and arrangement. The phrase "pH-reactive polymers" refers to polymers containing ionizable basic or acidic groups where ionization is affected by the pH of the solution. In the latest days, the topic of pH-reactive polymers has grown in popularity, with scientific research being published year after year. As either a result, pH-sensitive polymer systems are extremely helpful in a broad array of applications, including gene delivery, drug administration, surfaces, membranes receptors, and chromatography [37–39].

Polymers that respond to pH might be linear, branching, or networked. According to their architectures, polymers may have varied sensitivities to solution circumstances and variable self-assembly tendencies. A pH shift, for instance, might result in the (de)protonation of functional moiety in the polymeric chain. It can produce flocculation, strand collapse-extension, including deposition in homopolymers in certain situations. It also might produce self-assembly in the forms of micelles, unimers, gels, vesicles, swelling, and deswelling, among other things. Surface active behaviors are demonstrated by pH alteration in block (co)polymers, branching (co)polymers, and starry (co)polymers with pH-sensitive block(s). Furthermore, pH changes cause (de)swelling in hydrogel as well as dendrimer-like formations. Surfaces altered with polymers allow for the creation of ionic interfaces with thin/thick layers as a result of pH changes. **Figure 2** depicts the variations in polymers of various topologies caused by pH changes.

pH Adaptive polymers are polyelectrolytes with weakly basic or acidic moieties in their architecture that receive or liberate protons in reaction to variations in the pH of the surroundings. Polymers containing acidic or basic groups, such as carboxyl, pyridine, sulfonic, phosphate, and tertiary amines, are commonly referred to as pH adaptive polymers because of ionization of the molecules with pH variation causes a structural change. Their pH sensibility or ionization allows us to modify its self-assembly behavior, wettability phase segregation, polyelectrolyte character, and other properties, in complement to their biotechnological uses. It is feasible to make a polymer with a pKa ranging from 1 to 14. pH Reactive polymers having basic monomers behave like cationic polymers in acidic conditions, whereas polymers having acidic monomers behave like anionic polymers in basic conditions. Depending on the requirements, a few of these two types or a combination of the two with the appropriate composition is necessary. Natural polymers, as well as manmade polymers, have indeed been thoroughly investigated. Biopolymers are by far the most widely investigated because of their richness in ecology, rapid degradation, bio-compatibility, their potential to be modified. Polypeptides such as poly(histidine), poly(L-glutamic acid), and poly(aspartic acid) can be used to synthesize pH-reactive polymers. Such polymers are biodegradable and biocompatible, just like biopolymers. These biopolymers are quite significant among pH-sensitive polymers [38, 40, 41].

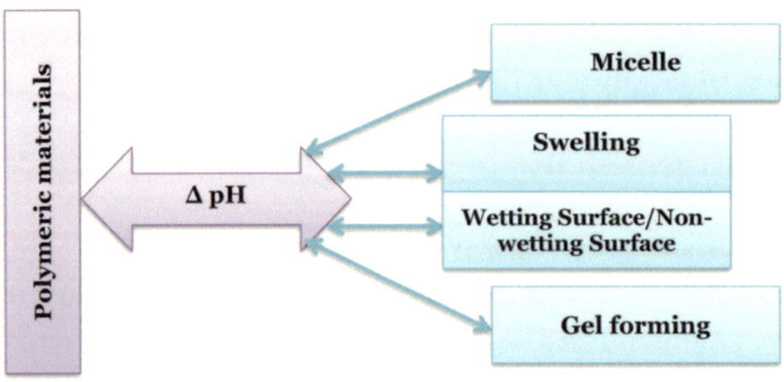

Figure 2.
Polymers that respond to pH in a variety of ways.

2.3 Polymers sensitive to two impulses (pH and temperature)

These really are polymeric frameworks that are thermal and pH-sensitive, but they are created by combining ionizable with lipophilic (inverse thermo-sensitive) moiety in a straightforward way [42]. Chitosan, acrylic acid, N,Ndime thylaminoethylmethacrylate, and other polymers that really are thermal and pH-responsive are instances. This is accomplished mostly by copolymerizing monomers with all these molecules, integrating thermally responsive polymers with polyelectrolytes, or developing novel monomers that adapt to both stimulation concurrently [43, 44].

2.4 Polymers that respond to glucose

Glucose-sensitive polymers can imitate typical internal insulin production, reducing diabetes problems and allowing for regulated delivery of the bioactive chemical. These really are sugar responsive and exhibit a wide range of responses to glucose. Although their applicability for both glucose monitoring and insulin administration, such polymers have gotten a lot of interest. Despite these benefits, the main drawbacks are the quick reaction time as well as the possibility of non-biocompatibility. The following techniques have been used to build glucose-sensitive polymeric-based formulations: enzymatic oxidation of glucose using glucose oxidase, glucose binding using lectin, or reversible covalent bond creation using phenylboronic acid molecules. Glucose responsiveness is caused by the polymer's reaction to the by-products produced either by oxidation (enzymatic) of glucose. Glucose oxidase (GOx) is oxidized to form glucose to produce gluconic acid with hydrogen peroxide (H2O2). Within the instance of poly (acrylicacid) coupled with GOx mechanism, for instance, when blood glucose levels rise, conversion of glucose to gluconic acid, causing a drop in pH enabling hydrogenation of PAA carboxylate groups, allowing insulin to be released more quickly. Because its release profile closely resembles that of internal insulin, this approach is gaining popularity [45, 46].

Another technique makes use of lectin's specific carbohydrate-binding characteristics to create a glucose-responsive system. Lectins are bifunctional proteins, and their glucose-biding function allows them to produce a variety of glucose-sensitive materials. The responses of these mechanisms were unique to glucose and mannose, with no reaction to certain other sugars. Concanavalin A is a 4 binding-site lectin that has been widely employed in insulin-containing medication delivery. The insulin component is chemically changed by inserting functional moieties (or glucose molecule) and afterward connected to a transporter or support via particular interactions that can only be disrupted by the glucose it in this sort of system. Concanavalin A competitive binding characteristic to glucose as well as glycosylated insulin is exploited in the glycosylated insulin-Concanavalin A combination. The bioactive unbound glucose moieties cause glycosylated Concanavalin A-insulin complex to be displaced inside the surrounding structures. The production of single-substituted glucosyl terminal PEG with insulin complex was also described in other investigations. The G-PEG–insulin complex was covalently coupled to Concanavalin A, which was connected to a PEG–poly(vinylpyrrolidone-co-acrylic acid) framework, and when the levels of sugar grew, the competitive attachment of glucose to Con A caused the G-PEG insulin complex to be displaced and released (**Figure 3**) [47].

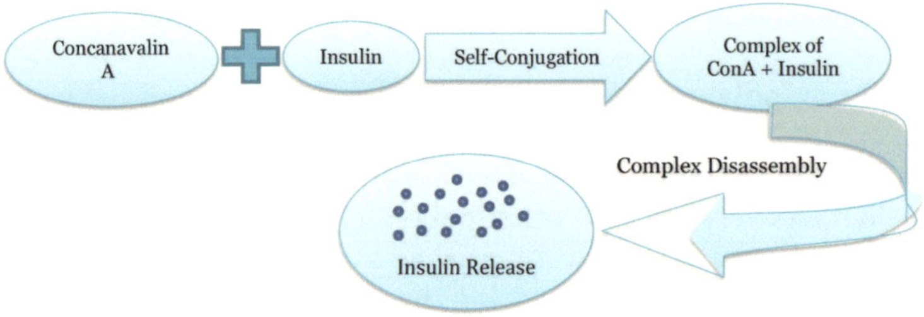

Figure 3.
Polymers that respond to glucose in a variety of ways.

2.5 Smart polymers with photo responsiveness

Photo-sensitive polymeric materials are useful in that they could transport bioactive substances in reaction to light, including drug release happening nearly instantly and with excellent precision due to photo-induced restructuring in nano-carriers [48]. Three primary strategies were used to do this: This non-invasive form of drug administration reacts to the lighting of a certain wavelength and depends on either a single or multiple on-off drug release patterns [49]: (1) photo-generated change of hydrophobic nature to hydrophilic nature, (2) photo splitting reaction, and (3) photo-induced warming. Whilst also electromagnetic radiations with wavelengths in the range from 250 to 380 nm (ultraviolet region) and 700–900 nm (near-infrared region) are being used to stimulate photo-sensitive responses, light with wavelengths greater than 900 nm is inappropriate for delivery of drugs to certain parts of the human body, including the posterior section of the ocular system, because it cannot permeate the ocular soft tissue. Despite the fact that various polymers have been explored for ocular administration, several have been ruled out owing to chromophore intolerance and tissue destruction from photostimulation [50]. In order to establish an osmolality of a gel system, UV-responsiveness polymeric materials have been used in the eye to trigger an ionization process in the exposed to UV light, culminating in drug release through an inflow of solvent [51]. In another study, Viger et al. [52] used light thermally release of drugs to show the liberation of aqueous nano-platforms from watered poly(lactic-co-glycolic acid) (PLGA) micro-particulate system. Whenever moisture was subjected to NIR light with a wavelength of 980 nm, the photo-energy was quickly converted into thermal energy. The PLGA changed to a rubbery condition as a result of the warming, allowing the Nile red or Nile blue to be released from the micro-particulate system more easily. When compared with untreated particulates, the substantial release was achieved, which was also shown in vitro [52].

At the minimum one aqueous soluble area, at minimum one biodegradable part, as well as at least minimum of two free radical polymerizable portions are included in the macromers. Free radical activators polymerize macromers in presence of UV irradiation, visible light stimulation, or heat energy. Poly (vinyl alcohol), PEG, polysaccharides like hyaluronan, or peptides like albumin can make up the core aqueous soluble area. Polymers consisting of polyglycolic acid, polylactic acid, poly(anhydrides), polylactones, and poly(amino acids), may be used in the biodegradable zones. Acrylates, methacrylates, diacrylates, and other physiologically acceptable polymerizable units are favored polymerizable areas. Ethyl eosin, camphorquinone, and acetophenone analogs, are examples of promoters that can be employed to generate free radicals [53].

2.6 Enzyme sensitive polymeric material

Some fundamental guidelines should be followed while synthesizing enzyme-sensitive polymers with biomedical utilization. Enzymes must work in certain settings (e.g., an aquatic milieu having multiple ions with a pH of 7.4 or mildly basic or acid), while enzyme-sensitive polymers must withstand these circumstances. Apart from the availability of a substrate/substrate-mimic molecule for such focused enzyme to respond, the focused enzymes' operations must cause a variation in the polymers' characteristics for the particular activities to occur. The activity of the enzyme and the reaction of the final substance can be performed concurrently or in a step-by-step manner. For instance, proteins were used as a crosslinking agent in the DNA nanoparticles, and proteases quickly degrade the protein, destroying the nanoparticles [54]. In some other cases, enzymatic dissociation of a protective moiety causes peptides generated from amyloid to fold, reorganize, and self-assemble forming fibrillar clumps [55].

In live organisms, enzymes govern the bond generation and breakage, substrate oxidation/reduction, as well as isomerization processes, with the first two chemical reactions being exploited in the development of enzyme-sensitive materials. The bond breakage process has been utilized to cleave protein as well as ester bonds with polymers and/or tiny moiety, which really is important in controlled medication delivery with implant biodegradation. The kinase/phosphatase combination, which catalyzes the dephosphorylation/phosphorylation events here on substrates, might be employed to build reversibly sensitive materials through enzymatic bond creation and breaking.

Chitosan, alginate, dextran, polyethylene glycol, polyacrylamide, and polyethylene oxide have all been investigated as polymer matrices for the creation of enzyme-sensitive systems (butyl methacrylate) (**Figure 4**) [56–58].

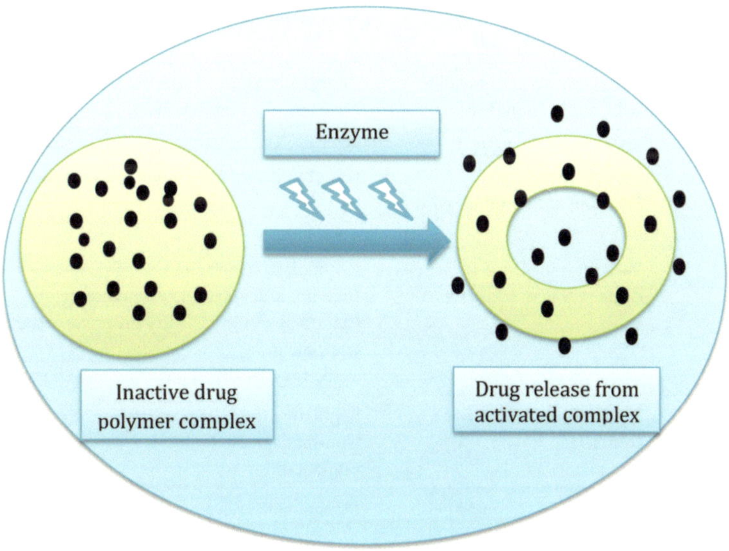

Figure 4.
Polymers that respond to enzymes in a variety of ways.

2.7 Oxidation and reduction sensitive polymeric material

Redox polymeric materials can be separated into reduction reactive systems and oxidation reactive processes depending on the nature of a reductive stimulus. Disulfide and diselenide connections are typically seen in the reduction reactive system, which will be disrupted by considerable growth in the cost of nearby reducing molecules such as GSH. Direct production of disulfide coupling and bridging with a disulphide-containing crosslinking agent are basically two strategies for incorporating disulfide coupling in the process. By live or regulated polymerization, disulfide could be incorporated into the polymer as the oligomer (e.g. Reversible addition-cleavage crosslinking polymerization and atomic transfer radical polymerization) [59]. The thiol-disulfide interchange process, which is commonly utilized to create reduction reactive prodrugs including genetic transporters, is another viable method with gentler circumstances (e.g. at room temperature) than the controlled/living polymerization [60]. To stop the drug leaking, polymeric micelles comprising substances can indeed be crosslinked with covalently crosslinking agents (using bis (2,2′-hydroxyethyl)disulfide, dithiodipropionic acid, and their derived products) and afterward the disulfide conduits split to discharge the substances after the micelles meet the goal [61]. Since the bond-breaking energies of the C-Se (244 kJ mol1) and Se-Se (172 kJ mol1) bond formation are lesser than those from the C-S (272 kJ mol1) and S-S (251 kJ mol1) bond formation, replacing the disulfide interconnection with the diselenide connection is a simple approach to strengthen the responsiveness of the redox-sensitive system. However, diselenide link insertion into a polymeric matrix is more difficult than disulfide link formation, and more research into effective synthetic techniques is needed (**Table 1**) [62].

Responsiveness	Merits	Constraints
Thermal	Introduction of active moieties is simple. Manufacturing and composition are easy.	Issues with injectability during application criteria. Weak mechanical sturdiness, biocompatibility problems, and thermolablile medicine instabilities.
pH	Drugs that are thermolabile will benefit from this.	There is a scarcity of data about toxicity. Mechanical strength is low.
Light	Managing the trigger procedure is simple. Controlling the stimuli with precision.	Gel has a poor mechanical strength, which increases the risk of noncovalently bound chromophores seeping off.
Electric field	Variations in electrical charge cause pulsative releasing.	Unpredictable behaviors to light. Implantation via surgery is necessary. External stimulus delivery necessitates the use of extra equipment. Perfecting the size of electric charge is challenging.
Ultrasound	Protein release that can be controlled.	Regulating the release using specialized equipment. Non-biodegradable delivery systems necessitate surgical implantation.
Mechanical abrasion	Possibility of obtaining medication release	Managing the release pattern is difficult.

Table 1.
Several smart polymeric drug delivery technologies are available [7].

The reactive oxygen system, the result of aerobic metabolism, is what activates oxidation reactive systems. Oxidation reactive materials include sulfur-based compounds. To accomplish the lipophilic-hydrophilic shift, reactive oxygen moiety can oxidize poly(propylene sulfide) (PPS) to generate sulphoxide [63]. The comparatively higher stability of sulfur in sulfur-containing substances is a fundamental restriction, and the reaction to reactive oxygen may not be as sensitive. The addition of selenium to the polymeric materials, which will be more sensitive than sulfur, improves the susceptibility of the reaction to reactive oxygen [64]. Owing to its own oxidation responsiveness, ferrocene-containing polymeric materials are another prominent family of oxidation reactive polymers [65, 66]. Ferrocene can be inserted in the framework, side chain, and terminal unit of the polymeric materials. Developing themes such as boronic ester moieties, oligoproline, and tetrathiafulvalene have been studied for the development of new oxidation-sensitive polymeric substances to broaden the uses [67, 68].

3. Applications of specialized polymeric system

3.1 Drug delivery

The majority of bio-sensitive systems, notably those used in cancer therapy, rely on regulated medication release. While significant advancements in chemotherapy have resulted in the development of a number of novel medications for treating cancer that has significantly improved patients' prognoses and standard of living, a key obstacle remains the treatments' lack of compassion for neoplastic cells [69]. The treatment impact of the anticancer treatment is harmed by the possibility of a deadly systemic adverse effect and the development of resistant strains [70]. Continued improvement of chemotherapy necessitates adequate drug release at the tumor site as well as the avoidance of drug-carrier endosomal sequestration, and the development of suitable stimulus-sensitive systems has shown tremendous promise in both areas. This is attributable to the fact that tumor tissues' milieu can produce a variety of natural signals. For instance, tumor cells contain moderate acidity, significant GSH (glutathione) levels, as well as a top-level of hyaluronidase [71], therefore pH-, redox-, and enzyme sensitive drug carriers, as well as their combinations (to optimize the release of drug efficiency), have been extensively studied. Blood serum albumin (HSA)-coatedMnO_2 nanomaterial's as an adaptive transporter of cis-platinum is a fresh example. The MnO_2 combines with internal H_2O_2 just at tumor site to produce O_2 in vivo, overcoming medicaments resistance caused by local hypoxic, while the nanoparticles disintegrate in an acidic medium, releasing cis-platinum [72]. In another layout, the water-soluble rhodamine B was covalently conjugated to the PDMAEMA (Poly((2-dimethylamino)ethyl methacrylate) and via disulphide bond formation with the lipophilic coumarin 102 physiologically encapsulated inside the nanogel, and the hydrophilic rhodamine B has been covalently linked to the PDMAEMA via disulfide bond formation with the lipophilic coumarin 102. The nano gel is swollen in an acidic medium and shrinks at increased temperature to liberate the coumarin 102, whereas decreasing DL-dithiothreitol cleaves the disulfide bridges to liberate the aqueous cargo medication [73]. The development of bio-sensitive drug carriers for controlled release has exploded in the past few decades, and additional improvements in release effectiveness have resulted in dual and numerous systems that can carry several medicines for programmable site-specific delivery of drugs. Pharmaceutical loading, persistence in a microenvironment, tumor-targetability, effective absorption of cancerous cells, and controlled intracellular release of the drug are among the fundamental difficulties in the delivery of drugs addressed by the many configurations of the bio-sensitive delivery mechanism. Even though there are a lot of good studies, most of it makes a specialty of the difficulties and still in the concept-proofing phase [74]. The challenges are associated with most existing bio-sensitive drug delivery mechanisms, such as poor drug loading efficiency, biodegradability, as well as the ability to remain circulatory and concentrate in the target organs, must be overcome in order to convert the study into practical practice (e.g. tumor). In contrast, more research into the subatomic scale in vivo behavior of bio-sensitive systems, as well as the influence of systemic physiological parameters on the release of the drug, is needed [74].

3.2 Biomaterials actuators and micro-fabrication

Designing microfluidic technologies for biochemical applications has proven to be a difficult task, and a properly working valve is a critical component in these technologies. Traditional micro-actuators are somewhat sophisticated components that needed additional electricity to operate. The use of sensitive smart polymer composites to govern flow eradicates this need for external power, output control, and complicated fabrication ploys, allowing them to be integrated within microfluidics streams and dwindle or perk up in response to an external stimulus, causing streams to open or close. Photo triggered polymerization inside the stream of a microfluidic chip that may be employed as a gate for changing; transmission, measuring, and closing of a PCR reaction vessel produced monolithic plugging PNiPAAm complexes using 5% methylenebisacrylamide. Because of their simple construction of sensors, the kinetic studies of the volume phase change process as a feature of gel structure and shape, the capacity of the sensors to thwart and supplant the transition between two fluids, anisotropic bulging of a polymer, as well as the ability to adapt to changing stimuli, responsive smart polymeric materials are the structural elements for microfluidic devices. Thermally sensitive smart polymeric materials have also been utilized to create "smart" affinities beads which can be transiently mounted on microfluidic walls of the channel just above MinCST in order to acquire the target biomaterials via its friendliness component. Proteomic functionalities, such as pre-concentration and isolation of soluble proteins on an embedded fluidics device, have been enabled by this technology. Many efforts were made to emulate live creatures' effective transition of chemical energy to mechanical energy. The bio-inspired actuators might be employed in future 'soft' technologies that are based on biological concepts rather than mechanical ones. Because bio-inspired actuators can tolerate extremely hostile conditions, they can also be utilized to pick up extremely small items in watery solutions. By contorting a barrier that subsequently occludes an opening, a system built on pH-sensitive smart polymeric discs of polymethacrylic acid-triethylene glycol dimethacrylate (PMAA-EG) has indeed been utilized to control medication delivery. The electronegative interpenetrating matrix (IPM) made of PVA with PNiPAAm was studied in aquatic NaCl solution for its moisture content and carrying behavior with electromagnetic current, with the goal of using it in bio-inspired sensors and devices that respond quickly to exterior electric fields. The immobilized smart polymer's prompted manipulation of interfacial characteristics at the solid-liquid interface has benefits in the development of microfluidics bio-analytical systems since they supply the actuation pressure necessary for both valving and dispensing functionalities in micro-dispensing gadgets [75–77].

3.3 Diagnostic uses

Biomedicine research involves advancing our understanding of biology and the processes behind physiological activity and disorders. As a result, in addition to illness therapy, one of the most significant goals is diagnostics, wherein bio-sensitive materials have shown promising potential in detecting low concentrations of biochemical, proteins, and genes that act as sickness-specific indicators. Those indicators are typically tested using high-cost chromatography techniques like high-performance liquid chromatography and gas chromatography-mass spectrometry, but using stimuli-sensitive systems, easy, rapid, precise, and low-cost detection procedures may be established.

For instance, metallic nanoparticles with a size of 4 nm may greatly boost T1 distinction in magnetic resonance imaging; however, their aggregation led in T2 contrasting augmentation owing to in uniform magnetic field around the aggregates. As a result, IONs like these have been employed as a T2 contrast media to diagnose liver disorders. They are, nevertheless, unsuitable for the identification of smaller hepatocellular carcinomas that requires a good detection to improve the individuals' average five-year rate of survival [78]. The fall in pH dispersed the aggregation of the functional metallic nanoparticles when they were treated using i-Motif DNAs that really can convert from unistranded to fused quadruple-helical structure in an acidic medium. Because acidification of the tumor encouraged the breakdown of the metallic nanoparticles aggregates and shifted the MRI signal between T2 to T1 augmentation to better the differentiation between hepatocyte and tiny hepatocytic carcinoma tissues, tiny hepatocytic carcinoma may be diagnosed with these bifunctional metallic nanoparticles [79]. pH-sensitive surfaces made comprised of nanoparticles with just an amino group having a silane layer are another intriguing instance. In an acidic medium, the amino groups are protonated, making the surfaces highly hydrophilic, whereas in a highly alkaline, the surfaces become really hydrophobic. The amount of glucose in the mouth and pee may be reliably determined in one second using this surface via measuring the contact area of the liquid specimen, which is dependent on the created gluconic acid following adding glucose oxidase to the specimen [80]. This non-invasive, economic approach of fast glucose measurement is useful for overcoming the drawbacks of standard intrusive diagnosis of diabetes, including such discomfort and infection hazard. While contemporary research has demonstrated the stimuli-sensitive system's potential and performance in preclinical testing for diagnostic uses, the majority of the built systems do not fulfill the standards for clinical usage. This is owing to the large variety of chemicals found in real specimens collected from individuals with varying situations (e.g., various diets, ethnicities, and lifestyles), which considerably affects the measurement's specificity and stability [81]. Aside from identifying biochemical levels, constant monitoring and distribution centres in human, both of which are challenging to perform, may be required. As a result, motivated monitoring technologies are still in the early stages of development, and more investigation is necessary before they can be used in clinical illness treatment.

3.4 Implants for cardiology

Creating actuators including such valves and levers out of the material, which could be utilized as blood artery implants, is one potential application. To modulate blood flow, the artery might be enlarged or constricted, also utilizing internal biochemical impulses. The valves would've been placed into the blood channels of the heart, or prosthetic muscular implants may be created [82].

3.5 Mucoadhesive delivery using polymers

Hydrophilic polymers must be employed to construct the liquid ophthalmic delivery mechanism since they may serve as a useful viscosity altering or boosting agent. In the ophthalmic mucoadhesive delivery method, polysaccharides are often employed. Hyaluronic acid, methylcellulose, hydroxypropyl methylcellulose, chitosan, gellan gum, carrageenan, xanthan gum, and guar gum are some of its variants. Chitosan is a polysaccharide polymer made up of polysaccharides. It is appropriate for usage in medication compositions due to its biodegradability, low toxicity, and biocompatibility [83]. Polyvinylpyrrolidone, poloxamer, and polyvinyl alcohol are among additional non-ionic polymers utilized for mucoadhesive characteristics [84].

3.6 Cancer treatment using a polymer drug combination

The medications as well as the polymer have a physiologically labile connection. Paclitaxel [poly(L-glutamic acid)] is a chemotherapeutic medication employed to treat cancers of the ovary, breast, as well as lung. Phase III studies have been conducted on it. Among its 2'hydroxyl unit and the carboxylic acid of poly(L-glutamic acid), it possesses an ester bond [83]. To improve its efficacy as an antitumor targeted drug delivery, Poly (amidoamine) and PEG is covalently attached with the chemotherapy medication Paclitaxel. Both improve the solubility of the substance. In an in vitro investigation of mankind ovarian cancer cells, it was discovered that PEG-based conjugates lowered paclitaxel activity by 25-fold, but the Poly (amidoamine)]-G4 dendrimer increased its efficacy by more than ten times [12]. The medication 5-fluorouracil induces cell death. Some researchers created PLA nanospheres as an encapsulating reagent for 5-fluorouracil [12].

3.7 Medicine and biotechnology

Smart polymeric materials may be chemically attached to bio-substances or physically combined with them to create a vast variety of polymeric materials and bio-molecular systems that really can adapt to physiological and chemical stimuli. Oligosaccharides, Polypeptides, glucose and polysaccharides, solitary as well as double-sided oligonucleotides, DNA plasmid, basic lipids and ligands, phospholipids, as well as synthesized medicine compounds are examples of bio-substances that can be polymer linked. Smart polymeric materials and sensitive surfaces that cope with environmental stimuli are made with these materials. Smart polymers with size-specific switches for turning proteins on and off were also studied. When a sensible polymer chain is connected to a protein complex that is further away from active site, the expanded polymer chain shields the active-locations, preventing bigger molecules from attaching. These polymers operate as a molecular gatekeeper, limiting the types of molecules that really can attach to proteins depending on their size [85].

3.8 Glucose level monitoring

The manufacture of insulin administration devices for the management of diabetic individuals is a prime utilization of smart polymeric materials. Several technologies have been used to give precise amounts of insulin at precisely the right moment, and all of them include a glucose sensor, sometimes known as a "biosensor," incorporated into

Stimuli	Drug	Polymer	Uses	Goal/outcome of the research
Thermal responsive	Exenatide	PLGA–PEG–PLGA	Diabetic type 2 treatment	To create an injectable composition with a long-acting effect [90].
	Leuprolide	Polybenzofulvene	For treatment of tumors	External warmth is used to preserve the oligopeptide medication and modulate the release rate [91].
pH responsive	Ketoprofen	Poly(acrylamide)-g-carrageenan and sodium alginate	Targeted distribution to the colon	Whenever the ph of the sample was changed from acidic to basic, ketoprofen release rose considerably [92].
	Dauxorubicin and paclitaxel	Poly(ethylene glycol)-block-poly (propylene glycol)-poly(ethylene glycol)	Survival time is extended as compared to single-drug treatment.	The rate of release can be enhanced by lowering the pH of the external surroundings from acidic to basic [93].
Glucose responsive	Insulin-Con A complex	Methacrylate derivatives of dextran and concanavellin	Insulin delivery that is self-controlled	The findings showed that insulin release was bidirectional in reaction to varying glucose level, and also that the insulin produced was effective [94].
	Sulphonamide	N,N(dimethylacrylamide) and sulfadimethoxine monomer	Glucose-responsive hydrogel made of sulphonamide	In such a buffered salt solution at pH 7.4, the gelatin displayed bidirectional expansion as a result of glucose content from 0 and 300 mg/dL [95].
Enzyme responsive	Amyloid	Chitosan	The amyloid-derived proteins are rearranged as a result of this.	In live organisms, enzymes govern binding and breakage, substrates oxidation / reduction, including isomerization processes, with the first two chemical reactions being exploited in the development of enzyme responsive substances [57].
Photo responsive	Cross linked hyalouronic acid hydrogel	Trisodium salt of copper chlorophyllin	The enzymatic reaction is what drives the prospective application of visible light-responsive hydrogels for temporal delivery of drugs.	Photosensitive compounds including such chromophores are used to make visible light-sensitive hydrogels [94].

Table 2.
Several uses of advanced drug delivery systems.

the mechanism. The word 'biosensor' refers to sensing devices that are used to detect the number of chemicals and other biologically relevant analytes. mGlucose oxidase (GluOx) is primarily employed in glucose monitoring and enables the use of various pH-sensitive smart polymeric materials for regulated insulin administration [86, 87].

3.9 Surfaces that react to stimuli

Tissue culture techniques have leveraged the shift in surface characteristics of thermally sensitive smart polymeric materials from hydrophilic well above threshold temperature to hydrophobic underneath it. Human cells are grown on hydrophobic solid culture plates and are normally separated from them using a protease therapy that causes the cells to be damaged. Because of the close connectivity among cells and cells, this allows for a high level of effectiveness whenever transplanted into individuals. The intensity of each molecule's reaction to variations in stimuli is a combination of single monomer unit modifications that are weak on their own, and these modest reactions combine to generate a force that drives biochemical mechanisms. Likewise, the chromatographic matrix has been modified using surfaces with thermally responsive hydrophobic/hydrophilic qualities. For protein-rich selectivity with minimal non-specific couplings, thermally responsive size-exclusion chromatography is utilized. Smart polymeric mats are distinguished by their non-linear behavior [88, 89]. A minor stimulus can cause a substantial change in structure and characteristics (**Table 2**). Once that shift happens, the polymer exhibits a predictable all-or-nothing reaction with full homogeneity throughout [96].

4. Conclusion and future trends

The topic of stimuli-sensitive polymeric materials is quickly evolving, with evidence of its pharmacokinetic and therapeutic usefulness in the delivery of drugs. Stimuli-sensitive polymeric materials, which constitute an adaptive delivery strategy, have been proven to effectively respond in the required manner to the associated stimuli and are interesting prospects as a specific drug delivery option. Despite the fact that most of these polymeric' multifunctionality qualities enable for a variety of health uses, stimuli sensitive polymeric substances have limited therapeutic potential due to cytocompatibility and toxicity concerns. The enormous progress and different benefits and prospects of stimuli-sensitive polymeric materials have been highlighted in this chapter. Despite the various options that are already available, additional research into healthier and much more biocompatible delivery mechanisms has still been needed.

Consent for publication

Not applicable.

Availability of data and materials

All the information in the manuscript has been referred from the included references and is available upon request from the corresponding author.

Competing interests

The authors declare no competing interest.

Authors' contributions

I declare that this work was done by the author named in this article. PS conceived, designed the study, carried out the literature collection of the data, writing, and corrected the manuscript. PS, MT, and VJ read and approved the final manuscript.

Abbreviations

MaxCST	Maximum crucial solution temperature
MinCST	Minimum crucial solution temperature
GOx	Glucose oxidase
PEG	Polyethylene Glycol
PPS	poly(propylene sulphide)
GSH	Glutathione
PDMAEMA	(Poly((2-dimethylamino)ethyl methacrylate)
PMAA-EG	Polymethacrylic acid-triethylene glycol dimethacrylate
IPM	Interpenetrating matrix

Author details

Pankaj Sharma[1*], Vinay Jain[1] and Mukul Tailang[2]

1 ShriRam College of Pharmacy, Banmore, Morena, Madhya Pradesh, India

2 SOS, Pharmaceutical Sciences, Jiwaji University, Gwalior, Madhya Pradesh, India

*Address all correspondence to: pankajsharma223@gmail.com

References

[1] Anderson JM, Kim SW. Advances in drug delivery systems (3), book review. Journal of Pharmaceutical Sciences. 1989;**78**:608-609

[2] Langer R, Peppas NA. Advances in biomaterials, drug delivery, and bio nanotechnology. AICHE Journal. 2003;**49**:2990-3006

[3] Heller A. Integrated medical feedback systems for drug delivery. AICHE Journal. 2005;**51**:1054-1066

[4] Martinho N, Damge C, Reis PC. Recent advances in drug delivery systems. Journal of Biomaterials and Nanobiotechnology. 2011;**2**:510-526

[5] Din F, Aman W, Ullah I, Quereshi OS, Mustapha O, Shafique S, et al. Effective use of nano-carriers as drug delivery systems for the treatment of selected tumors. International Journal of Nanomedicine. 2017;**12**:7291-72309

[6] Tiwari G, Tiwari R, Sriwastawa B, Bhati L, Pandey S, Pandey P, et al. Drug delivery systems: An updated review. International Journal of Pharmaceutical Investigation. 2012;**2**:2-11

[7] James HP, John R, Alex A, Anoop K. Smart polymers for the controlled delivery of drugs–a concise overview. Acta Pharmaceutica Sinica B. 2014;**4**(2):120-127

[8] Teleanu DM, Chircov C, Grumezescu AM, Volceanov A, Teleanu RI. Blood brain delivery methods using nanotechnology. Pharmaceutics. 2018;**10**:298-305

[9] Cacciatore I, Ciulla M, Fornasari E, Marinelli L, Di Stefano A. Solid lipid nanoparticles as a drug delivery system for the treatment of neurodegenerative diseases. Expert Opinion on Drug Delivery. 2016;**13**(8):1121-1131

[10] Patel M, Souto EB, Singh KK. Advances in brain drug targeting and delivery: Limitations and challenges of solid lipid nanoparticles. Expert Opinion on Drug Delivery. 2013;**10**:889-905

[11] Schmaljohann D. Thermo and pH responsive polymers in drug delivery. Advanced Drug Delivery Reviews. 2006;**58**:1655-1670

[12] Liechty WB et al. Polymers for drug delivery systems. Annual Review of Chemical and Biomolecular Engineering. 2010;**1**:149-173

[13] Langer RS, Peppas NA. Present and future applications of biomaterials in controlled drug delivery systems. Biomaterials. 1981;**2**:201-214

[14] Verma RK, Mishra B, Garg S. Osmotically controlled oral drug delivery. Drug Development and Industrial Pharmacy. 2000;**26**:695-708

[15] Hoffman AS. The origins and evolution of "controlled" drug delivery systems. Journal of Controlled Release. 2008;**132**(3):153-163

[16] Howard MD, Jay M, Dziubla TD, Lu X. PEGylation of nanocarrier drug delivery systems: State of the art. Journal of Biomedical Nanotechnology. 2008;**4**(2):133-148

[17] Knop K, Hoogenboom R, Fischer D, Schubert US. Poly (ethylene glycol) in drug delivery: Pros and cons as well as potential alternatives. Angewandte Chemie – International Edition is Angew. 2010;**49**:6288

[18] Bae Y, Kataoka. Intelligent polymeric micelles from functional poly(ethylene glycol)-poly(amino acid) block copolymers. Advanced Drug Delivery Reviews. 2009;**61**:768

[19] Marcucci F, Lefoulon F. Active targeting with particulate drug carriers in tumor therapy: Fundamentals and recent progress. Drug Discovery Today. 2004;**9**:219

[20] Torchilin VP. Passive and active drug targeting: Drug delivery to tumors as an example. Handbook of Experimental Pharmacology. 2010;**197**:3

[21] Bhadra D, Bhadra S, Jain P, Jain NK. Pegnology: A review of PEGylated systems. Die Pharmazie. 2002;**57**:65

[22] Lammers T, Kiessling F, Hennink WE, Storm G. Nanotheranostics and image-guided drug delivery: Current concepts. Molecular Pharmaceutics. 2010;**7**:1899

[23] Ahmed F, Pakunlu RI, Srinivas G, Brannan A, Bates F, Klein ML, et al. Shrinkage of a rapidly growing tumor by drug-loaded polymersomes: pH-triggered release through copolymer degradation. Molecular Pharmaceutics. 2006;**3**(3):340-350

[24] Ahmed F, Pakunlu RI, Brannan A, Bates F, Minko T, Discher DE. Biodegradable polymersomes loaded with both paclitaxel and doxorubicin permeate and shrink tumors, inducing apoptosis in proportion to accumulated drug. Journal of Controlled Release. 2006;**116**(2):150-158

[25] Ward MA, Georgiou TK. Thermoresponsive polymers for biomedical applications. Polymers. 2011;**3**:1215-1242

[26] Kikuchi A, Okano T. Intelligent thermoresponsive polymeric stationary phases for aqueous chromatography of biological compounds. Progress in Polymer Science. 2002;**27**:1165-1193

[27] Hoffman AS, Stayton PS, Bulmus V, Chen G, Chen J, Cheung C, et al. Really smart bioconjugates of smart polymers and receptor proteins. Journal of Biomedical Materials Research. 2000;**52**(4):577-586

[28] Al-Tahami K, Singh J. Smart polymer based delivery systems for peptides and proteins. Recent Patents on Drug Delivery & Formulation. 2007;**1**:65-71

[29] Kumar A, Srivasthava A, Galevey IY, Mattiasson B. Smart polymers: Physical forms and bioengineering applications. Progress in Polymer Science. 2007;**32**:1205-1237

[30] Bawa P, Viness B, Yahya EC, Lisa C. Stimuli-responsive polymers and their applications in drug delivery. Biomedical Materials. 2009;**4**:022001

[31] Diez-Pena E, Quijada-Garrido I, Barrales-Rienda JM. On the water swelling behaviour of poly(N-isopropylacrylamide) [P(N-iPAAm)], poly(methacrylic acid) [P(MAA)], their random copolymers and sequential interpenetrating polymer networks (IPNs). Polymer. 2002;**43**:4341-4348

[32] Varga I, Gilanyi T, Meszaros R, Filipcsei G, Zrinyi M. Effect of crosslink density on the internal structure of poly(N isopropylacrylamide) microgels. The Journal of Physical Chemistry. B. 2001;**105**:9071-9076

[33] Yan L, Zhu Q, Kenkare PU. Lower critical solution temperature of linear PNIPA obtained from a yukana potential chains. Journal of Applied Polymer Science. 2007;**78**:1971-1976

[34] Jones MS. Effect of pH on the LCST of random copolymers of

N-isopropylacrylamide and acrylic acid. European Polymer Journal. 1999;**35**:795-801

[35] Cao YL, Ibarra C, Vacanti C. Preparation and use of thermo responsive polymers. In: Morgan JR, Yarmush ML, editors. Tissue Engineering: Methods and Protocols. Totowa: Humana Press; 2006. pp. 75-84

[36] Spohr R, Reber N. Thermal control of drug release by a responsive ion track membrane observed by radio tracer flow dialysis. Journal of Controlled Release. 1988;**50**:1-11

[37] Hu J, Zhang G, Ge Z, Liu S. Stimuli-responsive tertiary amine methacrylate-based block copolymers: Synthesis, supramolecular self-assembly and functional applications. Progress in Polymer Science. 2014;**39**(6):1096-1143

[38] Hoffman AS. Hydrogels for biomedical applications. Progress in Polymer Science. 2012;**64**:18-23

[39] Dai S, Ravi P, Tam KC. pH-responsive polymers: Synthesis, properties and applications. Soft Matter. 2008;**4**(3):435-449

[40] Alvarez-Lorenzo C, Blanco-Fernandez B, Puga AM, Concheiro A. Crosslinked ionic polysaccharides for stimuli-sensitive drug delivery. Advanced Drug Delivery Reviews. 2013;**65**:1148-1171

[41] Jiang TY, Wang ZY, Tang LX, Mo FK, Chen C. Polymer micellar aggregates of novel amphiphilic biodegradable graft copolymer composed of poly (aspartic acid) derivatives: Preparation, characterization, and effect of pH on aggregation. Journal of Applied Polymer Science. 2006;**99**(5):2702-2709

[42] Gil ES, Hudson SM. Stimuli-responsive polymers and their bioconjugates. Progress in Polymer Science. 2004;**29**:1173-1222

[43] Lou L, Kato M, Tsuruta T, Kataoka K, Nagasaki Y. Stimuli-sensitive polymer gels that stiffen upon swelling. Macromolecules. 2000;**33**:4992-4994

[44] Gonalez N, Elvira C, San RJ. Novel dualstimuli- responsive polymers derived from ethylpyrrolidine. Macromolecules. 2005;**38**:9298-9303

[45] Ravaine V, Ancla C, Catargi B. Chemically controlled closed-loop insulin delivery. Journal of Controlled Release. 2008;**132**:2-11

[46] Roy VD, Cambre JN, Sumerlin BS. Future perspectives and recent advances in stimuli-responsive materials. Progress in Polymer Science. 2010;**35**:278-301

[47] Takemoto Y, Ajiro H, Asoh TA, Akashi M. Fabrication of surface modified. Hydrogels with polyion complex for controlled release. Chemistry of Materials. 2010;**22**:2923-2929

[48] Cabane E, Zhang X, Langowska K, Palivan CG, Meier W. Stimuli-responsive polymers and their applications in nanomedicine. Biointerphases. 2012;**7**(1):9

[49] Mura S, Nicolas J, Couvreur P. Stimuli-responsive nanocarriers for drug delivery. Nature Materials. 2013;**12**(11):991-1003

[50] Yasin MN, Svirskis D, Seyfoddin A, Rupenthal ID. Implants for drug delivery to the posterior segment of the eye: A focus on stimuli-responsive and tunable release systems. Journal of Controlled Release. 2014;**196**:208-221

[51] Mamada A, Tanaka T, Kungwatchakun D, Irie M. Photoinduced phase transition of gels. Macromolecules. 1990;**23**(5):1517-1519

[52] Viger ML, Sheng W, Doré K, Alhasan AH, Carling CJ, Lux J, et al. Near-infrared-induced heating of confined water in polymeric particles for efficient payload release. ACS Nano. 2014;**8**(5):4815-4826

[53] Gan LH, Gan YY, Roshan DG. Poly (N-acrylol-N propylpiperazine): A new stimuli responsive polymer. Macromolecules. 2000;**33**:7893-7897

[54] Santiana JJ, Sui B, GomezNand Rouge JL. Programmable peptide-cross-linked nucleic acid nanocapsules as a modular platform for enzyme specific cargo release. Bioconjugate Chemistry. 2017;**28**:2910-2914

[55] Dos Santos S, Chandravarkar A, Mandal B, Mimna R, Murat K, Saucède L, et al. Switch-peptides: Controlling self-assembly of amyloid β-derived peptides in vitro by consecutive triggering of acyl migrations. JACS. 2005;**127**:11888-11889

[56] Hu Q, Katti PS, Gu Z. Enzyme-responsive nanomaterials for controlled drug delivery. Nanoscale. 2014;**6**:12273-12286

[57] Hu J, Gand Z, Liu S. Enzyme-responsive polymeric assemblies, nanoparticles and hydrogels. Chemical Society Reviews. 2012;**41**:5933-5949

[58] Zelzer M, Todd SJ, Hirst AR, McDonald TO, Ulijn RV. Enzyme responsive materials: Design strategies and future developments. Biomaterials Science. 2013;**1**:11-39

[59] Siegwart DJ, Oh JK, Matyjaszewski K. ATRP in the design of functional materials for biomedical applications. Progress in Polymer Science. 2012;**37**:18-37

[60] Huo M, Yuan J, Tao L, Wei Y. Redox-responsive polymers for drug delivery: From molecular design to applications. Polymer Chemistry. 2014;**5**:1519-1528

[61] Zhang S, Zhao Y. Rapid release of entrapped contents from multi-functionalizable, surface cross-linked micelles upon different stimulation. JACS. 2010;**132**:10642-10644

[62] Xu H, Cao W, Zhang X. Selenium-containing polymers: Promising biomaterials for controlled release and enzyme mimics. Accounts of Chemical Research. 2013;**46**:1647-1658

[63] Napoli A, Valentini M, Tirelli N, Muller M, Hubbell JA. Oxidation-responsive polymeric vesicles. Nature Materials. 2004;**3**:183-189

[64] Liu J, Pang Y, Zhu Z, Wang D, Li C, Huang W, et al. Therapeutic nanocarriers with hydrogen peroxide-triggered drug release for cancer treatment. Biomacromolecules. 2013, 2013;**14**:1627-1636

[65] Zhang X, Han L, Liu M, Wang K, Tao L, Wan Q, et al. Recent progress and advances in redox-responsive polymers as controlled delivery nanoplatforms. Materials Chemistry Frontiers. 2017;**1**:807-822

[66] Staff RH, Gallei M, Mazurowski M, Rehahn M, Berger R, Landfester K, et al. Patchy nanocapsules of poly (vinylferrocene)-based block copolymers for redox-responsive release. ACS Nano. 2012;**6**:9042-9049

[67] Broaders KE, Grandhe S, Frechet JM. A biocompatible oxidation-triggered carrier polymer with potential in therapeutics. JACS. 2011;**133**:756-758

[68] de Gracia LC, Joshi-Barr S, Nguyen T, Mahmoud E, Schopf E, Fomina N, et al. Biocompatible polymeric nanoparticles degrade and release cargo in response to

biologically relevant levels of hydrogen peroxide. JACS. 2012;**134**:15758-15764

[69] Cao Y, DePinho RA, Ernst M, Vousden K. Cancer research: Past, present and future. Nature Reviews. Cancer. 2011;**11**:749-754

[70] Patel NR, Pattni BS, Abouzeid AH, Torchilin VP. Nanopreparations to overcome multidrug resistance in cancer. Advanced Drug Delivery Reviews. 2013;**65**:1748-1762

[71] Lu Y, Aimetti AA, Langer R, Gu Z. Bioresponsive materials. Nature Reviews Materials. 2016;**2**:16075

[72] Chen Q, Feng L, Liu J, Zhu W, Dong Z, Wu Y, et al. Intelligent albumin–MnO2 nanoparticles as pH-/H2O2-responsive dissociable nanocarriers to modulate tumor hypoxia for effective combination therapy. Advanced Materials. 2016;**28**:7129-7136

[73] Cao Z, Zhou X, Wang G. Selective release of hydrophobic and hydrophilic cargos from multi-stimuli-responsive nanogels. ACS Applied Materials & Interfaces. 2016;**8**:28888-28896

[74] Cheng R, Meng F, Deng C, Klok HA, Zhong Z. Dual and multi-stimuli responsive polymeric nanoparticles for programmed site-specific drug delivery. Biomaterials. 2013;**34**:3647-3657

[75] Zangmeister RA, Tarlov MJ. DNA displacement assay integrated into microfluidic channels. Analytical Chemistry. 2004;**76**:3655-3659

[76] Harmon ME, Tang M, Frank CW. A microfluidic actuator based on thermo responsive hydrogel. Polymer. 2003;**44**:4547-4556

[77] Huber DL, Manginell RP, Samara MA, Kim B, Bunker BC. Programmed adsorption and release of proteins in a microfluidic device. Science. 2003;**301**:352-354

[78] Llovet JM, Burroughs A, Bruix J. Hepatocellular carcinoma. Lancet. 2013;**362**:1907-1917

[79] Lu J, Sun J, Li F, Wang J, Liu J, Kim D, et al. Highly sensitive diagnosis of small hepatocellular carcinoma using pH-responsive iron oxide nanocluster assemblies. JACS. 2018;**140**:10071-10074

[80] Gao ZF, Sann EE, Lou X, Liu R, Dai J, Zuo X, et al. Naked-eye point-of-care testing platform based on a pHresponsive superwetting surface: Toward the non-invasive detection of glucose NPG. Asia Mater. 2018;**10**:177-189

[81] Jung IY, Kim JS, Choi BR, Lee K, Lee H. Hydrogel based biosensors for in vitro diagnostics of biochemicals, proteins, and genes. Advanced Healthcare Materials. 2017;**6**:1601475

[82] Mahajan A, Aggarwal G. Smart polymers: Innovations in novel drug delivery. International Journal of Drug Development and Research. 2011;**3**(3):16-30

[83] Vilar G, Tulla-Puche J, Albericio F. Polymers and drug delivery systems. Current Drug Delivery. 2012;**9**:367-394

[84] Javadzadeh Y, Hamedeyazdan S. Novel drug delivery systems for modulation of gastrointestinal transit time. In: Recent Advances in Novel Drug Carrier Systems. Rijeka: IntechOpen; 2012

[85] Cao X, Lai S, Lee LJ. Design of a self-regulated drug delivery device. Biomedical Microdevices. 2001;**3**:109-118

[86] Brahmin S, Narinesingh D, Gniseppi-elie A. Biosmart hydrogels: Conjoined molecular recognition and signal transduction in biosensor fabrication

and drug delivery. Biosensors & Bioelectronics. 2002;**17**:973-981

[87] Sheppard NF, Lesho MJ, Mc Nally P, Shaun FA. Microfabricated conductimetric pH sensor. Sensors & Actuators, B: Chemical. 1995;**28**:95-102

[88] Sharma P, Tailang M. Design, optimization, and evaluation of hydrogel of primaquine loaded nanoemulsion for malaria therapy. Future Journal of Pharmaceutical Sciences. 2020;**6**:26

[89] Sharma P, Tailang M. In-vivo study of orodispersible tablet of primaquine. International Journal of Pharmaceutical Sciences and Research. 2018;**9**(8):3506-3510

[90] Li K, Yu L, Liu XJ, Chen C, Chen Q, Ding J. A long-acting formulation of a polypeptide drug exenatide in treatment of diabetes using an injectable block copolymer hydrogel. Biomaterials. 2013;**34**:2834-2842

[91] Licciardi M, Amato G, Cappelli A, Paolino M, Giuliani G, Belmonte B, et al. Evaluation of thermo-responsive properties and biocompatibility of polybenzofulvene aggregates for leuprolide delivery. International Journal of Pharmaceutics. 2012;**438**:279-286

[92] Kulkarni RV, Boppana R, Krishna MG, Mutalik S, Kalyane NV. pHresponsive interpenetrating network hydrogel beads of poly(acrylamide)-g-carrageenan and sodium alginate for intestinal targeted drug delivery: Synthesis, in vitro and in vivo evaluation. Journal of Colloid and Interface Science. 2012;**367**:509-517

[93] Zhao LL, Zhu L, Liu FY, Liu CY, Shan-Dan WQ, et al. pH triggered injectable amphiphilic hydrogel containing doxorubicin and paclitaxel. International Journal of Pharmaceutics. 2011;**410**(83-91):26

[94] Yin R, Tong Z, Yang D, Nie J. Glucose and pH dual-responsive concanavalin A based microhydrogels for insulin delivery. International Journal of Biological Macromolecules. 2011;**49**:1137-1142

[95] Kang SI, Bae YH. A sulfonamide based glucose-responsive hydrogel with covalently immobilized glucose oxidase and catalase. Journal of Controlled Release. 2003;**86**:115-121

[96] Ruan C, Zeng K, Grimes CA. A mass-sensitive pH sensor based on a stimuli-responsive polymer. Analytica Chimica Acta. 2003;**497**:123-131

Chapter 3

Thin Films: A Promising Approach for Drug Delivery System

Ramakant Joshi, Wasim Akram, Rajendra Chauhan and Navneet Garud

Abstract

The prime goal of drug delivery through drug carrier system to the specific target site at the suitable concentration for therapeutic action. Recently thin films are acquiring attention as drug carrier and various scientists are working on the formulation and development of thin films as a novel drug delivery system. Because of its capacity to safely load medications and release them in a regulated manner, thin films have attracted increasing interest in the field of drug delivery, which improves drug efficacy. They are more patient compliance and alternative to oral drug delivery employing self-application, prolonged action and easily terminate if drug toxicity is produced. Oral, buccal, sublingual, ocular, and transdermal routes have all been employed to deliver this delivery mechanism for both systemic and local effects. The development of thin films comprises of various methods with keeping in mind the anatomical and physiological constraints, physicochemical properties and types of drug substance and use of various polymers (matrix, hydrophilic and hydrophobic) as well as the characterisation methods with recent trends.

Keywords: film, prolonged action, film formation polymers, self-administration, local and systemic effect

1. Introduction

Biotechnological developments in the field of biomedical science have become more widely publicised in recent years, as the relevance of life extension and quality of life has become more widely recognised. Drug delivery system research, in particular, has been identified as one of the most challenging problems in biomedical science. In general, drug delivery system research focuses on keeping drug concentrations in the blood at a minimum and avoiding drug toxicity in vivo [1]. Thin films, in general, are ideal for targeting sensitive regions that tablets or liquid formulations may not be able to reach. Thin films have been shown to increase pharmaceutical action onset, dose frequency reduction, and treatment efficacy. Consequently, thin films may be beneficial in reducing excessive proteolytic enzyme metabolism and eliminating pharmaceutical side effects [2].

Thin films have demonstrated their ability to improve medication action onset, reduce dose frequency, and improve treatment efficacy. Thin films may also be useful for decreasing excessive metabolism induced by proteolytic enzymes and removing the negative effects of medicine [3].

Penetration enhancers are substances that temporarily lessen the skin's impermeability, making it easier to absorb penetrant through the skin. These materials should be pharmacologically inert, non-toxic, non-irritating, non-allergenic, and compatible with the drug and excipients, odourless, tasteless, colourless, and inexpensive, as well as having good solvent properties. The enhancer must not provoke a loss of physiological fluids, ions, or other endogenous elements, and the skin should quickly regain its barrier properties after it has been removed [4]. Chemical penetration enhancers boost skin permeability by reversibly eroding or changing the physicochemical makeup of the stratum corneum to reduce diffusional resistance. Most chemical penetration enhancers irritate the skin, which is one of their drawbacks [5]. It's unsurprising that agents that interrupt ordered lipid patterns, cellular membranes, and components also disrupt ordered lipid structures, cell membranes, and constituents. The clinical utility of numerous chemical permeation enhancers has been limited due to the toxicity related to them. In recent years, the FDA has looked into essential oils, terpenes, and polymeric enhancers, all of which are GRAS (Generally Recognised as Safe) [6].

Polysaccharides, proteins, peptides, polyesters, and other substances are examples of natural polymers. Because of their biocompatibility and processability, the first two kinds of endogenous polymers were widely explored in the DDS. Because polysaccharides and proteins are more similar to the extracellular matrix, natural polymer-based medicament carriers are less intrusive. Furthermore, the polymers' backbones are plentiful in a variety of easy-to-change groups, such as amino groups, carboxyl groups, hydroxyl groups, and so on, allowing them to be easily modified [7]. Finally, as life science research developed, more specific connections between native polymers and organs or cells were uncovered. Natural polymers have been demonstrated to have a stronger affinity for cell receptors and to regulate cellular processes including adhesion, division, and migration, implying that they could be exploited to create more targeted and efficient high-efficiency applications [8]. Furthermore, their breakdown behaviour in the presence of enzymes in vivo ensures their potential to develop stimuli-responsive delivery in local locations.

The main objective of thin films delivers drugs topically, where they are absorbed by the skin and into the bloodstream. They provide consistent delivery of small amounts of a drug into the bloodstream over a long period. The duration of wear time and the amount of drug delivered is different from film to film.

2. Advantages and disadvantages over conventional dosage form

2.1 Advantages

First, there are biological advantages to delivering drugs through the skin:

1. Transdermal distribution avoids the stomach environment, where the medicine may decay and become ineffective, or where it may cause the patient to experience unpleasant gastrointestinal symptoms [9].

2. The first-pass effect, in which active medication molecules are transformed to inactive molecules or even molecules that cause side effects, is avoided with transdermal distribution [10].

3. Transdermal medication administration ensures consistent plasma concentrations. When a patch is applied for 24 hours or even 7 days, the plasma levels remain consistent once a steady state is attained since the rate of drug delivery from the patch is constant. When a medicine is given four times a day, or even once a day, the drug levels rise immediately after administration and then gradually fall until the following administration, resulting in peaks and troughs throughout treatment [10].

4. TDDS, in contrast to limited controlled release via oral and intravenous routes, provides a continuous infusion of the drug over an extended period, making it ideal for drugs with a short biological half-life that requires frequent dosing, resulting in increased patient compliance and decreased inter and intra-patient variability [11].

5. It is possible to avoid therapeutic failure or the side effects that are usually linked with intermittent dosage for chronic diseases [12].

6. When necessary, self-administration and removal are feasible [13].

7. This non-invasive and safe parenteral route of drug delivery helps take away the pain and inconvenience of injections [13].

2.2 Other advantages to delivering drugs through the skin

1. Transdermal medication delivery devices, particularly simple thin films, are simple to use and non-invasive, which patients prefer [14].

2. Thin films can improve compliance and lower medical expenditures because they are simple to use. Many studies suggest that increasing pharmacological compliance lowers a patient's overall healthcare costs. Furthermore, studies have shown that prescribing thin films improves patient compliance and lowers healthcare expenses [15].

3. Medical waste can be reduced by using a transdermal delivery device instead of a needle, lowering healthcare expenditures once again.

2.3 Disadvantages

1. Many drugs especially drugs with hydrophilic structures that permeate the skin too slowly may not achieve a therapeutic level.

2. The drug, the adhesive or other excipients in the thin film formulation can cause erythema, itching, and local oedema.

3. The barrier function of the skin changes from one site to another on the same person, from person to person and also with age.

4. Daily dose of more than 10 mg is not possible.

5. Local irritation is the major problem.

6. Drugs with a long half-life cannot be formulated in the thin film.

7. It May not be Economical.

8. Barrier function changes from person to person and within the same person.

9. Heat, cold, sweating (Perspective) and showering prevent the thin film from sticking to the surface of the skin for more than one day. A new thin-film has to be applied daily.

10. In case of any medical emergency, the thin film is not a good choice.

3. Routes of thin films administration

3.1 Oral route

The oral route has traditionally been chosen over other existing administrative methods due to its ease of administration, patient compliance, and possible formulation flexibility. The buccal area (buccal mucosa) of the oral cavity provides an appealing channel for medication delivery for both local and systemic activities. Buccal mucosa possesses morphological and physiological properties that make it a good drug delivery route, including the presence of smooth muscles with high vascular perfusion, high accessibility, minimal enzymatic activity, and escape of hepatic first-pass metabolism. However, the formulation's transit duration at an application location is limited by the constant salivary flush in the mouth cavity. More study into the use of bioadhesive polymers to prolong the residence time (RT) of formulations in living tissue has resulted as a result of this [16]. Drug delivery through to the buccal mucosa has been accomplished with tablets, lozenges, chewing gums, sprays, films, patches, hydrogels, pastes, ointments, solutions, microspheres, and other dosage forms, but buccal films have been reported to be the most favourable and successful strategy for delivering through the epithelium with greater patient compliance [17].

The microenvironment of the mucosa controls medication disintegration (release) and penetration through the mucosa. The environment of the mucosa can be modified or transformed with the help of well-designed mucoadhesive drug delivery devices [17]. These systems are designed and formulated with mucoadhesive polymers, which are generally of high molecular weight and high viscosity grades with improved flexibility and optimal chain length. A variety of mucoadhesive polymers have also been used to study buccal drug delivery. Buccal films are superior to oral gels and buccal tablets among mucoadhesive drug delivery systems due to their long residence time, more flexibility in covering the buccal mucosa, and improved comfort [18]. The major goal of this study was to create a buccal mucoadhesive patch that would maintain a stable miconazole level in the mouth for lengthy periods. The created patch's performance will be compared to that of a commercial oral gel. In addition, the effect of ageing on the produced patches' mucoadhesive function will be examined.

The oral route, which includes buccal mucosa, is the most suitable for both local and systemic drug delivery among the different locations accessible for mucoadhesive drug delivery. The created buccal mucosal membrane by Jacob S et al., 2021 presents an appealing drug-delivery channel to boost both systemic and local therapy. The advantages and disadvantages of buccal drug delivery, anatomical and physiological characteristics of the oral mucosa and several in vitro techniques often employed for assessing buccal drug-delivery systems are all discussed in this paper. The importance of mucoadhesive polymers, penetration enhancers, and enzyme inhibitors in overcoming formulation problems, including the salivary refurbishment cycle, masticatory effect, and limited absorption area, is discussed. Because of their flexibility, convenience, lightness, acceptability, ability to endure mechanical stress, and specific size, biocompatible mucoadhesive films and patches are preferred dosage forms for buccal administration. The methods of preparation, the scaling-up process, and the manufacturing of buccal films are discussed [19].

Furthermore, Semalty et al. develop mucoadhesive buccal films of enalapril maleate to increase therapeutic efficacy, patient compliance, and bioavailability. Using the solvent casting technique, five formulations of mucoadhesive drug delivery systems of enalapril maleate were created as buccal films in this study. Mucoadhesive polymers employed were sodium carboxymethylcellulose, hydroxypropylmethylcellulose, hydroxyethylcellulose, and polyvinyl pyrrolidone K-90. In permeation tests, films showed controlled release for more than 10 hours. The films containing 20 mg of enalapril maleate in sodium carboxymethylcellulose 2% w/v and hydroxyethylcellulose 2% w/v showed good swelling, a convenient residence time, and promising controlled drug release, and thus can be chosen for the development of buccal films for effective therapeutic uses [17].

3.2 Ocular route

The thin layer provides a variety of functions as the interface between the ocular surface and the external environment. It generates a refracting thin coating on the corneal surface that smooth's out the uneven topography. It maintains a somewhat constant extracellular environment for corneal and conjunctival epithelial cells in terms of pH, oxygen and carbon dioxide levels, nutrition, and growth factor concentrations. Microorganisms, which are also combated by a complex and powerful antibacterial system, are diluted and washed away by tears. The tear film changes its composition in response to physiological events. The human tear film appears to be quite stable and attached to the cornea while the eyes are maintained open, taking up to 60 seconds to disclose the initial break. When a contact lens is implanted, a stable tear film is not maintained throughout the lens, and the surface dries up between blinks. The tear film on the surface of a contact lens begins to break up in 4–6 seconds (hard) or 7–9 seconds (soft) when a human blinks once every 10 seconds on average. The single most critical element in deposit formation and long-term discomfort during contact lens usage is lens drying. Several theories have been presented to explain this phenomenon. A thin film containing surface-active molecules like those found in tears should not rupture as quickly from a curved surface, according to physical chemistry. Experiments with lenses in the lab have shown that certain lens surfaces may hold a water coating for up to 2 minutes. On-eye surface dryness is caused by many reasons. With a stiff lens, drainage is unavoidable due to the tear meniscus, which is evident around the lens periphery. With the lens on the eye, the structured layers of the tear film are unable to form up as they do on the cornea. Another explanation is that the lipid layer is thin or disturbed, leaving the tear film vulnerable to evaporation. Early tear components binding to lenses might also impair wettability [20].

It has various advantages for ocular distribution, including sanitation, ease of eye drop formulation, less irritation, increased precorneal residence duration, and improved ocular bioavailability of medications that are insoluble in tear fluid. In 2015,

Mahajan HS and Deshmukh SR investigated the use of xyloglucan, a polysaccharide polymer, as a new film-forming agent for ciprofloxacin ocular administration. Ciprofloxacin ocular films were made utilising xyloglucan and the solvent casting process (2%). The formulas were made following the unusual transport release mechanism. The formulation is safe for the ocular mucosa, according to an ocular irritancy study. As a result, this research proposes that xyloglucan could be used as a film-forming polymer for ciprofloxacin ocular administration [21].

3.3 Transdermal route

Topically given pharmaceuticals in the form of patches that, when placed to the skin distributes the drug through the skin at a predetermined and controlled pace are referred to as transdermal drug delivery systems. Transdermal patches distribute drugs via the skin in a controlled and predefined manner, resulting in increased therapeutic efficacy and fewer side effects. The medications must be able to permeate the skin and reach the target site to be effective in a transdermal drug delivery system. When compared to the oral route, TDDS improves patient compliance and reduces load [6].

Transdermal delivery of drugs through the skin to the systemic circulation is a useful methodology of administration for a variety of clinical indications. Transdermal delivery systems are available for scopolamine (hyoscine) for motion sickness, clonidine and nitroglycerin for cardiovascular disease, fentanyl for chronic pain, nicotine for cessation of smoking, oestradiol (alone or in combination with levonorgestrel or norethisterone) for hormone replacement, and testosterone for hypogonadism [22].

Some of the possible benefits of transdermal drug delivery include controlled absorption, more consistent plasma levels, increased bioavailability, decreased adverse effects, painless and uncomplicated application, and the flexibility of discontinuing drug administration by simply removing the patch from the skin. Padula et al. reported a novel drug delivery system consisting of a water-based, vapour permeable membrane for cutaneous and/or transdermal distribution. The goal of this study was to control the administration of the model drug lidocaine hydrochloride through rabbit ear skin using a transdermal film. On lidocaine transport over the skin, the effects of drug loading, film-forming polymer type and content, adhesive and plasticiser were studied [23]. Aside from that, Ammar HO et al. (2013) developed and tested a transdermal ketorolac film-forming polymeric solution for pain treatment employing Eudragits® RLPO, RSPO, and E100, as well as polyvinyl pyrrolidone K30 dissolved in ethanol as film-forming solutions. An improved transdermal ketorolac formulation has shown a significant potential to provide a rapid and enhanced analgesic impact, which is a critical requirement in pain treatment [24].

4. Film formation polymers

The FFS is built on a foundation of polymers, and a range of polymers are available for this purpose. These polymers can be employed alone or in conjunction with other film-forming polymers to get the necessary film characteristics at skin temperature, these polymers should produce a clear flexible film. The **Table 1** shows a list of polymers, along with their molecular weights and properties [15].

Polymer	Properties	Use	References
Hydroxypropyl methylcellulose (HPMC)	Moderate tensile strength, moisture and oxygen barrier characteristics, elasticity, transparency, and oil and fat resistance.	HPMC is used as a raw material for coatings with moderate strength and elasticity in Film, transparency.	[25, 26]
Hydroxypropyl cellulose (HPC)	HPC used for artificial tears, emulsion stabiliser, Binder, thicke ner, white to slightly yellow tinted, odourless, inert, and tasteless powder Absolute ethanol, methanol, isopropyl alcohol, and propylene glycol are all polar organic solvents that are soluble in both cold and hot temperatures. Mucoadhesive characteristics are moderate.	Used as an excipient, and topical ophthalmic protectant and lubricant and also used in ophthalmic films.	[27, 28]
Carboxymethyl cellulose (CMC)	Anionic, water-soluble cellulose derivative, rapid hydration, High swelling strength, Good bioadhesive properties.	Used as a flocculant, chelating agent, surfactant, thickening agent, water-retaining agent, sizing agent, and film-forming material, among other things.	[29]
Polyvinyl pyrrolidone	Solubility across a wide range, Non-ionic substances, Susceptibility to swelling, Used as a mucoadhesion enhancer as a co-adjuvant.	Food additive, stabilizer, in paints and also having film-forming property.	[30, 31]
Poly ethylene oxide	For the polymer that is not ionic, Mucoadhesion is high when the molecular weight is high.	Used to deliver drugs in the transdermal and transmucosal system.	[32, 33]
Pectin	Non-ionic, high swelling characteristics, a wide range of solubility To increase mucoadhesion, it's used as a co-adjuvant.	Food, beverages, pharmaceuticals, drug and vitamin capsules, photographic films, thin-film, and cosmetics all employ it as a gelling agent.	[34, 35]
Chitosan	Odourless white or creamy powder or flakes After chitin has been partially deacetylated, Biodegradable and biocompatible Water is sparingly soluble; ethanol (95 per cent), various organic solvents, and neutral or alkali solutions with pH more than 6.5 are practically insoluble.	Chitosan has the potential to be employed as a medication carrier, a tablet excipient, a Film Forming agent, and a delivery platform for parenteral formulations, among other applications.	[36, 37]
Sodium alginate	It appears as a white or buff powder with no odour or taste. Purified carbohydrate product obtained by dilute alkali extraction from brown seaweed, is insoluble in other organic solvents and acids. Anionic has a high mucoadhesive capacity, is Non-allergenic, biodegradable, and safe In water, rapid swelling and dissolution.	Stabilisers in emulsions, suspending agents, tablet binders, and tablet disintegrants are all examples of film-forming properties.	[36, 38]
Carrageenan	Lota, Kappa, and Lambda are three structural kinds with different	Used in the food technology and pharmaceutical industry for their	[39, 40]

Polymer	Properties	Use	References
	solubility and rheology. All three kinds of sodium are soluble in both cold and hot water. pH 6 to 10 provides the optimum solution stability. Mucoadhesive characteristics are moderate.	gelling, thickening, stabilising and also having film-forming properties.	
Gelatin	A powder that ranges in colour from light amber to pale yellow. The molecular weight ranges from 15,000 to 250,000. Glycerin, acid, alkali, and hot water are all soluble in it. 9–11 per cent (w/w) moisture content.	Giving flexibility, stability and prolonged life span for the thin film.	[41, 42]
Poly (vinyl alcohol) (PVA)	Molecular weight 20,000–200,000, white to cream-coloured granular powder Synthetic polymer that is water-soluble, Polymer that is not ionic, Mucoadhesive characteristics that are moderate.	As buccal films, nanotechnology, hydrogels, and transdermal patches.	[43, 44]

Table 1.
Film formation polymers.

5. Category of thin films

Thin film is not a new preparation; it was initially launched in the late 1970 to help people take tablets and capsules that were difficult to swallow. The oral film, oral thin film, orodispersible film, oral soluble film, wafer, oral strip, buccal film, mucoadhesive film, transmucosal film, ocular film, and transdermal and topical film are some of the names given to thin films [2].

5.1 Oral film (oral thin film)

Oral films are composite polymeric matrices that may be employed as drug delivery platforms effectively. To generate elegant drug delivery platforms, these polymeric matrices can be made up of a variety of components, however, hydrophilic polymers are frequently in the centre. The European Medicines Agency (EMA) and the Food and Drug Administration (FDA) both refer to a thin film that rapidly dissolves in the oral cavity as orodispersible film. Oral films originated as unique breath-freshening formulations, but they swiftly evolved to satisfy several commercial needs, including a convenient and easy-to-swallow medicine delivery method [15].

5.1.1 Orodispersible film/oral soluble films

Because of its simplicity of administration, non-invasiveness, flexibility, patient compliance, and acceptance, the oral route of medication administration is the most popular. When put on the tongue, orally disintegrating films quickly hydrate via soaked saliva after the breakup and/or dissolution, liberating the active pharmacological substance from the dosage form. Orodispersible films are a type of formulation that is often made with hydrophilic polymers and allows for fast disintegration when exposed to saliva. Oral disintegrating tablets and oral disintegrating films are two typical oral disintegrating medicine administration strategies. These systems were developed in the late 1970s as an alternative to standard dosage forms such as quick-dissolving tablets and capsules for elderly and paediatric patients who had difficulty swallowing traditional dosage forms [45].

Orodispersible films, on the other hand, are flexible while remaining resistant to mechanical stresses. While lyophilization is a standard method for creating oral disintegrating tablets, orodispersible films are made using a technology similar to that used to make transdermal patches, which is less costly than lyophilization. Orodispersible films are preferable to liquid dosage forms such as drops or syrups because they allow for precise dosage. A quick beginning of effect might be obtained since the medication is delivered into the oral cavity in seconds. Some medications can bypass first-pass metabolism if they are absorbed through the oral mucosa, which may boost bioavailability. To ensure a strong production and packaging process as well as ease of handling and administration, an ideal orally disintegrating film must be thin and flexible, yet sturdy. The films must be transportable, non-sticky, and maintain a level shape without rolling up. They should have a nice taste and a comfortable tongue feel. The time it takes for something to disintegrate should be as quick as feasible. Because of the inverse link between mechanical qualities and disintegration time, meeting all of these parameters is difficult [46].

5.1.2 Wafers

Wafers are paper-thin polymer sheets that are used to transport pharmaceuticals. The novel dosage form is taken orally and does not need the use of water or swallowing. The wafer dissolves fast in the mouth, allowing the active substance to be taken into the bloodstream through the oral mucosa. The active component escapes the liver's first-pass action once absorbed by the oral mucosa, improving bioavailability. Based on the chosen wafer type, the active substance delivery may also be delayed. In this situation, it is absorbed through the gastrointestinal tract after ingestion [47].

Wafers that have been lyophilized and positioned on the patient's tongue grip saliva fast and dissolve within seconds, releasing the medication. Developing a dose form that improves patient confidence and acquiescence, principally intended for oral/buccal drug delivery systems, is becoming increasingly difficult. Buccal wafers are preferred over other dosage forms because of their small dimensions, low dose, and thickness. For paediatric and geriatric patients, the lyophilized oral wafer medication delivery method offers a substitute for tablets, capsules, and liquid oral dosage forms. When compared to alternative dose forms, lyophilized wafers have a bigger surface area, ensuring improved patient compliance, particularly in geriatrics and paediatrics. A good buccal wafer ought to be flexible, elastic, and easy-going, as well as have good bioadhesive characteristics to stay in the mouth cavity for the specified amount of time [48].

5.1.3 Oral strip

The oral strip, a thin film made of hydrophilic polymers that liquefy quickly on the tongue or in the buccal cavity, is one such relatively recent dosage form [49]. Oral medication delivery has progressed from basic conventional tablets/capsules to modified-release tablets/capsules to oral disintegrating tablets to wafer to the newest creation of oral strips due to research and development. Essentially, an oral strip is a postage-stamp-sized ultra-thin strip containing an active agent or active medicinal component as well as additional excipients. The simplicity of administration and portability of oral strips have led to a greater acceptance of this dose form among both paediatric and geriatric patients [50].

However, because the oral strip technology's derived devices were easily available in the marketplace in the type of breath-freshening strips, no additional determinations were required to re-instruct the general public on how to administer this dosage form. With the release and well-known usage of Listerine pocket strips, a novel unveiling in the mouthwash line, oral strip tools was already popular among the public in the early 2000s. This delivery mechanism can accommodate a wide range of compounds. Cough/cold cures (antitussives, expectorants), sore throat, erectile dysfunction medications, antihistaminics, antiasthmatics, gastrointestinal issues, nausea, pain, and CNS stimulants are just a few examples (e.g. antiparkinson disease). Caffeine strips, snoring aids, multivitamins, and sleeping aids are some of the other applications [51].

5.1.4 Buccal film

The buccal films are designed to deliver drugs to the mouth mucosa. This aim may be supplementary difficult to achieve than it appears, as increased mouth residence duration is far from the sole influencing factor. In the direction of circumventing inter and intra-individual inconsistency, the oral mucosa drug saturation ought to be taken into account, as well as one-way absorption. As a result, multilayer films have been coined as an innovative term for buccal films. The benefits of this medication delivery technology are substantial. Beyond patient acceptance, the oral cavity has many advantages for medication administration [15].

Because the buccal mucosa has a small surface area meant for application of the buccal delivery system, device dimensions and drug load are constrained. The real region for medication absorption is determined by the dosage form's size. For buccal distribution, a device with a surface area of 1–3 cm2 and a daily dosage of 25 mg or a lesser amount is preferable. Because meal ingestion and/or drinking may necessitate the removal of the delivery device, the maximum duration of buccal medication administration is roughly 4–6 hours. The more rapid turnover of the buccal mucosal epithelium (3–8 days) compared to the skin (30 days) may alter medication absorption by altering penetrability properties regularly [52].

5.1.5 Mucoadhesive film

Mucoadhesive films are retaining dosage formulae that deliver the medication into the biological substrate directly. Furthermore, as compared to lozenges and tablets, films ensure greater patient acquiescence owing to their small dimensions in addition to compact thickness. Some of these benefits, as well as others, are shared by mucoadhesive buccal films. In comparison to tablets, they have increased patient compliance in line with their modest size and thickness. Furthermore, because mucoadhesion entails addition to the buccal mucosa, films can be designed to have either a systemic or local effect. Numerous mucoadhesive buccal films have been developed to release drugs locally in the mouth cavity to treat fungal diseases such as oral candidiasis. The release can be focused on either one towards the buccal mucosa or towards the oral cavity due to the adaptability of the production methods; in the latter instance, it can give controlled release via gastrointestinal (GI) tract administration. On the other hand, films that deliver the medicine to the buccal mucosa can be created. Using directing absorption through the venous system that drains from the cheek, films delivering medicine towards the buccal mucosa prevent the first-pass effect [53]. The majority of polymers utilised as mucoadhesives are hydrophilic polymers that expand and let for chain connections with the mucin molecules in the buccal mucosa [54]. Hydroxypropyl cellulose (HPC), hydroxypropylmethylcellulose (HPMC), hydroxyethylcellulose (HEC), sodium carboxymethyl cellulose (SCMC), poly(vinyl pyrrolidone) (PVP), and chitosan are examples of swellable polymers.

5.1.6 Transmucosal film

Oral transmucosal distribution, particularly buccal and sublingual delivery, has advanced well beyond the use of traditional dosage forms, with new techniques being developed regularly. These transmucosal drug delivery methods have several benefits above oral administration meant for systemic drug delivery, together with the ability to skip the first pass effect and avoid presystemic elimination inside the GI tract. The administration of medications to the oral cavity has gotten a lot of interest because of its high potential for patient compliance and unique physiological characteristics. The distribution of medications within the mouth mucosal cavity is divided into dual categories: local delivery and systemic administration by the buccal or sublingual mucosa. Another key physiological obstacle to oral transmucosal drug administration is drug permeability through the mouth (e.g. buccal/sublingual) mucosa. The thickness of the oral mucosa, as well as the makeup of the epithelium, varies depending on the location [55].

5.2 Ocular film

The prognosis for visual illnesses such as glaucoma, age-related macular degeneration, diabetic macular oedema, and retinal vascular occlusions has considerably improved because of recent improvements in pharmaceutical therapy. As a result of these advancements in pharmacological therapy, there is a lot of interest in less invasive delivery methods, which has resulted in significant progress in the field of ocular drug administration. Therapeutic substances are difficult to distribute due to the anatomy of the eye. Due to the blood-ocular barrier, which compartmentalises the eye, as well as the eyewall itself, the eye is resistant to substantial quantities of external chemicals (cornea and sclera). Pathogens are prevented from accessing ocular tissues by the blood-ocular barrier, which also inhibits systemic pharmacologic drugs from reaching potential ocular tissue targets [56].

Ocular film lengthens the contact period, allowing for a more controlled release, lowering administration frequency, enhancing patient compliance, and increasing therapeutic efficacy. The main goal of the ocular film is to improve the contact period between the film and the conjunctival tissue to create a long-lasting formulation suited for topical or systemic therapy [57].

5.3 Transdermal and topical film

A unique technique, the film-forming technology, can be employed as an alternative to traditional topical and transdermal formulations. It's a non-solid dose form that forms a film in situ, or after being applied to the skin or any other bodily surface.

These systems include the drug and film-forming excipients in a vehicle that, when it comes into contact with the skin, evaporates leaving a film of excipients and the drug behind. The produced film can be a solid polymeric substance that works as a matrix for drug release to the skin over time or a residual liquid film that is quickly absorbed in the stratum corneum [58, 59]. The purpose of medication administration through the skin is to treat skin illnesses on a topical level or to allow pharmaceuticals to enter the systemic circulation via transdermal absorption. The topical method provides a vast and diverse surface, as well as simplicity of application by self-administration, and is a viable option to both oral and hypodermic drug delivery [60, 61]. The rate and degree of medication absorption via the skin are influenced by skin physiology, drug physicochemical qualities, and delivery mechanism [62]. The avoidance of first-pass metabolism and other GI tract factors such as pH, stomach emptying time, and others are among the benefits of transdermal film. Deliveries that are consistent and managed over a lengthy period, Minimization of peaks and troughs in blood-drug concentrations to reduce adverse effects associated with systemic toxicity. Treatment of skin diseases such as psoriasis, eczema, and fungal infections, for example, requires direct access to the target or afflicted location. Dose cessation is simple in the case of any systemic or local adverse effects [63].

6. Methods of preparation

Solvent casting and hot melt extrusion are the two most common methods for making oral films. However, several new advancements and novel ways have developed in recent years. Semisolid casting and solid-dispersion extrusion are two versions of these industrial technologies of casting and extrusion that have been defined and utilised alone or in combination. **Figure 1** showing innovative manufacturing processes, such as rolling and printing, are also discussed.

6.1 Solvent evaporation

The most typical approach for preparing thin films utilising water-soluble excipients, polymers, and drugs that are dissolved in de-ionised water is solvent evaporation; as a result, a homogeneous mixture is formed by applying high shear forces generated by a shear processor. To get good quality films, the prepared solution is placed onto a Petri plate and the solvent is allowed to dry by exposing it to high temperatures. The film-forming polymer is normally immersed in a suitable solvent overnight in the solvent casting procedure. The type of API that must be included in the film determines the appropriate solvent based on essential physicochemical parameters of the API such as melting temperature, shear sensitivity, and polymorphic form. Before completing a formulation, the drug's compatibility with the solvent and other excipients is taken into account. Entrapment of air bubbles during formulation might affect the homogeneity of produced films. **Figures 2** and **3** indicating the deaeration of the mixture is therefore accomplished with the aid of a vacuum pump [45].

6.2 Semi-solid casting

When the film constituent is an acid-insoluble polymer, this approach is favoured. The water-soluble polymers are initially dissolved in water in this step. The resulting solution is mixed with an acid-insoluble polymer solution that has been prepared

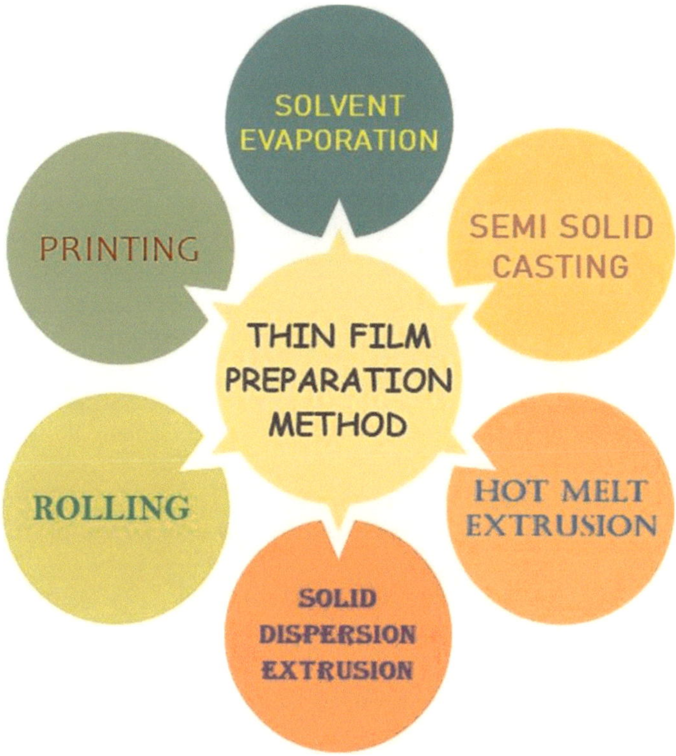

Figure 1.
Methods of preparation for thin films.

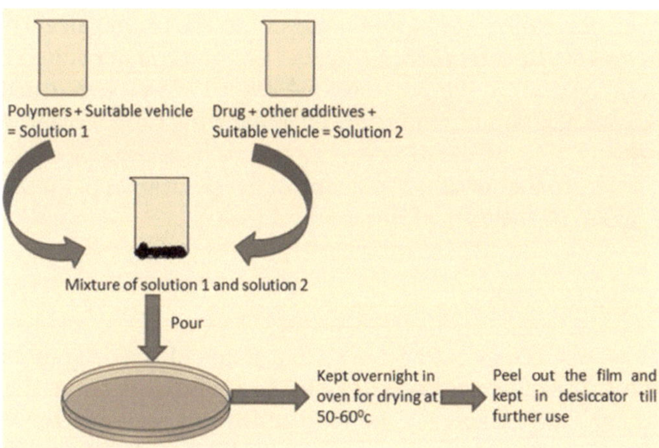

Figure 2.
Solvent evaporation method [64].

separately. Both solutions have been thoroughly combined. Following the mixing of the two solutions, a sufficient quantity of plasticiser is added to the final solution to get the gel's mass. Finally, using heat-controlled drums, the gel mass is cast onto the films or ribbons. The film thickness should be between 0.015 and 0.05 inches. The acid-insoluble polymer should be used at a 1:4 ratio with the film-forming polymer.

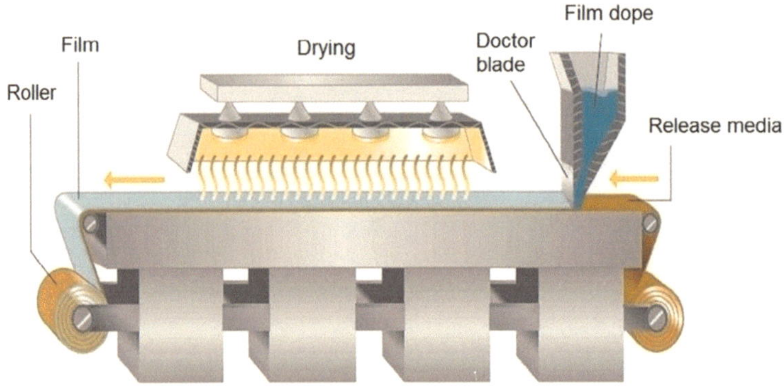

Figure 3.
Industrial machine for film formation by solvent evaporation [15].

Cellulose acetate phthalate and cellulose acetate butyrate are examples of acid-insoluble polymers [65].

6.3 Hot melt extrusion

Granules, prolonged-release tablets, transdermal and transmucosal drug delivery devices are all made with hot-melt extrusion shown in **Figure 4**. Rather than using the traditional solvent casting approach, this technique uses heating a polymer to shape it into a film. API and other components are combined in a dry state, then heated, and finally extruded out in a molten form in this procedure. There are no solvent systems involved in these operations. The film is cast from the molten mass that has resulted. The films are then cooled further before being cut to the proper size. Due to the utilisation of extremely high temperatures, this technique is not suited for thermolabile APIs. The casting and drying processes are crucial. Commercial-scale production necessitates the optimization of casting speed and drying time. Lower temperature and shorter residence time of the drug carrier mix, lack of organic solvents, continuous operation, little product waste, good control of operational parameters, and the ability to scale up are all features of this method [66].

6.4 Solid dispersion extrusion

The method entails incorporating a solid dispersion of the drug into a melted polymer solution to load the medication. To make a solid dispersion, the medication is dissolved in a suitable liquid solvent and then added to a melt of a suitable polymer that is attainable below 70°C without removing the liquid solvent. Finally, the dyes are used to form the solid dispersions into films [65].

6.5 Rolling

Water and a combination of water and alcohol are the most common solvents employed in this procedure. The active substance and other components are dissolved in a small amount of aqueous solvent using a high shear processor. Hydrocolloids that are water-soluble are dissolved in water to create a homogeneous viscous solution. The

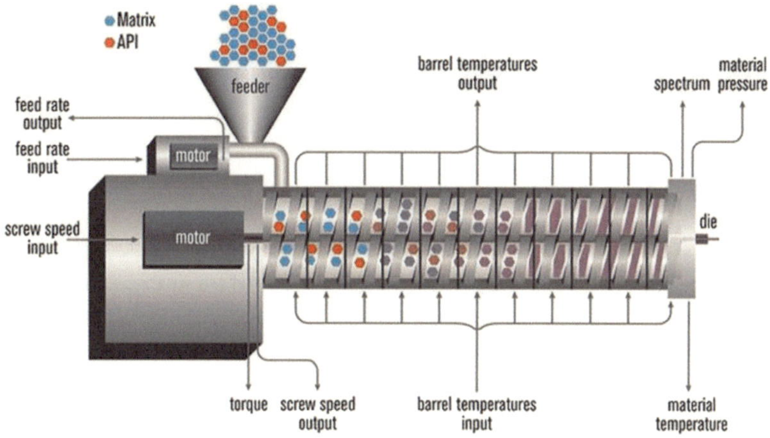

Figure 4.
Hot melt extrusion [67].

drug-containing solution or suspension is then rolled onto a carrier. After that, the film is cut into the proper shapes and sizes [68].

6.6 Printing

Polymeric thin films might be manufactured using novel technologies such as 3D printing. It might be a platform for developing the dose form that is most useful to the specific patient. Because of their versatility and cost-effectiveness, printing technologies are becoming increasingly popular. Printing technologies are extensively used in the pharmaceutical sector for identifying or labelling pharmaceutical dosage forms, especially to make the product more easily identifiable and to prevent counterfeit manufacture. However, this method has just lately been used to load drugs into medicinal dosage forms. The use of off-the-shelf consumer inkjet printers with drug-loaded inks to produce precisely dosed units of medicinal components is one example. Additionally, a hybrid of inkjet and flexographic technologies has been employed. Inkjet printing was utilised to print API on various substrates, while flexographic printing was used to cover the drug-loaded substrate with a thin polymeric coating [2].

In the all adopted method of preparation for thin films listed above like solvent evaporation, semisolid casting, hot-melt extrusion, solid dispersion extrusion, rolling and printing, the solvent evaporation method is more recommendable and mostly used. Evaporative systems provide passive and non-occlusive delivery of drugs. Therefore, this system is well tolerated and also demonstrates very low skin irritation rates. Compared to physical technologies they are having a simple working mechanism and more importantly they provide non-invasive drug delivery. Apart from that solvent evaporation method is more economical, reproducible and more efficient.

7. Characterisation aspects

Several attempts have been made to establish appropriate procedures for evaluating and characterisation of oral films, taking into account their unique properties. Certain essential criteria should be assessed for film quality control.

7.1 Surface morphology

Scanning Electron Microscopy (SEM) is used to examine the morphology of the films at various magnifications [69].

7.2 Thickness

Micrometre screw gauges or calibrated digital Vernier Callipers are used to determine the thickness of the film. The film thickness should be in the range of 5–200 μm. The thickness of the film should be measured at five distinct sites (four corners and one in the middle), and consistency in the thickness of the film is critical because it affects the accuracy of dosage distribution in the film [65].

7.3 Weight variation

The weight variation is usually calculated to guarantee that each film has the same quantity of a drug every time it is used. It's computed by weighing individual films and averaging the weights of a group of films. The individual weight of patches is deducted from the average weight of the film.

7.4 Elongation

The strain occurs when stress is given to a film ($2 \times 2\ cm^2$) sample, which causes it to stretch. Strain is the distortion of a strip before it breaks due to stress. The formula for calculating it is as follows-

$$\%Elongation = \frac{Increase\ in\ length\ of\ film}{Initail\ length\ of\ film} \times 100 \tag{1}$$

7.5 Tensile strength

The greatest stress applied to a point where the film specimen breaks are known as tensile strength. As shown in the equation below, it is computed by dividing the applied load at rupture by the cross-sectional area of the film.

$$Tensile\ strength = \frac{Load\ at\ failure}{Film\ thickness \times Film\ width} \times 100 \tag{2}$$

7.6 Tear resistance test

The complicated function of a film's final resistance to rupture is its tear resistance. The tear resistance value is the maximum force necessary to rip the film. The plastic industry is usually blamed for this test. The loading rate used is 2 in/min, which is intended to quantify the degree of force necessary to rip the film specimen. The highest amount of force required for tearing is usually observed around the tearing commencement, and this number is referred to as tear resistance value [70].

7.7 Young's modulus

Young's modulus, often known as elastic modulus, is a measure of a film's stiffness or elasticity. This reflects the films' resistance to deformation, which may be measured by graphing the stress–strain curve, where the slope denotes the modulus, i.e. the higher the slope, the higher the tensile modulus. The narrow slope, on the other hand, indicates a lower tensile modulus and deformation. Simply put, a film with higher tensile strength and greater Young's modulus values is rigid, brittle, and has little elongation. The Young's modulus may be measured with a texture analyser, with the slope acquired from the stress–strain curve [2]. Young's modulus is defined as the ratio of applied stress to strain in the elastic deformation area, which may be calculated using the formula below.

$$Young'smodulus = \frac{Slope}{Film\ thickness \times Cross\ head\ speed} \times 100 \quad (3)$$

7.8 Folding endurance

Folding endurance is another method for determining a film's mechanical qualities. It's calculated by folding a film at the same location over and over until it breaks. The number of times the film can be folded without breaking is known as the folding endurance value. A film with a higher folding endurance rating has better mechanical strength. The mechanical strength of films and their folding durability are inextricably linked. Because plasticiser concentration influences mechanical strength, it is apparent that plasticiser concentration also has an indirect effect on folding endurance.

7.9 Swelling index

Film swelling tests are carried out with a simulated saliva solution. Each film sample is weighed and put in a stainless steel wire mesh that has been pre-weighed. In a plastic container, the mesh containing the film sample is immersed in a 15 ml medium. The weight of the film was measured at predetermined intervals until it reached a consistent weight.

$$Swelling\ index = \frac{Increase\ in\ weight\ of\ film - Initial\ weight\ of\ film}{Initial\ weight\ of\ film} \times 100 \quad (4)$$

7.10 Moisture content and uptake

Films that have been previously weighed are kept in a desiccator for 24 hours. When the weight of each film does not change anymore, the final weight is recorded. The following formula may be used to calculate the percentage of moisture content.

$$\%Moisture\ content = \frac{Initial\ weight\ of\ film - Final\ weight\ of\ film}{Initial\ weight\ of\ film} \times 100 \quad (5)$$

The test is carried out by storing previously weighed film in desiccators at a certain temperature and relative humidity level. The film is removed after three days and reweighed to estimate the percentage of moisture absorption [66]. The following formula may be used to calculate the percentage of moisture uptake.

$$\%Moisture\ uptake = \frac{Final\ weight\ of\ film - Initial\ weight\ of\ film}{Initial\ weight\ of\ film} \times 100 \quad (6)$$

7.11 *In vitro* dissolution study

Under standardised circumstances of liquid/solid interface, temperature, and solvent concentration, dissolution is defined as the quantity of drug material that enters the solution per unit time. For dissolving testing, any of the pharmacopoeia's standard basket or paddle apparatus can be utilised. The dissolving medium will be chosen based on the sink circumstances and the greatest dosage of API. The temperature of the dissolving media should be kept at 37 ± 0.5°C and the rotational speed at 50. The paddle device has the problem of causing oral films to float above the dissolving liquid when used [71].

8. Conclusion

In recent years, medication formulation into various films has become increasingly popular. The development of innovative polymeric thin films as a drug delivery platform has been pushed by several unwanted problems associated with current dosage forms, such as inconvenient administration, poorer bioavailability, and patient non-compliance. Because of the versatility of this dissolvable film technology platform, it has the potential to be used in a variety of pharmaceutical, biopharmaceutical, and medical sectors in the future. It also allows current pharmaceuticals whose patents are about to expire and will shortly be subject to generic competition to extend their revenue life cycles. In other words, oral films provide product lifetime management. Furthermore, the bulk of the production processes is well-understood and controllable, resulting in a stable and efficient transition from bench to market. The businesses are working to develop a variety of thin films for use in the oral, buccal, sublingual, ophthalmic, and transdermal routes. As a result, polymeric thin films are predicted to stand out as a dosage form as an alternative to traditional dosage forms, overcoming the limits provided by existing dosage forms. Finally, the thin-film technology combined with the chosen medication component must obtain widespread public acceptability, paving the path for other medicines to adopt this portable, extremely handy pharmaceutical form. As new technologies for preparing thin films are quickly launched, the future of film technology appears to be bright.

Authors' contributions

I declare that this work was done by the authors named in this article. RJ conceived and designed the study, WA carried out the literature collection of the data, RC did the writing and NG corrected the manuscript. The authors read and approved the final manuscript.

Competing interests

The authors declare no competing interest.

Consent for publication

Not applicable.

Availability of data and materials

All the information in the manuscript has been referred from the included references and is available upon request from the corresponding author.

Abbreviations

FDA	Food and Drug Administration
GRAS	Generally Recognised as Safe
DDS	Drug delivery system
TDDS	Transdermal drug delivery system
RT	Residence time
HPMC	Hydroxypropyl methylcellulose
HPC	Hydroxypropyl cellulose
CMC	Carboxymethyl cellulose
PVA	Poly (vinyl alcohol)
EMA	European Medicines Agency
CNS	Central nervous system
GI	Gastrointestinal tract
HEC	Hydroxyethylcellulose
SCMC	Sodium carboxymethyl cellulose
PVP	Poly(vinyl pyrrolidone)
API	Active pharmaceutical ingredient
3D	Three-dimensional space
SEM	Scanning Electron Microscopy

Author details

Ramakant Joshi*, Wasim Akram, Rajendra Chauhan and Navneet Garud
School of Studies in Pharmaceutical Sciences, Jiwaji University, Gwalior, MP, India

*Address all correspondence to: joshiram78@gmail.com

References

[1] Park S, Han U, Choi D, Hong J. Layer-by-layer assembled polymeric thin films as prospective drug delivery carriers: Design and applications. Biomaterials Research. 2018;**22**(1):1-3. DOI: 10.1186/s40824-018-0139-5

[2] Karki S, Kim H, Na SJ, Shin D, Jo K, Lee J. Thin films as an emerging platform for drug delivery. Asian Journal of Pharmaceutical Sciences. 2016;**11**(5):559-574. DOI: 10.1016/j.ajps.2016.05.004

[3] Arora P, Mukherjee B. Design, development, physicochemical, and in vitro and in vivo evaluation of transdermal patches containing diclofenac diethylammonium salt. Journal of Pharmaceutical Sciences. 2002;**91**(9):2076-2089. DOI: 10.1002/jps.10200

[4] Sinha VR, Kaur MP. Permeation enhancers for transdermal drug delivery. Drug Development and Industrial Pharmacy. 2000;**26**(11):1131-1140. DOI: 10.1081/DDC-100100984

[5] Rajendra C, Naveen M, Anurekha J, Sanjay J, Kumar JA, Gupta MK. Optimization of plasticizer for diclofenac sodium transdermal film: Permeation enhancement. Asian Journal of Pharmaceutical and Clinical Research. 2011;**4**(Suppl. 2):1178-1180

[6] Benson HA. Transdermal drug delivery: Penetration enhancement techniques. Current Drug Delivery. 2005;**2**(1):23-33. DOI: 10.2174/1567201052772915

[7] Tong X, Pan W, Su T, Zhang M, Dong W, Qi X. Recent advances in natural polymer-based drug delivery systems. Reactive and Functional Polymers. 2020;**148**:104501. DOI: 10.1016/j.reactfunctpolym.2020.104501

[8] Qi X, Yuan Y, Zhang J, Bulte JW, Dong W. Oral administration of salecan-based hydrogels for controlled insulin delivery. Journal of Agricultural and Food Chemistry. 2018;**66**(40):10479-10489. DOI: 10.1021/acs.jafc.8b02879

[9] Gordon R. More than skin deep: Advances in transdermal technologies are opening up new avenues of exploration. Pharmaceutical Technology Europe. 2005;**17**(11):66

[10] Rios M. Advances in transdermal technologies-transdermal delivery takes up once-forbidden compounds, reviving markets and creating formulation opportunities. Pharmaceutical Technology. 2007;**31**(10):54-58

[11] Patel D, Chaudhary SA, Parmar B, Bhura N. Transdermal drug delivery system: A review. The Pharma Innovation. 2012;**1**(4, Part A):66

[12] Magnusson BM, Runn P, Karlsson K, Koskinen LO. Terpenes and ethanol enhance the transdermal permeation of the tripeptide thyrotropin releasing hormone in human epidermis. International Journal of Pharmaceutics. 1997;**157**(1):113-121. DOI: 10.1016/S0378-5173(97)00235-4

[13] Alkilani AZ, McCrudden MT, Donnelly RF. Transdermal drug delivery: Innovative pharmaceutical developments based on disruption of the barrier properties of the stratum corneum. Pharmaceutics. 2015;7(4):438-470. DOI: 10.3390/pharmaceutics7040438

[14] Han T, Das DB. Potential of combined ultrasound and microneedles for enhanced transdermal drug permeation: A review. European Journal

of Pharmaceutics and Biopharmaceutics. 2015;**89**:312-328. DOI: 10.1016/j.ejpb.2014.12.020

[15] Borges AF, Silva C, Coelho JF, Simões S. Oral films: Current status and future perspectives: I—Galenical development and quality attributes. Journal of Controlled Release. 2015;**206**: 1-9. DOI: 10.1016/j.jconrel.2015.03.006

[16] Kaur G, Singh D, Brar V. Bioadhesive okra polymer based buccal patches as platform for controlled drug delivery. International Journal of Biological Macromolecules. 2014;**70**: 408-419. DOI: 10.1016/j.ijbiomac.2014.07.015

[17] Semalty A, Semalty M, Nautiyal U. Formulation and evaluation of mucoadhesive buccal films of enalapril maleate. Indian Journal of Pharmaceutical Sciences. 2010;**72**(5):571. DOI: 10.4103%2F0250-474X.78522

[18] Nafee NA, Ismail FA, Boraie NA, Mortada LM. Mucoadhesive buccal patches of miconazole nitrate: in vitro/in vivo performance and effect of ageing. International Journal of Pharmaceutics. 2003;**264**(1–2):1-4. DOI: 10.1016/S0378-5173(03)00371-5

[19] Jacob S, Nair AB, Boddu SH, Gorain B, Sreeharsha N, Shah J. An updated overview of the emerging role of patch and film-based buccal delivery systems. Pharmaceutics. 2021;**13**(8): 1206. DOI: 10.3390/pharmaceutics13081206

[20] Pahuja P, Arora S, Pawar P. Ocular drug delivery system: A reference to natural polymers. Expert Opinion on Drug Delivery. 2012;**9**(7):837-861. DOI: 10.1517/17425247.2012.690733

[21] Mahajan HS, Deshmukh SR. Development and evaluation of gel-forming ocular films based on xyloglucan. Carbohydrate Polymers. 2015;**122**:243-247. DOI: 10.1016/j.carbpol.2015.01.018

[22] Darwhekar G, Jain DK, Patidar VK. Formulation and evaluation of transdermal drug delivery system of clopidogrel bisulfate. Asian Journal of Pharmacy & Life Science. 2011;**2231**: 4423

[23] Padula C, Nicoli S, Colombo P, Santi P. Single-layer transdermal film containing lidocaine: Modulation of drug release. European Journal of Pharmaceutics and Biopharmaceutics. 2007;**66**(3):422-428. DOI: 10.1016/j.ejpb.2006.11.014

[24] Ammar HO, Ghorab M, Mahmoud AA, Makram TS, Ghoneim AM. Rapid pain relief using transdermal film forming polymeric solution of ketorolac. Pharmaceutical Development and Technology. 2013; **18**(5):1005-1016. DOI: 10.3109/10837450.2011.627867

[25] Deshmukh K, Ahamed MB, Deshmukh RR, Pasha SK, Bhagat PR, Chidambaram K. Biopolymer composites with high dielectric performance: Interface engineering. In: Biopolymer Composites in Electronics. Amsterdam, Netherlands: Elsevier; 2017 Jan 1. pp. 27-128. DOI: 10.1016/B978-0-12-809261-3.00003-6

[26] Chandak AR, Verma PR. Development and evaluation of HPMC based matrices for transdermal patches of tramadol. Clinical Research and Regulatory Affairs. 2008;**25**(1):13-30. DOI: 10.1080/10601330701885066

[27] Gencturk A, Kahraman E, Güngör S, Özhan G, Özsoy Y, Sarac AS. Polyurethane/hydroxypropyl cellulose electrospun nanofiber mats as potential

transdermal drug delivery system: Characterization studies and in vitro assays. Artificial Cells, Nanomedicine, and Biotechnology. 2017;**45**(3):655-664. DOI: 10.3109/21691401.2016.1173047

[28] Godinho MH, Gray DG, Pieranski P. Revisiting (hydroxypropyl) cellulose (HPC)/water liquid crystalline system. Liquid Crystals. 2017;**44**(12–13): 2108-2120. DOI: 10.1080/02678292.2017.1325018

[29] Ermawati DE, Ambarwati DA, Dewi NR, Artanti AN, Rohmani S, Kundarto W. Optimization of hydroxymethylcellulose and sodium CMC of transdermal patch of antihypertension "Hortus Medicus" and transport through membrane using franz diffusion cell method. In: AIP Conference Proceedings. Vol. 2237, No. 1. Melville, NY, USA: AIP Publishing LLC; 2020 Jun 2. p. 020063. DOI: 10.1063/5.0005628

[30] Amnuaikit C, Ikeuchi I, Ogawara KI, Higaki K, Kimura T. Skin permeation of propranolol from polymeric film containing terpene enhancers for transdermal use. International Journal of Pharmaceutics. 2005;**289**(1–2):167-178. DOI: 10.1016/j.ijpharm.2004.11.007

[31] Bühler V. Polyvinylpyrrolidone Excipients for Pharmaceuticals: Povidone, Crospovidone and Copovidone. Berlin, Heidelberg, New York: Springer Science & Business Media; 2005

[32] Crowley MM, Fredersdorf A, Schroeder B, Kucera S, Prodduturi S, Repka MA, et al. The influence of guaifenesin and ketoprofen on the properties of hot-melt extruded polyethylene oxide films. European Journal of Pharmaceutical Sciences. 2004;**22**(5):409-418. DOI: 10.1016/j.ejps.2004.04.005

[33] Desai NP, Hossainy SF, Hubbell JA. Surface-immobilized polyethylene oxide for bacterial repellence. Biomaterials. 1992;**13**(7):417-420. DOI: 10.1016/0142-9612(92)90160-P

[34] Suksaeree J, Maneewattanapinyo P, Panrat K, Pichayakorn W, Monton C. Solvent-cast polymeric films from pectin and Eudragit® NE 30D for transdermal drug delivery systems. Journal of Polymers and the Environment. 2021 Oct;**29**(10):3174-3184. DOI: 10.1007/s10924-021-02108-3

[35] Suksaeree J, Karnsopa P, Wannaphruek N, Prasomkij J, Panrat K, Pichayakorn W. Transdermal delivery of nicotine using pectin isolated from durian fruit-hulls-based polymer blends as a matrix layer. Journal of Polymers and the Environment. 2018;**26**(8):3216-3225. DOI: 10.1007/s10924-018-1203-x

[36] Sonawane PR, Katti SA. Natural polymers: Carriers for transdermal drug delivery system. International Journal of Research in Pharmaceutical Chemistry. 2016;**6**(3):534-542

[37] Can AS, Erdal MS, Güngör S, Özsoy Y. Optimization and characterization of chitosan films for transdermal delivery of ondansetron. Molecules. 2013;**18**(5):5455-5471. DOI: 10.3390/molecules18055455

[38] Walker HL, Connick WJ. Sodium alginate for production and formulation of mycoherbicides. Weed Science. 1983; **31**(3):333-338. DOI: 10.1017/S0043174500069113

[39] Kaur R, Sharma A, Puri V, Singh I. Preparation and characterization of biocomposite films of carrageenan/locust bean gum/montmorrillonite for transdermal delivery of curcumin. BioImpacts: BI. 2019;**9**(1):37. DOI: 10.15171%2Fbi.2019.05

[40] Nesseem DI, Eid SF, El-Houseny SS. Development of novel transdermal self-adhesive films for tenoxicam, an anti-inflammatory drug. Life Sciences. 2011;**89**(13–14):430-438. DOI: 10.1016/j.lfs.2011.06.026

[41] Paul S, Jayan A, Sasikumar CS. Physical, chemical and biological studies of gelatin/chitosan based transdermal films with embedded silver nanoparticles. Asian Pacific Journal of Tropical Disease. 2015;**5**(12):975-986. DOI: 10.1016/S2222-1808(15)60968-9

[42] Maneewattanapinyo P, Yeesamun A, Watthana F, Panrat K, Pichayakorn W, Suksaeree J. Transdermal patches of lidocaine/aspirin ionic liquid drug-loaded gelatin/polyvinyl alcohol composite film prepared by freeze-thawed procedure. Anais da Academia Brasileira de Ciências. Jul 2020;**20**:92. DOI: 10.1590/0001-3765202020191073

[43] Seabra AB, De Oliveira MG. Poly (vinyl alcohol) and poly (vinyl pyrrolidone) blended films for local nitric oxide release. Biomaterials. 2004; **25**(17):3773-3782. DOI: 10.1016/j.biomaterials.2003.10.035

[44] Ngawhirunpat T, Opanasopit P, Rojanarata T, Akkaramongkolporn P, Ruktanonchai U, Supaphol P. Development of meloxicam-loaded electrospun polyvinyl alcohol mats as a transdermal therapeutic agent. Pharmaceutical Development and Technology. 2009;**14**(1):73-82. DOI: 10.1080/10837450802409420

[45] Irfan M, Rabel S, Bukhtar Q, Qadir MI, Jabeen F, Khan A. Orally disintegrating films: A modern expansion in drug delivery system. Saudi Pharmaceutical Journal. 2016;**24**(5): 537-546. DOI: 10.1016/j.jsps.2015.02.024

[46] Hoffmann EM, Breitenbach A, Breitkreutz J. Advances in orodispersible films for drug delivery. Expert Opinion on Drug Delivery. 2011;**8**(3):299-316. DOI: 10.1517/17425247.2011.553217

[47] Vibhooti P, Preeti K. Wafers technology-a newer approacah to smart drug dilevery system. Indian Journal of Research in Pharmacy and Biotechnology. May 1, 2013;**1**(3):428

[48] Mostafa DA, Hashad AM, Ragab MF, Wagdy HA. Comparison between the pharmacokinetics data of ketorolac Tromethamine wafer a novel drug delivery system and conventional ketorolac Tromethamine tablets to enhance patient compliance using a new LC-MS/MS method. BioNanoScience. 2020;**10**:745-757. DOI: 10.1007/s12668-020-00754-w

[49] Rathbone MJ, Hadgraft J. Absorption of drugs from the human oral cavity. International Journal of Pharmaceutics. 1991;**74**(1):9-24. DOI: 10.1016/0378-5173(91)90403-B

[50] Kunte S, Tandale P. Fast dissolving strips: A novel approach for the delivery of verapamil. Journal of Pharmacy & Bioallied Sciences. 2010;**2**(4):325. DOI: 10.4103%2F0975-7406. 72133

[51] Dixit RP, Puthli SP. Oral strip technology: Overview and future potential. Journal of Controlled Release. 2009;**139**(2):94-107. DOI: 10.1016/j.jconrel.2009.06.014

[52] Hao J, Heng PW. Buccal delivery systems. Drug Development and Industrial Pharmacy. 2003;**29**(8): 821-832. DOI: 10.1081/DDC-120024178

[53] Morales JO, McConville JT. Manufacture and characterization of mucoadhesive buccal films. European

Journal of Pharmaceutics and Biopharmaceutics. 2011;**77**(2):187-199. DOI: 10.1016/j.ejpb.2010.11.023

[54] Guo J, Cremer K. Development of bioadhesive buccal patches. In: Mathiowitz E, Chickering D, Lehr C, editors. Bioadhesive Drug Delivery Systems: Fundamentals, Novel Approaches, and Development. New York: Marcel Dekker, Inc.; 1999. pp. 541-562

[55] Patel VF, Liu F, Brown MB. Advances in oral transmucosal drug delivery. Journal of Controlled Release. 2011;**153**(2):106-116. DOI: 10.1016/j.jconrel.2011.01.027

[56] Kang-Mieler JJ, Osswald CR, Mieler WF. Advances in ocular drug delivery: Emphasis on the posterior segment. Expert Opinion on Drug Delivery. 2014;**11**(10):1647-1660. DOI: 10.1517/17425247.2014.935338

[57] Manvi FV, Patil MB, Mastiholimath VS, Rathod R. Development and evaluation of ocular films of cromolyn sodium. Indian Journal of Pharmaceutical Sciences. 2004;**66**(3):309

[58] McAuley WJ, Caserta F. Film-Forming and Heated Systems. Novel Delivery Systems for Transdermal and Intradermal Drug Delivery. Chichester, UK: John Wiley & Sons, Ltd; Jul 15, 2015. pp. 97-124

[59] Joshi R, Garud N. Development, optimization and characterization of flurbiprofen matrix transdermal drug delivery system using box–Behnken statistical design. Future Journal of Pharmaceutical Sciences. 2021;**7**(1): 1-8. DOI: 10.1186/s43094-021-00199-2

[60] Prausnitz MR, Langer R. Transdermal drug delivery. Nature Biotechnology. 2008;**26**(11):1261-1268. DOI: 10.1038/nbt.1504

[61] Chauhan R, Mehta N, Jain A, Jain S, Jain AK, Gupta MK. Optimization of plasticizer for diclofenac sodium transdermal film, permeation enhancement. Asian Journal of Pharmaceutical and Clinical Research. 2011;**4**:178-180

[62] Dhiman S, Singh TG, Rehni AK. Transdermal patches: A recent approach to new drug delivery system. International Journal of Pharmacy and Pharmaceutical Sciences. 2011;**3**(5):26-34

[63] Brown MB, Martin GP, Jones SA, Akomeah FK. Dermal and transdermal drug delivery systems: Current and future prospects. Drug Delivery. 2006; **13**(3):175-187. DOI: 10.1080/10717540500455975

[64] Kumar K, Teotia D. A comprehensive review on pharmaceutical Oral dissolving films. Journal of Drug Delivery and Therapeutics. 2019;**9**(5-s):170-174. DOI: 10.22270/jddt.v9i5-s.3641

[65] Bala R, Pawar P, Khanna S, Arora S. Orally dissolving strips: A new approach to oral drug delivery system. International Journal of Pharmaceutical Investigation. 2013;**3**(2):67. DOI: 10.4103%2F2230-973X.114897

[66] Panda BP, Dey NS, Rao ME. Development of innovative orally fast disintegrating film dosage forms: A review. International Journal of Pharmaceutical Sciences and Nanotechnology. 2012;**5**(2):1666-1674

[67] Patil H, Tiwari RV, Repka MA. Hot-melt extrusion: From theory to application in pharmaceutical formulation. AAPS PharmSciTech. 2016;

17(1):20-42. DOI: 10.1208/s12249-015-0360-7

[68] Arya A, Chandra A, Sharma V, Pathak K. Fast dissolving oral films: An innovative drug delivery system and dosage form. International Journal of ChemTech Research. 2010;**2**(1):576-583

[69] Mashru RC, Sutariya VB, Sankalia MG, Parikh PP. Development and evaluation of fast-dissolving film of salbutamol sulphate. Drug Development and Industrial Pharmacy. 2005;**31**(1): 25-34. DOI: 10.1081/DDC-43947

[70] Bhyan B, Jangra S, Kaur M, Singh H. Orally fast dissolving films: Innovations in formulation and technology. International Journal of Pharmaceutical Sciences Review and Research. 2011; **9**(2):9-15

[71] Dinge A, Nagarsenker M. Formulation and evaluation of fast dissolving films for delivery of triclosan to the oral cavity. AAPS PharmSciTech. 2008;**9**(2):349-356. DOI: 10.1208/s12249-008-9047-7

Chapter 4

Drug Delivery Applications of Metal-Organic Frameworks (MOFs)

Ashi Mittal, Indrajit Roy and Sona Gandhi

Abstract

There has been substantial progress in the field of metal–organic frameworks (MOFs) and their nanoscale counterparts (NMOFs), in recent years. Their exceptional physicochemical properties are being constantly and actively exploited for various applications such as energy harvesting, gas storage, gas separation, catalysis, etc. Due to their porous framework, large surface area, tunability and easy surface functionalization, MOFs and NMOFs have also emerged as useful tools for biomedical applications, specifically for drug delivery. As drug carriers, they offer high drug loading capacity and controlled release at the target site. This chapter aims to give a panorama of the use of these MOFs as drug delivery agents. A brief overview of the structure and composition of MOFs, along with various methods and techniques to synthesize NMOFs suitable for drug delivery applications are mentioned. In addition, the most commonly employed strategies to associate drugs with these NMOFs are highlighted and methods to characterize them are also briefly discussed. The last section summarizes the applications of MOFs and NMOFs as carriers of therapeutic drugs, biomolecules, and other active agents.

Keywords: metal–organic frameworks, synthesis, drug encapsulation, characterization, drug delivery, biomolecules, photosensitizers

1. Introduction

The use of nanomaterials as carriers for the administration of drugs and therapeutic agents is gaining increased attention. These nanocarriers are facilely taken up by the cells and are able to deliver the drug to the target site and prevent its rapid clearance or degradation [1]. Although several inorganic (such as iron oxide NPs, noble metal NPs, quantum dots, etc.) and organic (such as liposomes, polymers, dendrimers) nanomaterials have been produced as nanocarriers, each of these classes of nanomaterials has its own set of merits and demerits [2, 3]. Only a few of these nanosized drug carriers have been approved by the US Food and Drug Administration (FDA); though still, they have some limitations [4].

Metal–organic frameworks (MOFs) also referred to as porous coordination polymers (PCPs) are a crystalline class of coordination polymers and were first reported by Bernard F. Hoskins and Richard Robson in 1989 [5, 6]. MOFs are being synthesized in a building block fashion, in which inorganic building units (metal ion vertices or clusters) are interconnected by organic building units (organic linker molecules) by a self-assembly process, to form highly tailorable crystalline materials having pores in the nanometer range [7]. Their unique combination of high porosity, large surface areas, lack of non-accessible bulk volume, a wide range of pore sizes (micro- or mesopores), shapes (cages, channels, etc.) and topologies, tunable and rigid frameworks, easy surface functionalization, and a limitless number of possible combinations of metals and ligands have resulted in a large number of their potential applications [8, 9].

Nanoscale Metal–organic frameworks or Metal–organic framework nanoparticles (NMOFs or MOF NPs), nanoscale counterparts of MOFs are an attractive class of hybrid nanomaterials. These NMOFs not only exhibit the unique features of porous nanomaterials, but they also have benefits over analogous bulk MOFs for a variety of biomedical applications due to their small size. They can offer many advantages over conventional nanocarriers. (i) First, they can be designed to form desired structures with different shapes, sizes and chemical properties allowing for the loading of various therapeutic agents with different functionalities; (ii) next, their large surface area, high porosity, uniform pore size and volume results in high loading efficiency and selective transport; (iii) further, as a result of their somewhat labile metal and ligand coordination bonds, they are intrinsically biodegradable, which prevents their accumulation in the body after their task is achieved; (iv) finally, their surface functionalization by post-synthetic modifications can improve their colloidal stability, thereby prolonging their blood circulation time [10–12]. Thus, the miniaturization of MOFs to NMOFs has resulted in the development of nanomaterials with great potential to be used as drug delivery systems. The structural flexibility (referred to as "breathing") and switchability of MOFs is a unique feature not found in other porous materials [13].

This chapter will give the readers an overview of the use of MOFs and NMOFs as potential drug carriers. In the succeeding sections, the basic composition and structure of these porous frameworks and general synthetic routes adopted for their preparation shall be discussed. Commonly used drug incorporation techniques and characterization methods to verify drug association will also be presented. In the final section, a summary of some of the MOFs and NMOFs reported as carriers and for application in the delivery of therapeutic drugs, biomolecules such as proteins, nucleic acids, carbohydrates, and other active agents employed for light and magnetic field activated therapies, shall be provided.

2. Structure of MOFs

The design principles of reticular chemistry suggest that deconstruction of a MOF results in four levels of structure [14].

- The primary structure reveals the chemical composition of MOF, comprising of a metal ion (generally multivalent) and a polydentate organic linker molecule (topicity i.e., points of extension varying between 2 and 12) [15].

- Secondary building units or SBUs, which are mostly formed *in situ,* are obtained at the secondary level. These are basically polynuclear metal clusters locking the metal ion into a fixed geometry thereby giving directionality and rigidity to the final MOF structure [16].

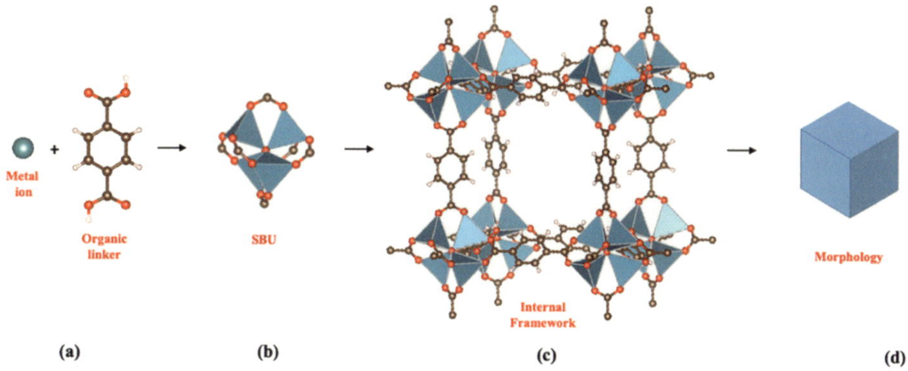

Figure 1.
Structure of MOF-5. (a) Primary structure showing composition: metal ion (Zn^{2+}) and linker (terephthalic acid), (b) secondary structure: SBU, $Zn_4O(-COO)_6$, (c) tertiary structure: internal framework formed showing linking of SBUs by the terephthalic acid linker, (d) quaternary structure: overall morphology.

- The tertiary level involves stitching of multiple SBUs together or two metal ions by bridging linkers (having binding groups like phosphates, carboxylates, imidazolates, etc.), giving rise to an internal framework comprising of pores and channels [15].

- The outer morphology (size and shape) or quaternary structure of MOF depends on the synthesis procedure dictating the growth of the internal framework [17].

Figure 1 depicts the above four levels of MOF structure concerning MOF-5.

3. Synthesis of NMOFs

Specialized synthetic routes are a prerequisite to obtaining MOFs in the nano-range, ideal for drug administration. The choice of synthesis protocol determines the final size, crystallinity, morphology, uniformity and stability of NMOF. **Figure 2** shows a summary of the most often used approaches.

- Nanoprecipitation is based on the premise that although the precursors (metal ion and linker) are miscible in the original solvent, the formed nanoparticles are either immiscible or can be precipitated out by adding another solvent in which it is not soluble [18].

- Solvothermal synthesis, performed at higher temperatures results in highly crystalline particles and can be used in combination with surfactants to form surfactant-coated stable particles [19].

- Reverse microemulsions (sometimes called nanoreactors), which are water-in-oil systems stabilized by appropriate surfactants, can be used as templates to produce monodisperse particles, and size control can be achieved by varying the w_0 (water: surfactant ratio) value [20].

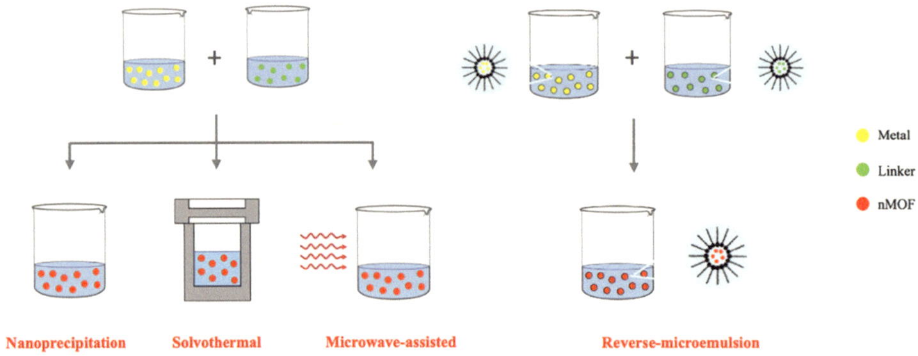

Figure 2.
Schematic representation of various synthetic methods used for the synthesis of NMOFs.

Other, less commonly used methods include the use of microwaves, ultrasounds, etc. [21, 22]. NMOFs are generally post-synthetically modified or altered to impart them with extra stability, targeting ability, and biocompatibility [23].

4. Drug incorporation strategies

Some MOFs possess rigid and permanent pores, whereas others are flexible and can respond to external/internal stimuli such as temperature, light, pH, etc. by changing their pore size [24]. In addition, MOFs have distinct features such as breathing, linker rotation, swelling, and subnetwork displacements, which are important for drug loading and release management [25]. There are many ways to associate a drug with MOF, which may be a medicine, a gene, a protein, an enzyme, or any other agent of therapeutic importance.

- The first approach is to carry out the encapsulation of the drug/therapeutic agent during the synthesis of MOF; this method is referred to as one-pot synthesis [26, 27]. This method can be used to entrap one or more drugs larger than the pore size of MOF and prevents its premature leaching.

- Another approach is to directly incorporate the prodrug or drug into the framework by using it as a ligand giving higher loading efficiency [28, 29]. The only limitation of this method is that it can lead to loss of therapeutic activity of the incorporated drug.

- Smaller drugs/cargos can also be post-synthetically encapsulated by introducing them into a dispersion of MOF in a suitable solvent in which they can subsequently diffuse through channels inside MOF pores [30]. This way the drug can also be physically adsorbed on the outer surface by electrostatic interactions.

- Another method is to post-synthetically associate the drug through covalent bonding with functional groups of organic linkers or by the formation of coordination bonds to metal ions present at coordinatively-unsaturated sites (CUSs) [21, 31–34]. These CUSs present on the MOF surface behave as Lewis acids and solvent molecules at these sites can be replaced by drugs.

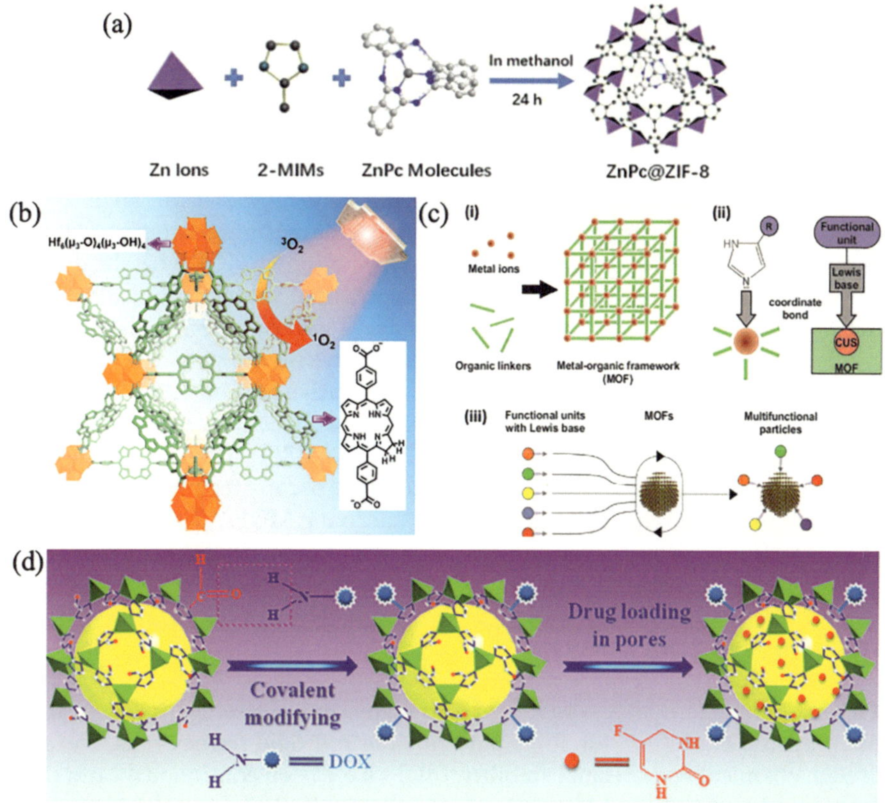

Figure 3.
(a) One-pot synthesis of ZIF-8 NMOF encapsulating zinc phthalocyanine, a photosensitizer used for PDT. Reproduced with permission from [26]. Copyright 2018 American Chemical Society. (b) Direct assembly of porphyrin-based DBC ligand in DBC-UiO NMOF for PDT application. Reproduced with permission from [29]. Copyright 2015 American Chemical Society. (c) Coordinative interaction of His-tags with CUS of MOF: (i) basic MOF molecular composition; (ii) formation of coordinate bond between CUS metal ion (Lewis acid) and imidazolate group of histidine (Lewis base); (iii) generation of multifunctional MOFs by attachment of multiple His-tags. Reproduced with permission from [33]. Copyright 2017 American Chemical Society. (d) Post-synthetic covalent attachment of amino group of DOX to aldehyde of ICA linker in ZIF-90, followed by loading of 5-Fluoro uracil into the pores of NMOF. Reproduced with permission from [34]. Copyright 2017 American Chemical Society.

Figure 3 gives a schematic illustration of some of these drug-loading techniques. Multimodal and theranostic systems can also be obtained by using one or more loading techniques to incorporate multiple drugs.

5. Characterization

Loading of drugs by MOFs can be confirmed by various methods. Spectroscopic techniques such as UV–visible and fluorescence spectroscopy are useful to confirm encapsulation/loading of chromophoric and fluorescent drugs. Encapsulation of zinc phthalocyanine (ZnPc), which shows characteristic absorbance peaks at 605 and 670 nm was confirmed by the presence of these peaks in the absorbance spectrum of ZnPc@ZIF-8 but absence in the spectrum of only ZIF-8 [26]. This technique is also helpful to quantify the loaded drug. Determination of Brunauer–Emmett–Teller

(BET) surface area and pore volume can also help in verifying successful encapsulation of drug. Nitrogen adsorption analysis of ZIF-90, ZIF-90-DOX, and 5-FU@ ZIF-90-DOX showed BET surface areas 1045.7, 890.4, and 48.3 m^2/g, respectively. A decrease in BET surface area validated drug loading [34]. Deviations in the TGA curve of drug incorporated MOF are also indicative of drug loading. TGA curve of ZIF-90 showed no significant loss in weight between 300 and 500° C, whereas ZIF-90-DOX showed much larger weight loss in the same temperature range. Zeta potential and hydrodynamic size measurement by dynamic light scattering (DLS) experiments can also confirm the nature of the association of MOF with the drug. Pure ZIF-8 nanospheres had a more positive zeta potential value of +31.4 mV, as compared to +22.9 mV for fluorescein adsorbed ZIF-8 nanospheres. This indicated surface adsorption of negatively charged fluorescein dye on the surface of positively charged nanospheres [35]. A very small change in negative zeta potential value for MIL-100 and DM NPs (DOX loaded MIL-100 NPs) confirmed encapsulation of DOX majorly inside the particle with some surface adsorption [36]. Other techniques such as FT-IR spectroscopy, PXRD, NMR, and electron microscopy techniques such as SEM and TEM are also frequently used for characterizing MOFs, with and without drugs [30, 37–39].

6. Applications in drug delivery

MOFs are unique inorganic–organic hybrid materials possessing ultrahigh surface area and porosity. They are crystalline, have flexible and rigid frameworks, and also exhibit high chemical and thermal stability. MOFs have been continuously and thoroughly explored and reviewed for numerous applications. Several applications related to MOFs have been reported such as for gas storage and separation, [40–42] catalysis, [43, 44] sensing, [45] magnetism, [46] and energy [47]. In addition, various biomedical applications have also been reported, including biological sensing, [48] molecular imaging, targeted drug delivery, [21, 49] among others [11].

A large number of side effects are associated with uncontrolled and non-specific drug delivery by direct administration of a free drug inside the body. Great efforts have been made by researchers for the development of methods for targeted, systemic, and controlled drug administration. Nanocarriers have provided a simple and effective solution to this problem. Both organic (such as dendrimers, liposomes, etc.) and inorganic (such as noble metal and metal oxide nanoparticles, quantum dots, silica nanoparticles, etc.) nanocarriers have been reported as potential drug delivery vehicles. Organic nanocarriers such as liposomes are less stable and easily captured by the reticuloendothelial system (RES) once inside the body [50]. Inorganic nanocarriers such as gold, silver, and silica nanoparticles have been reported to be cytotoxic [51]. Inorganic–organic hybrid nanocarriers, such as porous NMOFs, offer many advantages over their pure organic and inorganic counterparts and have established themselves as optimal drug delivery vehicles. In the following subsections, the applications of NMOFs for the delivery and as carriers of therapeutic drugs, biomolecules such as proteins, enzymes, carbohydrates, nucleic acids, and other active agents, shall be discussed briefly.

6.1 Therapeutic drugs

MOFs, owing to their porous structure have been frequently reported for delivery of therapeutic agents such as analgesics, antibiotics, anti-inflammatory and anti-cancer drugs, based on both *in vitro* and *in vivo* experiments. In 2006, Horcajada et al. were the first ones to report the ability of MOFs to act as efficient drug delivery agents. They prepared two mesoporous cubic MOFs, namely MIL-100 and MIL-101. They employed them to adsorb ibuprofen, a commonly used anti-inflammatory drug and found that MIL-101 with a larger cage size was able to adsorb more amount of drug (1.4 g/g of MOF) [30]. Nasrabadi et al. reported the use of UiO-66 NMOF with surface area 1196 m^2/g to post-synthetically load ciprofloxacin (CIP), an antibiotic. The resulting CIP-UiO-66 NMOF showed a very high drug loading percentage of about 84%, with significant antibacterial activity against *Escherichia coli* (Gram-negative) and *Staphylococcus aureus* (Gram-positive) bacteria in comparison to free CIP [52]. ZIF-8 is a pH-responsive MOF, which disintegrates in an acidic environment, and thus is a promising drug carrier especially for anti-cancer applications because of acidic nature of tumor micro-environment. Sun et al. for the first time reported the use of ZIF-8 for the controlled and pH-triggered release of 5-fluorouracil (5-FU), an anticancer drug with high loading capacity (660 mg/g of MOF) [53]. **Table 1** summarizes some of the NMOFs and MOFs reported for the delivery of therapeutic agents.

6.2 Biomolecules

MOFs have proven themselves as effective carriers for the delivery of large biomolecules such as proteins, enzymes, DNA, RNA, and carbohydrates and small biomolecules such as amino acids, peptides and nucleotides [73]. These biomolecule-MOF composites protect the biodegradation of these biomolecules inside physiological systems and offer a pathway for their safe delivery. Many diseases are a result of protein deficiencies in the body. Also, nucleic acid and carbohydrates based therapies are gaining increasing interest. Intracellular delivery of these biomolecules using MOFs will help in preserving their bioactivity and they will be able to reach their targets avoiding unwanted side effects. There are many methods to form biomolecule-MOF composites. Post-synthetic pore entrapment is the most used method, in which biomolecules smaller than the cavity size of MOF directly diffuse into the pores of the MOF. Chen et al. have demonstrated the use of mesoporous NU-1000 MOF for the entrapment of insulin with high loading (approximately 40%) to treat diabetes mellitus (type 2) [74]. Surface attachment/adsorption is another method that is relatively easy, and biomolecules of all sizes can be attached/adsorbed on the surface *via* non-covalent interactions such as hydrogen bonding, π-π interactions, Van-der waals interaction, etc. Ni et al. have reported Hf-DBP NMOF for the delivery of αCD47 antibody attached to its surface [75]. Biomolecules can also be covalently linked to MOFs. Wang et al. immobilized dibenzylooctyne (DBCO) appended DNA on UiO-66-N_3 through click reaction between DBCO and azide (N_3) group [76]. Co-precipitation or one-pot synthesis is another method for biomolecule-MOF composites. The biomolecule is encapsulated during the synthesis of MOF giving high loading and preventing leakage. Shieh et al. used this *de novo* approach to encapsulate catalase enzyme into the pores of ZIF-90 [77]. Biomimetic mineralization is another *in situ* encapsulation method in which biomolecules act as templates and nucleation sites for the growth of MOF around them, dictating their final size and morphology. Liang et al. demonstrated the use of various protein, enzyme and DNA templates for the synthesis of MOFs by biomimetic mineralization [38]. Bio-MOFs can also be synthesized by incorporating biomolecules into the framework. Biomolecules have reactive functional groups. They can act as organic linkers and react with metal ions to form bio-MOFs. An et al. synthesized bio-MOF-1 made up of zinc-adeninate

S.No.	MOFs/ NMOFs	Metal ion	Organic linker	Therapeutic drug	Drug encapsulation method	Reference
a. Analgesics and anti-inflammatory drugs						
1.	MIL-100	Cr^{3+}	1,3,5-benzene tricarboxylic acid	Ibuprofen	Post-synthetic encapsulation	[30]
2.	MIL-101	Cr^{3+}	1,4-benzene dicarboxylic acid	Ibuprofen	Post-synthetic encapsulation	[30]
3.	MIL-53	Fe^{3+}, Cr^{3+}	1,4-benzene dicarboxylic acid	Ibuprofen	Post-synthetic encapsulation	[54]
4.	MOF-5	Zn^{2+}	1,4-benzene dicarboxylic acid	Curcumin, Sulindac	Post-synthetic encapsulation	[55]
5.	ZJU-800	Zr^{2+}	F-H_2PDA	Diclofenac sodium	Post-synthetic encapsulation	[56]
6.	M_2(olz)	Fe^{2+}, Co^{+2},Ni^{+2}, Zn^{2+},Mg^{2+}	Olsalazine acid	Olsalazine	Direct assembly	[57]
b. Antibacterial and antiviral drugs						
1.	MIL-101-NH_2	Fe^{3+}	2-amino-1,4-benzene dicarboxylic acid	Cidofovir	Post-synthetic encapsulation	[49]
2.	UiO-66	Zr^{4+}	1,4-benzene dicarboxylic acid	Ciprofloxacin	Post-synthetic encapsulation	[52]
3.	MIL-53	Fe^{3+}	1,4-benzene dicarboxylic acid	Vancomycin	Post-synthetic encapsulation	[58]
4.	ZIF-8	Zn^{2+}	2-methyl imidazolate	Gentamicin	Post-synthetic encapsulation	[59]
				Ciprofloxacin	Post-synthetic encapsulation	[60]
				Ceftazidime	One-pot synthesis	[61]
				Tetracycline	One-pot synthesis	[62]

S.No.	MOFs/ NMOFs	Metal ion	Organic linker	Therapeutic drug	Drug encapsulation method	Reference
5.	γ-CD-MOF	K^+	Cyclodextrin	Enrofloxacin, Florfenicol	Post-synthetic encapsulation	[63]
6.	Bio-MOF	Mg^{2+}, Mn^{2+}	Nalidixic acid	Nalidixic acid	Direct assembly	[64]
c. Anti-cancer drugs						
1.	MIL-100	Fe^{3+}	1,3,5-benzene tricarboxylic acid	Busulfan	Post-synthetic encapsulation	[49]
				Doxorubicin	Post-synthetic encapsulation	[65]
2.	PCN-221	Zr^{4+}	TCPP	Methotrexate	Post-synthetic encapsulation	[66]
3.	NCP-1	Tb^{3+}	Disuccinatocisplatin	Cisplatin	Direct assembly	[28]
4.	MIL-89	Fe^{3+}	Muconic acid	Doxorubicin	Post-synthetic encapsulation	[49]
5.	Zn(bix)	Zn^{2+}	bix	Doxorubicin, Camptothecin, Daunomycin	One-pot synthesis	[67]
6.	UiO-66	Zr^{4+}	1,4-benzene dicarboxylic acid	Alendronate	Covalent bonding	[32]
7.	HKUST-1	Cu^{2+}	1,3,5-benzene tricarboxylic acid	Nimesulide	Post-synthetic encapsulation	[68]
8.	ZJU-64	Zn^{2+}-adenine	Terphenyl dicarboxylic acid	Methotrexate	Post-synthetic encapsulation	[69]
9.	ZIF-67	Co^{2+}	2-methyl imidazolate	Doxorubicin	One-pot synthesis	[70]
10.			Imidazole-2-carboxaldehyde	5-Fluoro uracil	Post-synthetic encapsulation	[34]
				Doxorubicin	Covalent bonding	
11.	ZIF-8	Zn^{2+}	2-methyl imidazolate	5-Fluoro uracil	Post-synthetic encapsulation	[53]

S.No.	MOFs/ NMOFs	Metal ion	Organic linker	Therapeutic drug	Drug encapsulation method	Reference
				Camptothecin Doxorubicin 3-Methyl adenine	One-pot synthesis One-pot synthesis One-pot synthesis	[35] [71] [27]
12.	MOF-5	Zn^{2+}	1,4-benzene dicarboxylic acid	Oridonin	Post-synthetic encapsulation	[72]

Table 1.
Examples of MOFs and NMOFs employed as carriers for therapeutic agents.

S.No.	MOFs/ NMOFs	Metal ion	Organic Linker	Biomolecule	Incorporation method	Reference
a. Peptides, Proteins, and enzymes						
1.	NU-1000	Zr^{4+}	4,4′,4″,4‴-(pyrene-1,3,6,8-tetrayl) tetrabenzoic acid	Insulin	Post-synthetic entrapment	[74]
2.	Tb-meso MOF	Tb^{3+}	Triazine-1,3,5-tribenzoic acid	Cytochrome c	Post-synthetic entrapment	[79]
				Microperoxidase-11	Post-synthetic entrapment	[80]
3.	MOF-74	Zn^{2+}, Mg^{2+}	2,5-dioxido terephthalate	Myoglobin	Post-synthetic entrapment	[81]
4.	PCN-333	Al^{3+}	TATB	Tyrosinase	Post-synthetic entrapment	[82]
5.	ZIF-90	Zn^{2+}	Imidazole-2-carboxaldehyde	Catalase	One-pot synthesis	[77]
6.	ZIF-8	Zn^{2+}	2-methyl imidazolate	Glucose oxidase, Horseradish peroxidase	One-pot synthesis	[83]
				Hemoglobin	One-pot synthesis	[84]
				Glucose oxidase	Biomimetic Mineralization	[85]
				Melittin	One-pot synthesis	[86]
7.	Cu-TCCP(Fe)	Cu^{2+}	TCPP(Fe)	Glucose oxidase	Surface attachment	[87]
8.	MIL-100	Fe^{3+}	1,3,5-benzene tricarboxylic acid	Insulin	Post-synthetic encapsulation	[88]
b.*Antibodies and antigens*						
1.	Hf-DBP	Hf^{4+}	5,15-di(p-benzoato) porphyrin	αCD47	Surface attachment	[75]
2.	ZIF-90	Zn^{2+}	Imidazole-2-carboxaldehyde	H-IgG, G-IgG	One-pot synthesis	[89]
3.	ZIF-8	Zn^{2+}	2-methyl imidazolate	Nivolumab	Biomimetic mineralization	[90]
				Ovalbumin	One-pot synthesis	[91]

S.No.	MOFs/ NMOFs	Metal ion	Organic Linker	Biomolecule	Incorporation method	Reference
4.	MIL-100	Fe^{3+}	1,3,5-benzene tricarboxylic acid	anti-EpCAM	Surface attachment	[92]
5.	UiO-AM	Zr^{4+}	1,4-benzene dicarboxylic acid, 2-amino-1,4-benzene dicarboxylic acid	Ovalbumin	Surface attachment	[93]
6.	Al-MOF	Al^{3+}	2-amino-1,4-benzene dicarboxylic acid	Ovalbumin	One-pot synthesis	[94]
c. Nucleotides and Nucleic Acids						
1.	IRMOF-74-II	Ni^{2+}	3,3′-dihydroxy-[1,1′-biphenyl]-4,4′-dicarboxylic acid	ss-DNA	Post-synthetic encapsulation	[95]
2.	UiO-66-N_3	Zr4^{+}	2-azido-1,4-benzene dicarboxylic acid	DBCO-DNA	Covalent linkage	[76]
3.	UiO-66	Zr^{4+}	1,4-benzene dicarboxylic acid	Terminal phosphate modified oligo-nucleotides	Covalent linkage	[31]
4.	ZIF-8	Zn^{2+}	2-methyl imidazolate	Plasmid DNA	One-pot synthesis	[96]
5.	MIL-101	Fe^{3+}	1,4-benzene dicarboxylic acid	siRNA	Covalent-linkage	[97]
c. Carbohydrates						
1.	ZIF-8	Zn^{2+}	2-methyl imidazolate	Meglumine, Carboxylate dextran Heparin, Hyaluronic acid	Biomimetic mineralization One-pot synthesis	[98] [99]
2.	MAF-7	Zn^{2+}	3-methyl-1,2,4-triazole	Heparin, Hyaluronic acid, Chondroitin sulfate, Dermatan sulfate	One-pot synthesis	[100]

Table 2.
Examples of biomolecule-MOF composites incorporating biomolecules of biological importance.

clusters and biphenyl dicarboxylic acid. The adenine nucleobase consists of ring N atoms and an amino group that can coordinate with metal ions [78]. **Table 2** lists some of the biomolecule-MOF composites.

6.3 Other active agents

Targeted delivery of photoactive compounds such as photosensitizers (dyes, metal nanoparticles/clusters, quantum dots, etc.) incorporated with MOFs and NMOFs can be achieved, preventing their degradation and accumulation in the physiological

S. No.	MOFs/NMOFs	Metal ion	Organic linker	Active agent	Incorporation method	Reference
a. Photodynamic therapy						
1.	ZIF-8	Zn^{2+}	2-methyl imidazolate	Zinc phthalo-cyanine Chlorin e6 Au nano-clusters	One-pot synthesis One-pot synthesis One-pot synthesis	[26] [103] [104]
2.	MIL-101-NH_2	Fe^{3+}	2-amino-1,4-benzene dicarboxylic acid	Black P quantum dots	One-pot synthesis	[105]
3.	DBC-UiO	Hf^{4+}	5,15-di(p-benzoato) chlorin	DBC	Direct assembly	[29]
4.	Cu-GA	Cu^{2+}	Gallic acid	Methylene blue	Post-synthetic encapsulation	[101]
b. Photothermal therapy						
1.	ZIF-8	Zn^{2+}	2-methyl imidazolate	Cyanine Graphene quantum dots Au nano-stars	One-pot synthesis Surface attachment One-pot synthesis	[106] [107] [108]
2.	UiO-66	Zr^{4+}	1,4-benzene dicarboxylic acid	Polyaniline	Surface attachment	[109]
3.	MIL-53	Fe^{3+}	1,4-benzene dicarboxylic acid	Polypyrrole nano-particles	Post-synthetic encapsulation	[110]
c. Magneto-cytolytic therapy						
1.	ZIF-8	Zn^{2+}	2-methyl imidazolate	Fe_3O_4 nano-particles	One-pot synthesis	[102]
2.	Fe-MOF	Fe^{3+}	1,4-benzene dicarboxylic acid	Fe_3O_4 nano-particles	Surface attachment	[111]

Table 3.
Examples of NMOFs and MOFs as carriers of active agents for novel therapies.

systems. These compounds are essential for light-activated novel therapies such as photodynamic therapy (PDT) and photothermal therapy (PTT). Xu et al. incorporated a hydrophobic porphyrin-based dye, zinc phthalocyanine inside the pores of ZIF-8 for PDT [26]. Sharma et al. synthesized a bioactive MOF, MB/Cu-GA, for simultaneous PDT and drug delivery. Gallic acid (GA), an anti-cancer agent was directly incorporated into the MOF framework, and the photosensitizer, methylene blue (MB) was post-synthetically encapsulated [101]. Magnetic nanoparticles can also be encapsulated or decorated on the surface of MOF for magneto-cytolytic therapy (magnetic hyperthermia). Chen et al. prepared Fe_3O_4@PDA@ZIF-90 loaded with DOX nanocomposites for combined magnetic hyperthermia and chemotherapy [102]. **Table 3** summarizes some of the examples of MOFs employed for the delivery of photosensitizers and magnetic nanoparticles.

7. Conclusion

This chapter gives a general perspective regarding the use of metal–organic frameworks as drug carriers, in terms of their composition, structure, synthesis, procedures to incorporate drugs and characterization techniques. MOFs are highly porous frameworks with large surface area, made up of repeating units, and generally synthesized by solvothermal and non-solvothermal methods. Therapeutic agents and drugs can be encapsulated, post synthetically attached on the surface, or directly incorporated into the framework. Apart from these compounds, functional biomolecules can also be incorporated with MOFs for the possible treatment of various diseases and therapies. Due to their distinct physicochemical properties, MOFs and NMOFs are gaining prominence for various applications. MOFs have already established themselves as efficient systems for gas storage and separation. Their use as potential drug carriers is relatively new. The available work done by researchers around the world for utilizing these porous frameworks as carriers for drugs will help in synthesizing and designing MOF-drug composites in the future, that can successfully be used for real-world applications.

Acknowledgements

Ashi Mittal acknowledges fellowship support from the University Grants Commission (UGC), Government of India.

Conflict of interest

The authors declare no conflict of interest.

Nomenclature

bix	1,4-bis(imidazole-1-ylmethyl)benzene
DBC	5,15-di(p-benzoato) chlorin
DBCO	dibenzyl cyclooctyne
DBP	5,15-di(p-benzoato)porphyrin

F-H2PDA	(2E,2′E)- 3,3′-(2-fluoro-1,4-phenylene) diacrylic acid
HKUST	Hong Kong University of Science and Technology
ICA	Imidazole-2-carboxaldehyde
IRMOF	Isoreticular Metal Organic Framework
MAF	Metal Azolate Framework
MIL	Materials Institute Lavoisier
NCP	Nanoscale coordination polymers
TATB	4,4′,4″-s-triazine-2,4,6-triyl-tribenzoic acid
TCPP	tetrakis (4- carboxyphenyl) porphyrin
UiO	University of Oslo
ZIF	Zeolitic Imidazolate Framework
ZJU	Zhejiang University

Author details

Ashi Mittal, Indrajit Roy* and Sona Gandhi*
Department of Chemistry, University of Delhi, Delhi, India

*Address all correspondence to: indrajitroy11@gmail.com and gandhi7hd@gmail.com

References

[1] Wilczewska AZ, Niemirowicz K, Markiewicz KH, Car H. Nanoparticles as drug delivery systems. Pharmacological Reports. 2012;**64**:1020-1037. DOI: 10.1016/s1734-1140(12)70901-5

[2] Wu MX, Yang YW. Metal-organic framework (mof)-based drug/cargo delivery and cancer therapy. Advanced Materials. 2017;**29**:e1606134. DOI: 10.1002/adma.201606134

[3] Davis ME, Chen ZG, Shin DM. Nanoparticle therapeutics: An emerging treatment modality for cancer. Nature Reviews. Drug Discovery. 2008;**7**:771-782. DOI: 10.1038/nrd2614

[4] Anselmo AC, Mitragotri S. Nanoparticles in the clinic: An update. Bioeng Translational Medicine. 2019;**4**:e10143. DOI: 10.1002/btm2.10143

[5] Luo Z, Fan S, Gu C, Liu W, Chen J, Li B, et al. Metal-organic framework (MOF)-based nanomaterials for biomedical applications. Current Medicinal Chemistry. 2019;**26**:3341-3369. DOI: 10.2174/0929867325666180214123500

[6] Hoskins BF, Robson R. Infinite polymeric frameworks consisting of three dimensionally linked rod-like segments. Journal of the American Chemical Society. 1989;**111**:5962-5964. DOI: 10.1021/ja00197a079

[7] Peller M, Böll K, Zimpel A, Wuttke S. Metal-organic framework nanoparticles for magnetic resonance imaging. Inorganic Chemistry Frontiers. 2018;**5**:1760-1779. DOI: 10.1039/C8QI00149A

[8] Eddaoudi M, Li H, Yaghi OM. Highly porous and stable metal-organic frameworks: structure design and sorption properties. Journal of the American Chemical Society. 2000;**122**:1391-1397. DOI: 10.1021/ja9933386

[9] Horcajada P, Gref R, Baati T, Allan PK, Maurin G, Couvreur P, et al. Metal-organic frameworks in biomedicine. Chemical Reviews. 2012;**112**:1232-1268. DOI: 10.1021/cr200256v

[10] Simon-Yarza T, Mielcarek A, Couvreur P, Serre C. Nanoparticles of metal-organic frameworks: on the road to in vivo efficacy in biomedicine. Advanced Materials. 2018;**30**:e1707365. DOI: 10.1002/adma.201707365

[11] Zhang S, Pei X, Gao H, Chen S, Wang J. Metal-organic framework-based nanomaterials for biomedical applications. Chinese Chemical Letters. 2020;**31**:1060-1070. DOI: 10.1016/j.cclet.2019.11.036

[12] Riccò R, Liang W, Li S, Gassensmith JJ, Caruso F, Doonan C, et al. Metal-organic frameworks for cell and virus biology: A perspective. ACS Nano. 2018;**12**:13-23. DOI: 10.1021/acsnano.7b08056

[13] Alhamami M, Doan H, Cheng CH. A review on breathing behaviors of metal-organic-frameworks (MOFs) for gas adsorption. Materials (Basel). 2014;**7**:3198-3250. DOI: 10.3390/ma7043198

[14] Yaghi OM, O'Keeffe M, Ockwig NW, Chae HK, Eddaoudi M, Kim J. Reticular synthesis and the design of new materials. Nature. 2003;**423**:705-714. DOI: 10.1038/nature01650

[15] Yaghi OM, Kalmutzki MJ, Diercks CS. Introduction to Reticular

Chemistry: Metal-Organic Frameworks and Covalent Organic Frameworks. Wiley; 2019. DOI: 10.1002/9783527821099. Available from: https://onlinelibrary.wiley.com/doi/book/10.1002/9783527821099

[16] Kalmutzki MJ, Hanikel N, Yaghi OM. Secondary building units as the turning point in the development of the reticular chemistry of MOFs. Science Advances. 2018;**4**:eaat9180. DOI: 10.1126/sciadv.aat9180

[17] Lawson HD, Walton SP, Chan C. Metal-organic frameworks for drug delivery: A design perspective. ACS Applied Materials & Interfaces. 2021;**13**:7004-7020. DOI: 10.1021/acsami.1c01089

[18] Rocca JD, Liu D, Lin W. Nanoscale metal-organic frameworks for biomedical imaging and drug delivery. Accounts of Chemical Research. 2011;**44**:957-968. DOI: 10.1021/ar200028a

[19] Butova VV, Soldatov MA, Guda AA, Lomachenko KA, Lamberti C. Metal-organic frameworks: Structure, properties, methods of synthesis and characterization. Russian Chemical Reviews. 2016;**85**:280-307. DOI: 10.1070/RCR4554

[20] Rieter WJ, Taylor KM, An H, Lin W, Lin W. Nanoscale metal-organic frameworks as potential multimodal contrast enhancing agents. Journal of the American Chemical Society. 2006;**128**:9024-9025. DOI: 10.1021/ja0627444

[21] Taylor-Pashow KM, Della Rocca J, Xie Z, Tran S, Lin W. Postsynthetic modifications of iron-carboxylate nanoscale metal-organic frameworks for imaging and drug delivery. Journal of the American Chemical Society. 2009;**131**:14261-14263. DOI: 10.1021/ja906198y

[22] Safarifard V, Morsali A. Applications of ultrasound to the synthesis of nanoscale metal-organic coordination polymers. Coordination Chemistry Reviews. 2015;**292**:1-14. DOI: 10.1016/j.ccr.2015.02.014

[23] Yang B, Shen M, Liu J, Ren F. Post-synthetic modification nanoscale metal-organic frameworks for targeted drug delivery in cancer cells. Pharmaceutical Research. 2017;**34**:2440-2450. DOI: 10.1007/s11095-017-2253-9

[24] Uemura K, Matsuda R, Kitagawa S. Flexiblemicroporouscoordinationpolymers. Journal of Solid State Chemistry. 2005;**178**:2420-2429. DOI: 10.1016/j.jssc.2005.05.036

[25] Nasrollahi M, Nabipour H, Valizadeh N, Mozafari M. The Role of Flexibility in MOFs. Elsevier Inc; 2020. DOI: 10.1016/B978-0-12-816984-1.00006-8. Available from: https://www.sciencedirect.com/science/article/pii/B9780128169841000068?via%3Dihub

[26] Xu D, You Y, Zeng F, Wang Y, Liang C, Feng H, et al. Disassembly of hydrophobic photosensitizer by biodegradable zeolitic imidazolate framework-8 for photodynamic cancer therapy. ACS Applied Materials & Interfaces. 2018;**10**:15517-15523. DOI: 10.1021/acsami.8b03831

[27] Chen X, Tong R, Shi Z, Yang B, Liu H, Ding S, et al. MOF nanoparticles with encapsulated autophagy inhibitor in controlled drug delivery system for antitumor. ACS Applied Materials & Interfaces. 2017;**10**:2328-2337. DOI: 10.1021/acsami.7b16522

[28] Rieter WJ, Pott KM, Taylor KM, Lin W. Nanoscale coordination polymers

for platinum-based anticancer drug delivery. Journal of the American Chemical Society. 2008;**130**:11584-11585. DOI: 10.1021/ja803383k

[29] Lu K, He C, Lin W. A chlorin-based nanoscale metal-organic framework for photodynamic therapy of Colon cancers. Journal of the American Chemical Society. 2015;**137**:7600-7603. DOI: 10.1021/jacs.5b04069

[30] Horcajada P, Serre C, Vallet-Regí M, Sebban M, Taulelle F, Férey G. Metal-organic frameworks as efficient materials for drug delivery. Angewandte Chemie (International Ed. in English). 2006;**45**:5974-5978. DOI: 10.1002/anie.200601878

[31] Wang S, McGuirk CM, Ross MB, Wang S, Chen P, Xing H, et al. General and direct method for preparing oligonucleotide-functionalized metal-organic framework nanoparticles. Journal of the American Chemical Society. 2017;**139**:9827-9830. DOI: 10.1021/jacs.7b05633

[32] Zhu X, Gu J, Wang Y, Li B, Li Y, Zhao W, et al. Inherent anchorages in UiO-66 nanoparticles for efficient capture of alendronate and its mediated release. Chemical Communications. 2014;**50**:8779-8782. DOI: 10.1039/C4CC02570A

[33] Röder R, Preiß T, Hirschle P, Steinborn B, Zimpel A, Höhn M, et al. Multifunctional nanoparticles by coordinative self-assembly of his-tagged units with metal-organic frameworks. Journal of the American Chemical Society. 2017;**139**:2359-2368. DOI: 10.1021/jacs.6b11934

[34] Zhang FM, Dong H, Zhang X, Sun XJ, Liu M, Yang DD, et al. Postsynthetic modification of ZIF-90 for potential targeted codelivery of two anticancer drugs. ACS Applied Materials & Interfaces. 2017;**9**:27332-27337. DOI: 10.1021/acsami.7b08451

[35] Zhuang J, Kuo CH, Chou LY, Liu DY, Weerapana E, Tsung CK. Optimized metal-organic-framework nanospheres for drug delivery: Evaluation of small-molecule encapsulation. ACS Nano. 2014;**8**:2812-2819. DOI: 10.1021/nn406590q

[36] Xue T, Xu C, Wang Y, Wang Y, Tian H, Zhang Y. Doxorubicin-loaded nanoscale metal-organic framework for tumor-targeting and combined chemotherapy and chemodynamic therapy. Biomaterials Science. 2019;7:4615-4623. DOI: 10.1039/C9BM01044K

[37] Lei B, Wang M, Jiang Z, Qi W, Su R, He Z. Constructing redox-responsive metal-organic framework nanocarriers for anticancer drug delivery. ACS Applied Materials & Interfaces. 2018;**10**:16698-16706. DOI: 10.1021/acsami.7b19693

[38] Liang K, Ricco R, Doherty CM, Styles MJ, Bell S, Kirby N, et al. Biomimetic mineralization of metal-organic frameworks as protective coatings for biomacromolecules. Nature Communications. 2015;**6**:7240. DOI: 10.1038/ncomms8240

[39] Yang Y, Hu Q, Zhang Q, Jiang K, Lin W, Yang Y, et al. A large capacity cationic metal-organic framework nanocarrier for physiological pH responsive drug delivery. Molecular Pharmaceutics. 2016;**13**:2782-2786. DOI: 10.1021/acs.molpharmaceut.6b00374

[40] Eddaoudi M, Kim J, Rosi N, Vodak D, Wachter J, O'Keeffe M, et al. Systematic deign of pore size and functionality in isoreticular MOFs and their application in methane storage.

Science. 2002;**295**:469-472. DOI: 10.1126/science.1067208

[41] Suh MP, Park HJ, Prasad TK, Lim DW. Hydrogen storage in metal-organic frameworks. Chemical Reviews. 2012;**112**:782-835. DOI: 10.1021/cr200274s

[42] Sumida K, Rogow DL, Mason JA, McDonald TM, Bloch ED, Herm ZR, et al. Carbon dioxide capture in metal-organic frameworks. Chemical Reviews. 2012;**112**:724-781. DOI: 10.1021/cr2003272

[43] Seo JS, Whang D, Lee H, Jun SI, Oh J, Jeon YJ, et al. A homochiral metal-organic porous material for enantioselective separation and catalysis. Nature. 2000;**404**:982-986. DOI: 10.1038/35010088

[44] Lv XL, Wang K, Wang B, Su J, Zou X, Xie Y, et al. A base-resistant metalloporphyrin metal-organic framework for C-H bond halogenation. Journal of the American Chemical Society. 2017;**139**:211-217. DOI: 10.1021/jacs.6b09463

[45] Li K, He K, Li Q, Xia B, Wang Q, Zhang Y. A zinc(II) MOF based on secondary building units of infinite wavy-shaped chain exhibiting obvious luminescent sense effects. Chinese Chemical Letters. 2019;**30**:499-501. DOI: 10.1016/j.cclet.2018.05.001

[46] Kurmoo M. Magnetic metal-organic frameworks. Chemical Society Reviews. 2009;**38**:1353-1379. DOI: 10.1039/B804757J

[47] Zhang T, Lin W. Metal-organic frameworks for artificial photosynthesis and photocatalysis. Chemical Society Reviews. 2014;**43**:5982-5993. DOI: 10.1039/C4CS00103F

[48] Ling P, Lei J, Zhang L, Ju H. Porphyrin-encapsulated metal-organic frameworks as mimetic catalysts for electrochemical DNA sensing via allosteric switch of hairpin DNA. Analytical Chemistry. 2015;**87**:3957-3963. DOI: 10.1021/acs.analchem.5b00001

[49] Horcajada P, Chalati T, Serre C, Gillet B, Sebrie C, Baati T, et al. Porous metal-organic frameworks nanoscale carriers as a potential platform for drug delivery and imaging. Nature Materials. 2010;**9**:172-179. DOI: 10.1038/nmat2608

[50] Ishida T, Harashima H, Kiwada H. Liposome Clearance. Bioscience Reports. 2002;**22**:197-224. DOI: 10.1023/A:1020134521778

[51] Soenen SJ, Parak WJ, Rejman J, Manshian B. (Intra) cellular stability of inorganic nanoparticles: effects on cytotoxicity, particle functionality, and biomedical applications. Chemical Reviews. 2015;**115**:2109-2135. DOI: 10.1021/cr400714j

[52] Nasrabadi M, Ghasemzadeh MA, Zand Monfared MR. The preparation and characterization of UiO-66 metal-organic frameworks for the delivery of the drug ciprofloxacin and an evaluation of their antibacterial activities. New Journal of Chemistry. 2019;**43**:16033-16040. DOI: 10.1039/C9NJ03216A

[53] Sun CY, Qin C, Wang XL, Yang GS, Shao KZ, Lan YQ, et al. Zeolitic imidazolate framework-8 as efficient pH-sensitive drug delivery vehicle. Dalton Transactions. 2012;**41**:6906-6909. DOI: 10.1039/C2DT30357D

[54] Horcajada P, Serre C, Maurin G, Ramsahye NA, Balas F, Vallet-Regí M, et al. Flexible porous metal-organic frameworks for a controlled drug delivery. Journal of the American Chemical Society. 2008;**130**:6774-6780. DOI: 10.1021/ja710973k

[55] Suresh K, Matzger AJ. Enhanced drug delivery by dissolution of amorphous drug encapsulated in a water unstable metal-organic framework (MOF). Angewandte Chemie (International Ed. in English). 2019;**58**:16790-16794. DOI: 10.1002/anie.201907652

[56] Jiang K, Zhang L, Hu Q, Zhao D, Xia T, Lin W, et al. Pressure controlled drug release in a Zr-cluster-based MOF. Journal of Materials Chemistry B. 2016;**4**:6398-6401. DOI: 10.1039/C6TB01756H

[57] Levine DJ, Runčevski T, Kapelewski MT, Keitz BK, Oktawiec J, Reed DA, et al. Olsalazine-based metal-organic frameworks as biocompatible platforms for H2 adsorption and drug delivery. Journal of the American Chemical Society. 2016;**138**:10143-10150. DOI: 10.1021/jacs.6b03523

[58] Lin S, Liu X, Tan L, Cui Z, Yang X, Yeung KWK, et al. Porous iron-carboxylate metal-organic framework: A novel bioplatform with sustained antibacterial efficacy and nontoxicity. ACS Applied Materials & Interfaces. 2017;**9**:19248-19257. DOI: 10.1021/acsami.7b04810

[59] Soltani B, Nabipour H, Nasab NA. Efficient storage of gentamicin in nanoscale zeolitic imidazolate framework-8 nanocarrier for pH-responsive drug release. Journal of Inorganic and Organometallic Polymers and Materials. 2018;**28**:1090-1097. DOI: 10.1007/s10904-017-0745-z

[60] Nabipour H, Sadr MH, Bardajee GR. Synthesis and characterization of nanoscale zeolitic imidazolate frameworks with ciprofloxacin and their applications as antimicrobial agents. New Journal of Chemistry. 2017;**41**:7364-7370. DOI: 10.1039/C7NJ00606C

[61] Sava Gallis DF, Butler KS, Agola JO, Pearce CJ, McBride AA. Antibacterial countermeasures via metal-organic framework-supported sustained therapeutic release. ACS Applied Materials & Interfaces. 2019;**11**:7782-7791. DOI: 10.1021/acsami.8b21698

[62] Zhang X, Liu L, Huang L, Zhang W, Wang R, Yue T, et al. The highly efficient elimination of intracellular bacteria via a metal organic framework (MOF)-based three-in-one delivery system. Nanoscale. 2019;**11**:9468-9477. DOI: 10.1039/C9NR01284B

[63] Wei Y, Chen C, Zhai S, Tan M, Zhao J, Zhu X, et al. Enrofloxacin/florfenicol loaded cyclodextrin metal-organic-framework for drug delivery and controlled release. Drug Delivery. 2021;**28**:372-379. DOI: 10.1080/10717544.2021.1879316

[64] André V, da Silva ARF, Fernandes A, Frade R, Garcia C, Rijo P, et al. Mg- and Mn-MOFs boost the antibiotic activity of nalidixic acid. ACS Applied Bio Materials. 2019;**2**:2347-2354. DOI: 10.1021/acsabm.9b00046

[65] Anand R, Borghi F, Manoli F, Manet I, Agostoni V, Reschiglian P, et al. Host-guest interactions in Fe(III)-trimesate MOF nanoparticles loaded with doxorubicin. The Journal of Physical Chemistry. B. 2014;**118**:8532-8539. DOI: 10.1021/jp503809w

[66] Lin W, Hu Q, Jiang K, Yang Y, Yang Y, Cui Y, et al. A porphyrin-based metal-organic framework as a pH-responsive drug carrier. Journal of Solid State Chemistry. 2016;**237**:307-312. DOI: 10.1016/j.jssc.2016.02.040

[67] Imaz I, Rubio-Martínez M, García-Fernández L, García F, Ruiz-Molina D, Hernando J, et al. Coordination polymer particles as potential drug delivery systems. Chemical

Communications. 2010;**46**:4737-4739. DOI: 10.1039/C003084H

[68] Ke F, Yuan YP, Qiu LG, Shen YH, Xie AJ, Zhu JF, et al. Facile fabrication of magnetic metal-organic framework nanocomposites for potential targeted drug delivery. Journal of Materials Chemistry. 2011;**21**:3843-3848. DOI: 10.1039/C0JM01770A

[69] Lin W, Hu Q, Yu J, Jiang K, Yang Y, Xiang S, et al. Low cytotoxic metal-organic frameworks as temperature-responsive drug carriers. ChemPlusChem. 2016;**81**:804-810. DOI: 10.1002/cplu.201600142

[70] Gao S, Jin Y, Ge K, Li Z, Liu H, Dai X, et al. Self-supply of O2 and H2O2 by a nanocatalytic medicine to enhance combined chemo/chemodynamic therapy. Advancement of Science. 2019;**6**:1902137. DOI: 10.1002/advs.201902137

[71] Zheng H, Zhang Y, Liu L, Wan W, Guo P, Nyström AM, et al. One-pot synthesis of metal-organic frameworks with encapsulated target molecules and their applications for controlled drug delivery. Journal of the American Chemical Society. 2016;**138**:962-968. DOI: 10.1021/jacs.5b11720

[72] Chen G, Luo J, Cai M, Qin L, Wang Y, Gao L, et al. Investigation of metal-organic framework-5 (MOF-5) as an antitumor drug oridonin sustained release carrier. Molecules. 2019;**24**:3369. DOI: 10.3390/molecules24183369

[73] An H, Li M, Gao J, Zhang Z, Ma S, Chen Y. Incorporation of biomolecules in metal-organic frameworks for advanced applications. Coordination Chemistry Reviews. 2019;**384**:90-106. DOI: 10.1016/j.ccr.2019.01.001

[74] Chen Y, Li P, Modica JA, Drout RJ, Farha OK. Acid-resistant mesoporous metal-organic framework toward oral insulin delivery: Protein encapsulation, protection, and release. Journal of the American Chemical Society. 2018;**140**:5678-5681. DOI: 10.1021/jacs.8b02089

[75] Ni K, Luo T, Culbert A, Kaufmann M, Jiang X, Lin W. Nanoscale metal-organic framework co-delivers TLR-7 agonists and anti-CD47 antibodies to modulate macrophages and orchestrate cancer immunotherapy. Journal of the American Chemical Society. 2020;**142**:12579-12584. DOI: 10.1021/jacs.0c05039

[76] Morris W, Briley WE, Auyeung E, Cabezas MD, Mirkin CA. Nucleic acid-metal organic framework (MOF) nanoparticle conjugates. Journal of the American Chemical Society. 2014;**136**:7261-7264. DOI: 10.1021/ja503215w

[77] Shieh FK, Wang SC, Yen CI, Wu CC, Dutta S, Chou LY, et al. Imparting functionality to biocatalysts via embedding enzymes into nanoporous materials by a de novo approach: size-selective sheltering of catalase in metal-organic framework microcrystals. Journal of the American Chemical Society. 2015;**137**:4276-4279. DOI: 10.1021/ja513058h

[78] An J, Geib SJ, Rosi NL. Cation-triggered drug release from a porous zinc-adeninate metal-organic framework. Journal of the American Chemical Society. 2009;**131**:8376-8377. DOI: 10.1021/ja902972w

[79] Chen Y, Lykourinou V, Vetromile C, Hoang T, Ming LJ, Larsen RW, et al. How can proteins enter the interior of a MOF? investigation of cytochrome c translocation into a MOF consisting of mesoporous cages with microporous windows. Journal of the American

Chemical Society. 2012;**134**:13188-13191. DOI: 10.1021/ja305144x

[80] Lykourinou V, Chen Y, Wang XS, Meng L, Hoang T, Ming LJ, et al. Immobilization of MP-11 into a mesoporous metal-organic framework, MP-11@mesoMOF: A new platform for enzymatic catalysis. Journal of the American Chemical Society. 2011;**133**:10382-10385. DOI: 10.1021/ja2038003

[81] Deng H, Grunder S, Cordova KE, Valente C, Furukawa H, Hmadeh M, et al. Large-pore apertures in a series of metal-organic frameworks. Science. 2012;**336**:1018-1023. DOI: 10.1126/science.1220131

[82] Lian X, Huang Y, Zhu Y, Fang Y, Zhao R, Joseph E, et al. Enzyme-MOF nanoreactor activates nontoxic paracetamol for cancer therapy. Angewandte Chemie (International Ed. in English). 2018;**57**:5725-5730. DOI: 10.1002/anie.201801378

[83] Wu X, Ge J, Yang C, Hou M, Liu Z. Facile synthesis of multiple enzyme-containing metal-organic frameworks in a biomolecule-friendly environment. Chemical Communications. 2015;**51**:13408-13411. DOI: 10.1039/C5CC05136C

[84] Peng S, Liu J, Qin Y, Wang H, Cao B, Lu L, et al. Metal-organic framework encapsulating hemoglobin as high-stable and long-circulating oxygen carriers o treat hemorrhagic shock. ACS Applied Materials & Interfaces. 2019;**11**:35604-35612. DOI: 10.1021/acsami.9b15037

[85] Zhang X, Zeng Y, Zheng A, Cai Z, Huang A, Zeng J, et al. A fluorescence based immunoassay for galectin-4 using gold nanoclusters and a composite consisting of glucose oxidase and a metal-organic framework. Microchimica Acta. 2017;**184**:1933-1940. DOI: 10.1007/s00604-017-2204-5

[86] Li Y, Xu N, Zhu W, Wang L, Liu B, Zhang J, et al. Nanoscale Melittin@Zeolitic imidazolate frameworks for enhanced anticancer activity and mechanism analysis. ACS Applied Materials & Interfaces. 2018;**10**:22974-22984. DOI: 10.1021/acsami.8b06125

[87] Liu X, Yan Z, Zhang Y, Liu Z, Sun Y, Ren J, et al. Two-dimensional metal-organic framework/enzyme hybrid nanocatalyst as a benign and self-activated Cascade reagent for in vivo wound healing. ACS Nano. 2019;**13**:5222-5230. DOI: 10.1021/acsnano.8b09501

[88] Zhou Y, Liu L, Cao Y, Yu S, He C, Chen X. A nanocomposite vehicle based on metal-organic framework nanoparticle incorporated biodegradable microspheres for enhanced oral insulin delivery. ACS Applied Materials & Interfaces. 2020;**12**:22581-22592. DOI: 10.1021/acsami.0c04303

[89] Feng Y, Wang H, Zhang S, Zhao Y, Gao J, Zheng Y, et al. Antibodies@MOFs: An in vitro protective coating for preparation and storage of biopharmaceuticals. Advanced Materials. 2018;**31**:1805148. DOI: 10.1002/adma.201805148

[90] Alsaiari SK, Qutub SS, Sun S, Baslyman W, Aldehaiman M, Alyami M, et al. Sustained and targeted delivery of checkpoint inhibitors by metal-organic frameworks for cancer immunotherapy. Science Advances. 2021;7:eabe7174. DOI: 10.1126/sciadv.abe7174

[91] Zhang Y, Wang F, Ju E, Liu Z, Chen Z, Ren J, et al. Metal-organic framework-based vaccine platforms

for enhanced systemic immune and memory response. Advanced Functional Materials. 2016;**26**:6454-6461. DOI: 10.1002/adfm.201600650

[92] Xie W, Yin T, Chen YL, Zhu DM, Zan MH, Chen B, et al. Capture and "self-release" of circulating tumor cells using metal-organic framework materials. Nanoscale. 2019;**11**:8293-8303. DOI: 10.1039/C8NR09071H

[93] Qi Y, Wang L, Guo H, Pan Y, Xie Z, Jin N, et al. Antigen-enabled facile preparation of MOF nanovaccine to activate the complement system for enhanced antigen-mediated immune response. Biomaterials Science. 2019;**7**:4022-4026. DOI: 10.1039/C9BM01145E

[94] Miao YB, Pan WY, Chen KH, Wei HJ, Mi FL, Lu MY, et al. Engineering a nanoscale Al-MOF-armored antigen carried by a "Trojan Horse"-like platform for oral vaccination to induce potent and long-lasting immunity. Advanced Functional Materials. 2019;**29**:1904828. DOI: 10.1002/adfm.201904828

[95] Peng S, Bie B, Sun Y, Liu M, Cong H, Zhou W, et al. Metal-organic frameworks for precise inclusion of single-stranded DNA and transfection in immune cells. Nature Communications. 2018;**9**:1293. DOI: 10.1038/s41467-018-03650-w

[96] Li Y, Zhang K, Liu P, Chen M, Zhong Y, Ye Q, et al. Encapsulation of plasmid DNA by nanoscale metal-organic frameworks for efficient gene transportation and expression. Advanced Materials. 2019;**31**:1901570. DOI: 10.1002/adma.201901570

[97] Chen Q, Xu M, Zheng W, Xu T, Deng H, Liu J. Se/Ru-decorated porous metal-organic framework nanoparticles for the delivery of pooled siRNAs to reversing multidrug resistance in taxol-resistant breast cancer cells. ACS Applied Materials & Interfaces. 2017;**9**:6712-6724. DOI: 10.1021/acsami.6b12792

[98] Astria E, Thonhofer M, Ricco R, Liang W, Chemelli A, Tarzia A, et al. Carbohydrates@MOFs. Materials Horizons. 2019;**6**:969-977. DOI: 10.1039/C8MH01611A

[99] Zheng J, Li B, Ji Y, Chen Y, Lv X, Zhang X, et al. Prolonged release and shelf-life of anticoagulant sulfated polysaccharides encapsulated with ZIF-8. International Journal of Biological Macromolecules. 2021;**183**:1174-1183. DOI: 10.1016/j.ijbiomac.2021.05.007

[100] Velásquez-Hernández MDJ, Astria E, Winkler S, Liang W, Wiltsche H, Poddar A, et al. Modulation of metal-azolate frameworks for the tunable release of encapsulated glycosaminoglycans. Chemical Science. 2020;**11**:10835-10843. DOI: 10.1039/D0SC01204A

[101] Sharma S, Mittal D, Verma AK, Roy I. Copper-gallic acid nanoscale metal-organic framework for combined drug delivery and photodynamic therapy. ACS Applied Bio Materials. 2019;**2**:2092-2101. DOI: 10.1021/acsabm.9b00116

[102] Chen J, Liu J, Hu Y, Tian Z, Zhu Y. Metal-organic framework-coated magnetite nanoparticles for synergistic magnetic hyperthermia and chemotherapy with pH-triggered drug release. Science and Technology of Advanced Materials. 2019;**20**:1043-1054. DOI: 10.1080/14686996.2019.1682467

[103] Sun Q, Bi H, Wang Z, Li C, Wang C, Xu J, et al. O2-generating metal-organic framework-based hydrophobic photosensitizer delivery system for enhanced photodynamic therapy.

ACS Applied Materials & Interfaces. 2019;**11**:36347-36358. DOI: 10.1021/acsami.9b11607

[104] Zhang L, Gao Y, Sun S, Li Z, Wu A, Zeng L. pH-Responsive metal-organic framework encapsulated gold nanoclusters with modulated release to enhance photodynamic therapy/chemotherapy in breast cancer. Journal of Materials Chemistry B. 2020;**8**:1739-1747. DOI: 10.1039/C9TB02621E

[105] Liu J, Liu T, Du P, Zhang L, Lei J. Metal-organic framework (MOF) hybrid as a tandem catalyst for enhanced therapy against hypoxic tumor cells. Angewandte Chemie (International Ed. in English). 2019;**58**:7808-7812. DOI: 10.1002/anie.201903475

[106] Li Y, Xu N, Zhou J, Zhu W, Li L, Dong M, et al. Facile synthesis of a metal-organic framework nanocarrier or NIR imaging-guided photothermal therapy. Biomaterials Science. 2018;**6**:2918-2924. DOI: 10.1039/C8BM00830B

[107] Tian Z, Yao X, Ma K, Niu X, Grothe J, Xu Q, et al. Metal-organic framework/graphene quantum dot nanoparticles used for synergistic chemo- and photothermal therapy. ACS Omega. 2017;**2**:1249-1258. DOI: 10.1021/acsomega.6b00385

[108] Deng X, Liang S, Cai X, Huang S, Cheng Z, Shi Y, et al. Yolk-shell structured Au nanostar@metal-organic framework for synergistic chemo-photothermal therapy in the second near-infrared window. Nano Letters. 2019;**19**:6772-6780. DOI: 10.1021/acs.nanolett.9b01716

[109] Wang W, Wang L, Li Y, Liu S, Xie Z, Jing X. Nanoscale polymer metal-organic framework hybrids for effective photothermal therapy of Colon cancers. Advanced Materials. 2016;**28**:9320-9325. DOI: 10.1002/adma.201602997

[110] Huang J, Li N, Zhang C, Meng Z. Metal-organic framework as a microreactor for in situ fabrication of multifunctional nanocomposites for photothermal-chemotherapy of tumors in vivo. ACS Applied Materials & Interfaces. 2018;**10**:38729-38738. DOI: 10.1021/acsami.8b12394

[111] Xiang Z, Qi Y, Lu Y, Hu Z, Wang X, Jia W, et al. MOF-derived novel porous Fe3O4@C nanocomposites as smart nanomedical platforms or combined cancer therapy: magnetic-triggered synergistic hyperthermia and chemotherapy. Journal of Materials Chemistry B. 2020;**8**:8671-8683. DOI: 10.1039/D0TB01021A

Chapter 5

Advances in Graphene Platforms for Drug Delivery in Cancer and Its Biocompatibility

Juan Pablo González-Castillo, Esdras Alfredo Zamora-Morán and Lourdes Rodriguez-Fragoso

Abstract

In the past decade, studies on the biomedical applications of graphene quantum dots (GQDs) have increased substantially, especially those related to cancer therapy. Experimental evidence has shown that GQD platforms do not merely serve for drug delivery but have multifunctional properties: their surface also allows several types of molecules to be joined and has photothermal properties that, when combined, make therapies more effective. Most studies have shown evidence of this specificity and therapeutic efficacy at the in vitro level. There is also evidence for potential use in the monitoring of cellular events given the high-quality bioimages that can be obtained with this type of nanomaterial. However, the application of this nanotechnology has stalled due to the lack of available biosafety and biocompatibility studies. This chapter addresses the advances in the use of GQD platforms for drug delivery and the biocompatibility studies reported so far.

Keywords: graphene, quantum dots, platforms, drug delivery, biocompatibility, cancer

1. Introduction

The major health problems currently afflicting the world population have spurred both research and the development of several medicines meant to treat historical diseases as well as more recent ones, such as the severe acute respiratory syndrome coronavirus-2 (SARS-CoV-2). The range of systems and approaches that can be used to deliver therapies is therefore growing and advancing at an accelerated rate. However, the development of any drug involves a research phase, during which several iterative tests and trials provide important information on the characteristics of the therapeutic target, the biological context, and possible physiological implications [1, 2]. These types of studies provide information on the formulation, efficacy, dosage, and safety of drugs. Products obtained from nanobiotechnology require very rigorous studies due to the great chemical diversity and toxicity said products can produce. These studies must be designed to provide detailed information on the biocompatibility of the nanomaterial and reveal any functional effect on the main

Model	Target	Result	References
***In vitro* models**			
MDAMB-231 cells	Genes	Suppression of gene expression and the reduction of the metastatic potential	Huang et al., [14]
MCF-7 and MDA-MB-231 cells	Genes	Induction of cell death	Imani et al., [15] Liyanage et al., [16]
MCF-7, MDA-MB-231 and MCF-10 cells	Genes	Induction of apoptosis and inhibition of the growth	Assali et al., [17]
MCF-7, MDA-MB-231 and MCF-10 cells	siRNA and pDNA	Protection of enzymatic degradation	Cheang et al., [18]
MCF-7 and MDA-MB-231 cells	P-gp/MDR-1	Reversal of multidrug resistance (MDR), anticancer drugs mediated by ATP-binding cassette (ABC) transporters	Luo et al., [19]
Huh-7 hepatocarcinoma cells	mRNA	Delivery intact mRNA	Liu et al., [20]
HeLa cells	miRNAs	Regulation of miRNAs	Dong et al., [21]
Myeloma cells and ovarian cancer cells	Enzymes	For the delivery of enzyme inhibitors to the nucleus for inducing cytotoxicity and cell death	Felix et al., [22]
4T1 cells, MFC7/ADR cells	miRNA-21	Reversal of multidrug resistance (MDR)	Tian et al., [23] Bukowski et al., [24]
Colorectal carcinoma cells	Mitochondria	Cellular stress and apoptosis	Ruan et al., [25]
Oral squamous cell carcinoma		Cytotoxic effect	Zhang et al., [26]
A549 cells	DNA	Cytotoxicity induced by doxorubicin	Iannazzo et al., [27]
Leukemia cells	DNA	Cytotoxicity induced by daunorubicin	Sinha et al., [28]
A549 cells	DNA	Cytotoxicity induced by doxorubicin	Ko et al., [29]
***In vivo* models**			
Mice/BALBc	DNA	Apoptosis of tumor cells and antitumoral effect induced by doxorubicin	Zhu et al., [30]
Breast tumor-bearing mice	Immune cells	Elimination of the tumor mass in a subcutaneous mammary tumor	Li et al., [31]
A549 tumor xenografts.	Tumor cells	Ablation of tumor	Gazzi et al., [32]
MDA-MB-231 triple-negative breast cancer (TNBC) model	miRNA-21i	Phototherapeutic efficiency of indocyanine green	Wu et al., [33]

Table 1.
Graphene quantum dots for cancer-targeted drug delivery.

physiological systems in order to decide whether a nanobiotechnological product should be tested in humans [3, 4].

The incorporation of nanomaterials into biological systems requires strategies for manipulating the ligands bound to the surface to make them more polar and biocompatible [5]. Nanomaterials must be soluble to have the biological application, and this is achieved by adding functional groups (functionalization). An ideal ligand must meet the following requirements: (1) provide stability and solubility to the nanomaterial in biological buffers; (2) maintain high resistance to photobleaching and other photophysical properties in aqueous media; (3) have functional groups that can conjugate biomolecules (conjugation), and (4) minimize the overall hydrodynamic

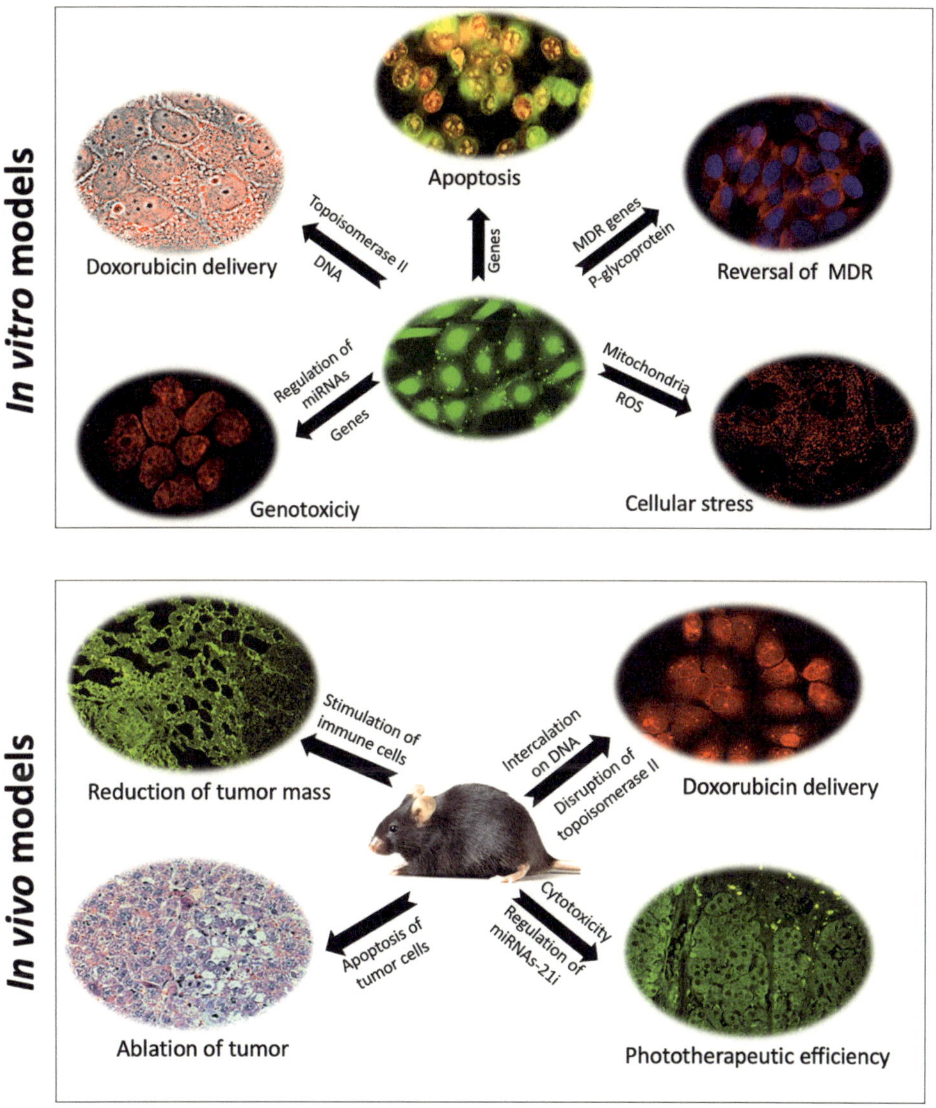

Figure 1.
Application of GQDs platforms for cancer treatment. Cellular targets and effects of GQDs platforms in cell lines and experimental animals.

size [6, 7]. Quantum dots (QDs) are among the most popular nanomaterials: they are semiconductor nanoparticles with photoluminescent properties and a wide variety of applications.

Functionalized QDs are very useful in biomedicine because they can be modified with a great variety of molecules and small biological polymers, which help improve their bioactivity and reduce their toxic effects [8–10]. Thanks to these characteristics, QDs can bind effectively to cell membranes, meaning they can be employed as excellent probes for cell detection, diagnosis, imaging, and delivery of therapeutic agents. Due to the great coupling achieved between QDs and biomolecules, today these are used as a tool for biological goals, to improve the efficacy of drug release control and significantly reduce toxicity [11–13]. At present, a wide range of studies on GQD platforms are mainly focused on cancer treatment (**Table 1** and **Figure 1**). This chapter will review the advances in all these areas, as well as aspects related to the toxicity and biocompatibility of GQDs.

2. Application of graphene platforms for drug delivery

GQDs are carbon-based nanomaterials. Their structure consists of one or more graphene sheets with lateral dimensions of 10 nm [34]. GQDs have a large π-conjugated aromatic structure and a large surface area that allows them to be easily conjugated with various molecules to generate hybrid nanomaterials, but they can also be conjugated with antibodies, proteins, and nucleic acids due to their dimensional similarity with these molecules [35–38]. They also have a high capacity for loading drugs containing aromatic groups, such as camptothecin, paclitaxel, and doxorubicin through π -π stacking interactions between layers of GQDs and drug molecules. Currently, a variety of synthesis methods allow for size, structure, and optical profile design, depending on the intended application. Even green synthesis has been used to protect the environment [39]. Given the properties of GQDs, the biomedical sector has found several applications in the prevention, diagnosis, and treatment of diseases. Recent studies report that GQDs are less toxic, show greater biocompatibility than other nanomaterials, and also have stable and strong fluorescence. All these characteristics make these nanomaterials ideal for use in cancer treatment.

Targeted therapy is a cancer treatment employing drugs that target specific genes and proteins involved in the growth and survival of cancer cells. Targeted therapy can affect tissue conditions that help cancer grow and survive, or it can target cells related to cancer growth, such as cells in blood vessels. To develop targeted therapies, researchers first identify the genetic changes that contribute to a tumor's growth and change [40]. A possible target can be a protein present in cancer cells but not healthy ones. Specificity is required. Targeted therapies are a rapidly growing field of cancer research, and researchers are studying many new targets and drugs in clinical trials. Hence, multifunctional nanoparticles directed at specific targets of the tumor cell are also being developed in the field of nanobiotechnology. GQD platforms have been studied in gene-based therapies across various breast cell lines, where a variety of effects have been discovered. These include the suppression of gene expression and the reduction of the metastatic potential of MDAMB-231 cells [14]; induction of cell death in MCF-7 and MDA cells [15, 16]; the induction of apoptosis and inhibition of the growth of MCF-7, MDA-MB-231, and MCF-10 cells [17]; protection of small interference RNA (siRNA) and DNA plasmids (pDNA) from enzymatic degradation [18]; and reversal of multidrug resistance (MDR) [19]. These same methodologies have been studied in animal models with good results. For example, in mice/BALBc, GQD platforms can induce apoptosis of tumor cells and have an antitumoral effect [30]. Furthermore, it has been observed that they can eliminate the tumor mass in a subcutaneous mammary tumor model [31].

Messenger ribonucleic acid (mRNA) delivery systems are another type of targeted therapy having a recent boom because of advantages such as biocompatibility and low genotoxicity. Stable graphene platforms functionalized with polyethyleneimine were used in one study, achieving successful delivery of intact mRNA to hepatocarcinoma cells [20]. Let us remember that mRNA has been widely used in the study of gene function and has become popular in the development of new therapeutic strategies for cancer immunotherapy and vaccines. GQDs have also been used as platforms for the delivery of nucleic acids for the regulation of microRNA (miRNAs), negative regulators of gene expression, with great therapeutic effectiveness in HeLa cells [21]. Various investigations indicate that the expression of some miRNAs is altered in some cancers; achieving their regulation would be useful in oncology. And while one would expect targeted cancer therapy to be less toxic than traditional chemotherapy drugs because tumor cells are more dependent on targets than normal cells, this is not the case. Clinical observation indicates that targeted therapies can also produce significant side effects.

Another approach to targeted therapy is for the delivery of enzyme inhibitors to the nucleus. For example, in one study, GQDs were conjugated to imatinib, successfully achieving cytotoxicity and apoptotic cell death in myeloma cells and ovarian cancer cells [22]; imatinib is an inhibitor of the protein tyrosine kinase, which potently and specifically inhibits breakpoint cluster region-Abelson (bcr-abl) tyrosine kinase. However, genetic manipulation and treatments directed at nuclear targets have numerous technical difficulties that are not yet fully resolved. Targeted therapy is complex and does not always work. One of the limitations of this type of therapy is that the drugs for some identified targets are difficult to formulate due to the structure of the target or the way its function is regulated in the cell. An example of this is Ras, a signaling protein that has mutations in up to a quarter of all cancers, but for this type of therapy to work, one would have to know what mutation the gene has [41]. In short, using nanotechnological platforms does not guarantee patient safety, given that side effects of drugs as well as those of the nanomaterial have yet to be assessed.

The lack of response to treatment and the recurrence of initially chemosensitive tumors are responsible for a significant number of deaths in cancer patients. Treatment options used as salvage, such as alternating chemotherapy, dose-escalation, or regional chemotherapy, have yet to yield the expected results. Most cancer patients who initially respond to chemotherapy have relapses because of the so-called acquired resistance to multiple antineoplastic drugs (MDR) [24]. Today, combination therapies seek to address different therapeutic targets using nanobiotechnology. GQD platforms can exhibit all the desirable characteristics of a combination therapy since, as previously mentioned, their surface can be conjugated with different molecules. Their physical, chemical, electrical, and optical properties, however, confer additional functions. As shown, GQDs have a high photothermal modification power under near-infrared radiation (NIR), which allows for their use as photothermal therapy [42–44]. Graphene platforms can also be employed for photodynamic therapy, the goal of which is to generate highly cytotoxic reactive oxygen species (ROS) [45]. A great variety of experimental studies involving different types of cancer have been carried out on animals, in most cases resulting in complete ablation of the tumor [32].

Both photothermic and photodynamic therapy show selectivity toward hyperthermic processes typical of cancer cells, but this is rare with normal cells. GQD platforms with more than one therapeutic effect have been used for the treatment of breast cancer; these include chemothermal therapy [46], chemogenic therapy [23, 47], chemo-photothermal therapy [33], and gene therapy [48]. With these platforms, it has been possible to induce greater cytotoxicity, apoptosis, and reverse drug resistance in breast cancer cells. Moreover, inhibition of tumor growth in an animal model of breast cancer MDA-MB-231 triple-negative has been achieved. Graphene platforms have also been employed as nano radiosensitizers to improve the effectiveness of radiotherapy. Oxidized GOQDs with high phototoxicity has been built to induce a cellular stress response via the production of the reactive oxygen species that would be generated during a tumor's exposure to radiation [49]. Important effects, such as mitochondrial damage and apoptotic death have been observed in colorectal carcinoma cells treated with graphene platforms and radiation therapy [25]. Based on this same principle and thanks to their photodynamic properties, GQDs have also been employed to induce phototoxicity and synergize the cytotoxic effect of radiation in oral squamous cell carcinoma [26].

In addition to these novel uses, GQD platforms are good for the delivery of multiple antineoplastic drugs. A multifunctional platform of GQDs for synergistic breast cancer therapy with controlled release of doxorubicin, methotrexate, and paclitaxel, showed a significant synergistic effect in killing tumor cells with improved efficacy [50]. The advantage of combination therapies is that a therapeutic effect is achieved while reducing drug resistance. On some occasions, however, and as happens in the clinic, the side effects could be considerable. Another method that has been tried for therapeutic efficacy is the conjugation of GQD with a ligand that directs it toward the therapeutic target while additionally carrying the antineoplastic drug. This methodology has been carried out in A549 cells treated with GQDs-biotin-doxorubicin and demonstrates GQDs may have multifunctional effects for cancer treatment [27].

As previously noted, graphene platforms can be built according to the needs of cancer therapy. The construction of ultra-small QDs makes them ideal for achieving not only cell penetration and drug delivery to target sites, but also visualization within the cell. Recently, a graphene platform was used in microspheres with daunorubicin. The small size allowed to monitor drug delivery and the intercalation of daunorubicin in DNA, exerting a better pharmacological effect [28]. Several studies have taken advantage of the fluorescence emitted by QDs to image neoplastic tissues so that, at the same time, drug delivery can be tracked and controlled [51]. In this sense, GQD platforms have become ideal candidates for such purposes due to the high quality of image formation obtained thanks to their fluorescence emission [52]. Additionally, drug/gene delivery in tumor cells has been achieved with greater efficiency both *in vitro* and *in vivo* [53]. For example, GQDs have proved an optimal multifunctional nanocarrier for delivering doxorubicin to specific cancer cells, allowing for the monitoring of intracellular anticancer drug release via imaging and therapeutic efficacy [29, 54, 55]. Ge et al. employed these properties for imaging and the application of dynamic phototherapy for the treatment of breast cancer and induced melanoma in female BALB/c nude mice with favorable results [56]. Other groups have performed functionalization studies of GQDs with silica, hypocrelin A, and porphyria derivatives, managing to obtain multi-color images and antitumor effects in cervical, lung, and breast cancer [57–59]. The results obtained to date appear promising, though they usually depend on the biological variability of the experimental animals.

The growth of solid tumors is characterized not only by the uncontrolled proliferation of cells but also by changes in the tumoral microenvironment. In solid tumors, hypoxic areas generally have a low pH. There may be low levels of glucose and other nutrients, as well as changes in temperature, all associated with various alterations in tumor cell metabolism [60]. While the heterogeneity of the tumor microenvironment sometimes makes it difficult to adequately characterize tumors [61], this has spawned interest in developing new nanotechnology therapeutic strategies to improve not only drug delivery conditions and directly destroy tumor cells, but also alter the balance between neoplastic cells and their microenvironment. Therefore, intelligent systems have been developed for the administration of drugs that respond to stimuli, and therapeutic agents can be activated by endogenous or exogenous stimuli [62, 63]. Platforms based on graphene have proven excellent due to their physicochemical properties since, according to the functional groups that are attached to them, they can be sensitive to changes in the tumor microenvironment or to intracellular signals in response to physical stimulus factors. Graphene platforms have been conjugated with functional chemical groups that allow the drug to be released when there are changes in pH and temperature [64]. For example, it has been observed that when pH-sensitive functional groups (COOH, $-NH_2$, and SO_3H) are added to graphene platforms, controlled drug release can be achieved in tumor areas [65]. The functionalization allows the pH of the platform to change in the bloodstream and, with this, remain in circulation for longer and favor the delivery and effectiveness of the treatment. This same effect has been achieved by changes in the loading of the platform. This was the case with the construction of the graphene platform with polymers such as polyethylene glycol and doxorubicin, where it was observed that the release of the drug is accelerated in an acidic environment [66]. Or with the construction of graphene microspheres conjugated with a dendrimer and maltose (Fe_3O_4@C@TDG) as a potential transporter to promote the release of doxorubicin and improve its therapeutic efficacy at specific pH [67]. Polymer aggregation has also served to make photoluminescence more stable at different pH for imaging tumor cells, which, as already mentioned, is part of the multifunctionality of the graphene platform.

3. Evidence regarding the biocompatibility and toxicity of graphene platforms

The available literature indicates that research on GQDs has grown widely in relation to their uses, and that is why we now know their biomedical applications include the elimination of bacteria, the administration of drugs, the development of nanocarriers, cancer therapy, and tissue engineering [35–37, 68]. The therapeutic applications of nanomaterials remain quite limited, and there is no safe and effective formulation yet that can be administered in humans [69–71]. While QDs produce a series of morphological and functional alterations that lead to tumor cell death, what happens to healthy cells is unknown [72]. Therefore, the toxicological profile of each nanomaterial is needed to make decisions regarding potential risks vs. benefits. However, what is known about the biocompatibility of GQDs and what evidence is there of the toxicity of drug delivery platforms?

GQDs and their derivatives have variable toxicity in biological systems ranging from prokaryotic to eukaryotic, depending on the dose and the functional groups with which they are coated [34]. They have also been evaluated in a series of human cell lines. For example, studies carried out on leukocytes showed that there was significant uptake of GQDs in monocytic and granulocytic cells, suggesting that phagocytic cells can incorporate GQDs. The toxicity observed in this study was relatively low (10%) after a 36-hour exposure period at concentrations of 500 μg/mL [73]. In another study using GQDs functionalized with NH_2, COOH, and $CO-N(CH_3)_2$ it was observed that A549 and C6 cells showed a slight increase in their proliferation at concentrations of 200 μg/mL, but no death due to apoptosis [74]. GQDs have also produced toxic effects on mesenchymal stem cell self-renewal and differentiation [75]. Several studies have pointed to the toxic effects of graphene derivatives [76–81]. These functionalized QDs can produce a variety of toxic effects at the cellular level and in vivo due to the series of impurities produced during the oxidation process. The same happens in the coating process with other molecules [82]. However, when GQDs are coated with polyethylene glycol at concentrations of 320 μg/mL, they do not affect the viability and differentiation capacity of neural stem/progenitor cells (NSPCs) [83]. Also, reduced toxicity, absence of ROS production, absence of apoptosis, and lack of morphological changes have been observed in HeLa and A549 tumor cells under concentrations of 100 μg/mL [84, 85].

The cellular and nuclear effects that GQDs produce are due to their high permeability in biological membranes. It is known that the uptake and localization of GQDs are highly dependent on size, shape, coating, and pH, among other factors. Previous studies have shown that GQDs use membrane lipid rafts for their transport across the cell membrane. This process is better, the smaller the QDs are [86]. However, protein-coated GQDs enter mainly by phagocytosis and with smaller coatings by clathrin-mediated endocytosis [87, 88]. GQDs with amide groups enter the cell through energy-dependent mechanisms by endocytosis, mediated by caveolae and phagocytosis [89]. Within the cell, GQDs are distributed in different organelles producing a variety of cellular effects. They are later distributed through endosomal trafficking and reach lysosomes, mitochondria, and the nucleus, and can produce autophagy, apoptosis, and DNA damage [90–92]. At the nuclear level, the NPC Kap2 and Nup98 genes can participate in the uptake of GQDs and can produce morphological and functional alterations associated with genotoxicity, including oxidative stress and DNA damage [93, 94].

There are many reports in the literature regarding the toxic effects of both GQDs and their derivatives in a variety of human cell lines and it is impossible to mention them all in this chapter. What is evident is the ease with which they penetrate cells, position themselves and participate in strategic cellular processes, thus potentially affecting cell functionality and leading to cell death. However, of the studies reviewed so far, most were done in tumor cell lines where physiological processes are altered and there are specific survival and adaptation mechanisms. To date, there are no studies carried out on cell lines from healthy tissue, so we cannot rule out the fact that GQDs could produce morphological and functional modifications associated with toxicity in healthy cells.

What effects do they produce in higher organisms and experimental animals? What is known about the processes of absorption, distribution, metabolism, and excretion (ADME) of GQDs? The information so far is limited. Previous studies in nematodes have shown that nitrogen-bound GQDs (N-GQDs) produce degeneration of dopaminergic and glutamatergic neurons at concentrations of 100 μg/mL [95]. A series of studies on the biocompatibility and biodistribution of GQDs in adult and embryonic zebrafish have been reported and provide important information on embryos' developmental delays, pigmentation inhibition, pericardial edema, and delayed hatching among other things. In adults, GQDs showed high biocompatibility and accumulation in the digestive tract [96]. Apparently, the accumulation of QDs depends on the stage of development of the zebrafish (embryo, larva, adult). Studies in adult zebrafish using GQDs at different concentrations (0.1 ng/mL to 100 μg/mL) and exposure times (8 h to 6 days) showed distribution in the heart, blood vessels, brain, intestine, head, and tail [97–101]. The effects that have been found in zebrafish are morphological and functional alterations, while mortality is attributed to the generation of ROS, oxidative stress, and, finally, apoptosis [102]. On the other hand, studies carried out in chicken embryos have also shown evidence of GQDs-induced toxicity. It was found this affected survival but did not produce morphological or biochemical alterations in the embryo [103]. However, another study found morphological alterations and hemolysis of erythrocytes [104], as well as ultrastructural alterations of the brain, suggesting neurotoxicity [105]. These results suggest that GQDs can alter key processes, not only in adulthood but also during embryonic development.

Biodistribution studies in rodents have shown that GQDs are distributed in various tissues and produce certain toxic effects as well. For example, in mice that received GQDs in a single dose of 10 mg/kg intravenously, it was found that 6 hours after inoculation the QDs were distributed in several organs. Clearance began after 3 days and, at 14 days, the QDs had been completely removed. Histological and biochemical studies did not reveal alterations, only weight loss [106]. However, in another biodistribution study carried out in rodents treated with a single dose of 5 and 15 mg/kg of GQDs intravenously, they produced morphological alterations compatible with inflammation and biochemical damage in the lungs after 7 days of exposure [107]. Additionally, yet another study using repeated doses of 5, 10, and 15 mg/kg every third day for 30 days, showed a reduction in blood cells, morphological alterations in the liver, lipofuscin deposits in the kidney, and the presence of inflammatory infiltrate in the lungs. These alterations were dose-dependent [108]. Taken together, these data suggest that GQDs produce acute toxicity at both single and repeated doses in mammals.

Today there are no reports of long-term studies (chronic toxicity), studies on reproduction and development, or of any other type that allow a general overview of the toxicological profile of GQDs. However, there is experimental evidence showing that other materials derived from graphene can produce a series of toxic effects that must be considered. For example, studies of the distribution of graphene and its derivatives after aerial exposure showed toxic effects in the lungs of rodents [109, 110]. In a chronic inhalation toxicity study of graphene nanoplates, deposits of the nanomaterial were observed in the lungs and pulmonary lymph nodes in mice [111]. In a distribution study in rats using doses of 10, 20, and 40 mg/kg of graphene oxide orally, it was found that it produced nephrotoxic effects due to oxidative stress [112]. While in another study, the administration of multiple doses of oxidized graphene (4 mg/kg) for 4 weeks showed deposits of the material in different tissues in rats [113]. Mutagenic effects have been observed in rats when exposed to graphene oxide at a dose of 4 mg/kg for 4 weeks [114]. Likewise, toxic effects on the reproductive capacity and development of offspring have also been reported after the administration of oxidized graphene to mice with doses from 6.25 mg/kg [115]. Unfortunately, when reviewing the subject, we noted there are no toxicity studies regarding the GQDs platforms employed for drug delivery in cancer research. In fact, all the studies have focused on evaluating its efficiency and specificity toward the tumor cell. That is, what has mattered so far is to demonstrate their possible therapeutic applications in cancer, but not the possible toxic effects they may produce. Therefore, we could say that biosafety studies on GQDs platforms are null.

To date, GQDs have been widely studied as carriers with a large surface area favoring drug transport and particular interest has been placed on characterizing their therapeutic bio properties *in vitro*. However, the preclinical studies carried out so far are hardly enough. Most of the studies in cells and animals have focused on evaluating the efficiency of drug/gene delivery at the site of interest. The dosage of the treatments used in animals has been empirical, since no study has demonstrated the real drug/QD concentration within the body, and it is not known if there could be pharmacological interactions between these platforms and other therapies used in the clinic. One aspect that has been completely neglected is the bioavailability of GQDs. What will be the appropriate route of administration? Do they bind to plasma proteins? Do they accumulate? Where do they metabolize? In the route of excretion? There are many questions that remain unanswered. In addition, long-term toxicity studies are required in different species of animals to test the effects on reproduction, carcinogenicity, and teratogenicity, among others. Many preclinical studies are still needed if GQDs are to be used for diagnosis and treatment in humans.

Concern regarding the toxicity of graphene not only stems from the findings mentioned above, but also from the long-standing concern about environmental and occupational exposure to graphene [116]. Inhalation toxicity data of graphene analyzed in experimental animals suggest that acute exposure by repeated inhalation to graphene-derived materials could induce inflammatory/fibrotic reactions, suggesting that it could also induce fibrotic disease in humans [117, 118]. Hence the importance of conducting preclinical biosafety studies of graphene nanomaterials and their derivatives using specific criteria, for these are not necessarily the same as those used for chemical products. The toxicological evaluation must be extrapolated with special care due to the size of the nanomaterials and the chemical groups they contain. If there is no complete toxicological profile that meets the standards required by the guidelines of administrative agencies such as the US Food and Drug Administration (FDA), the European Medicines Agency (EMA) or the European Medicines Evaluation Agency (EMEA), and the Japanese Agency for Pharmaceutical and Medical Devices Agency (PMDA), the research will not leave the laboratory.

4. Disadvantages of using graphene platforms

Drug delivery through nanocarriers has been used successfully in recent years; however, there are still certain challenges that must be addressed to achieve successful drug delivery to target sites. Each of these nanocarrier drug systems has its own chemical, physical and morphological characteristics, and may have an affinity for the different polarities of drugs through chemical or physical interactions, in addition to its own toxicity [119–123]. One of the goals of using GQDs platforms is to transport and deliver ligands to specific tumor targets and improve antitumor therapy by taking advantage of the supposedly low toxicity of this nanomaterial. However, and as was discussed above, one of the main problems with GQDs and GQD platforms is the lack of toxicological studies that effectively demonstrate their safety and biocompatibility. We have nothing to indicate that they have low toxicity, if there is no evidence to prove this. Additionally, there are several issues inherent to GQDs, the therapeutic targets to be reached and the drugs to be delivered that we must take into consideration.

One of the main problems with small nanomaterials, including GQDs, is the tendency toward aggregation. The lack of dispersion of a nanomaterial can result in transportation problems through the blood, the binding to the plasma protein corona, and the deposition of QDs in biological fluids and tissues [124]. Due to their size, they can go undetected by the immune system and, if they are not biocompatible, could induce toxicity. The dispersion of these QDs has been achieved with the use of some polymers. However, this can sometimes make the QDs larger and thus recognizable by the immune system [125]. Covalent functionalization of GQDs platforms is easy and simple, given their properties and the high surface area for their functionalization. On the other hand, the binding of non-covalent GQDs is more complicated and unstable and can lead to loss of important functional groups that can, in turn, lead to loss of electronic properties. It is also possible to obtain a wide area of functionalization [126] but the presence of a large, functionalized surface area can have adverse consequences, especially if it is a biologically active ligand that can impact cellular physiological processes. There are currently no studies on real-time monitoring and distribution of GQDs in animal models, so the effect of these platforms remains unknown.

If we want to direct GQD platforms toward specific tumor targets, we must know the molecular biology of the tumor. That is, where they need to be directed and with what do we intend them to interact. To achieve this, we require platforms that can specifically locate and access the tumor and not reach healthy tissue. Unfortunately, as we saw in the previous section, very few of the studies on animal models provide any information on this, since the studies only focus on the effects of GQD platforms at the tumor site but do not mention whether neighboring or distant tissues were affected, if systemic toxic effects were observed, or if there was mortality. The great disadvantage of most nanomaterial platforms, including GQDs, animal models have not yielded enough information about them. All nanomaterials are widely known to be cytotoxic, and so not a single one has been identified as harmless. Therefore, it is important that we obtain detailed information regarding the effects they produce *in vivo*. Additionally, we must remember that inter-individual biological variability is considerable, and it is not always possible to extrapolate data obtained directly from experimental animals to human beings.

Furthermore, all drugs used in clinical oncology are in themselves toxic and produce a variety of adverse effects. While GQD platforms have been used to target specific cells and molecules, most of the studies have been carried out using cells cultured *in vitro*, where the conditions and cellular response are more controlled. Also, only tumor cell lines have been used. There are currently no studies using cell lines from healthy tissue to determine the effect GQDs platforms may have on healthy tissue, either that adjacent to the tumor or healthy cells at a distance. The response of the tumor cell can vary greatly, as well as sensitivity to the GQDs platform and to the delivered drug. One of the big problems when extrapolating these findings to animal models is the dosage and exposure time, since we need to consider the different compartments where the platform will be distributed and the nanomaterial that will be lost during the ADME processes. Another important problem is the scaling of the product: it is not the same to produce the amounts to be used in *in vitro* models, than those needed to treat a laboratory animal, which is generally more complex and expensive. One of the characteristics of GQDs platforms is their large surface area for drug loading. However, more than an advantage, this can have adverse consequences given the large amounts of a certain drug that will be delivered to the cells. One of the great problems of nanobiotechnology is that it has not been possible to determine the exact amount of drug that can be attached to the QDs, nor how much of this actually reaches the target site. We could say that GQDs platforms have a great advantage insofar as they could have high therapeutic efficacy, but what about safety and specificity? Are they so efficient that they will only target tumor tissue? During the ADME processes, will they not affect other healthy tissues? At most, only five drugs have been used in the production of antitumor drug delivery platforms. Why? Can they not be viably employed with any type of antitumor drug? There are still questions that need to be clarified. If this information is not available, the lack of answers will remain one of the main limitations to these platforms vis-à-vis other nanomaterials.

5. Conclusions and future perspectives

GQDs hold great promise as a platform for multifunctional drug/gene delivery as well as an excellent tool for quality bioimaging. Current studies of drug delivery systems based on nanotechnology are expected to facilitate advanced forms of this kind of delivery. However, they are currently limited by the lack of preclinical pharmacological and toxicological studies, and their unknown biosafety and biocompatibility. A detailed understanding of how GQDs interact with blood components, the immune system, and aspects related to ADME processes is of vital importance. If the regulatory requirements requested by pharmacovigilance agencies are not addressed and resolved, the biotechnological and biomedical potential of GQDs cannot be employed in clinical studies. There is no doubt that, in the past decade, there have been great advances in drug delivery methods. GQD platforms have advantages over other platforms, including their surface area, size variability, their ability to functionalize with different ligands, and their photothermal and photodynamic properties. All these features make these platforms into ideal tools, not only as intelligent and multifunctional platforms for cancer therapy but also to monitor drug delivery and therapeutic effectiveness via their fluorescent emission. All these qualities could open up new pathways toward improved technological knowledge on nanoparticle-based therapies, particularly those aimed at a variety of cancers currently affecting the human population.

Acknowledgements

This work was supported by the Universidad Nacional Autónoma de México (UNAM) project DGAPA-PAPIIT-IG100920; as well as by the Consejo Nacional de Ciencia y Tecnología (CONACYT) México through grant FORDECYT-PRONACES No. Project 74884.

Conflict of interest

The authors declare no conflict of interest.

Author details

Juan Pablo González-Castillo, Esdras Alfredo Zamora-Morán
and Lourdes Rodriguez-Fragoso*
Facultad de Farmacia, Universidad Autónoma del Estado de Morelos, Cuernavaca,
Mexico

*Address all correspondence to: mrodriguezf@uaem.mx

References

[1] Masara B, van der Poll JA, Maaza M. A nanotechnology-foresight perspective of South Africa. Journal of Nanoparticle Research. 2021;**23**(4):92. DOI: 10.1007/s11051-021-05193-6

[2] Darrow JJ, Avorn J, Kesselheim AS. The FDA breakthrough-drug designation—four years of experience. New England Journal of Medicine. 2018;**378**(15):1444-1453. DOI: 10.1056/nejmhpr1713338

[3] Beaudrie CEH, Satterfield T, Kandlikar M, Harthorn BH. Expert views on regulatory preparedness for managing the risks of nanotechnologies. PLoS One. 2013;**8**(11):e80250. DOI: 10.1371/journal.pone.0080250

[4] Bayda S, Adeel M, Tuccinardi T, Cordani M, Rizzolio F. The history of nanoscience and nanotechnology: From chemical–physical applications to nanomedicine. Molecules. 2019;**25**(1):112. DOI: 10.3390/molecules25010112

[5] Shafique M, Luo X. Nanotechnology in transportation vehicles: An overview of its applications, environmental, health and safety concerns. Materials. 2019;**12**(15):2493. DOI: 10.3390/ma12152493

[6] Magro M, Venerando A, Macone A, Canettieri G, Agostinelli E, Vianello F. Nanotechnology-based strategies to develop new anticancer therapies. Biomolecules. 2020;**10**(5):735. DOI: 10.3390/biom10050735

[7] Mohd Nurazzi N, Asyraf MRM, Khalina A, et al. Fabrication, functionalization, and application of carbon nanotube-reinforced polymer composite: An overview. Polymers. 2021;**13**(7):1047. DOI: 10.3390/polym13071047

[8] Fusco L, Gazzi A, Peng G, et al. Graphene and other 2D materials: A multidisciplinary analysis to uncover the hidden potential as cancer theranostics. Theranostics. 2020;**10**(12):5435-5488. DOI: 10.7150/thno.40068

[9] Dasari Shareena TP, McShan D, Dasmahapatra AK, Tchounwou PB. A review on graphene-based nanomaterials in biomedical applications and risks in environment and health. Nano-Micro Letters. 2018;**10**(3):53. DOI: 10.1007/s40820-018-0206-4

[10] Bai Y, Xu T, Zhang X. Graphene-based biosensors for detection of biomarkers. Micromachines (Basel). 2020;**11**(1):60. DOI: 10.3390/mi11010060

[11] Wang J, Li Y, Nie G. Multifunctional biomolecule nanostructures for cancer therapy. Nature Reviews Materials. 2021;**6**(9):766-783. DOI: 10.1038/s41578-021-00315-x

[12] Zhang J, Lan T, Lu Y. Molecular engineering of functional nucleic acid nanomaterials toward in vivo applications. Advanced Healthcare Materials. 2019;**8**(6):1801158. DOI: 10.1002/adhm.201801158

[13] RDuangrat R, Udomprasert A, Kangsamaksin T. Tetrahedral DNA nanostructures as drug delivery and bioimaging platforms in cancer therapy. Cancer Science. 2020;**111**(9):3164-3173. DOI: 10.1111/cas.14548

[14] Huang Y-P, Hung C-M, Hsu Y-C, et al. Suppression of breast cancer cell migration by small interfering rna delivered by polyethylenimine-functionalized graphene oxide. Nanoscale Research Letters. 2016;**11**(1):247. DOI: 10.1186/s11671-016-1463-0

[15] Imani R, Shao W, Taherkhani S, Emami SH, Prakash S, Faghihi S. Dual-functionalized graphene oxide for enhanced siRNA delivery to breast cancer cells. Colloids and Surfaces B: Biointerfaces. 2016;**147**:315-325. DOI: 10.1016/j.colsurfb.2016.08.015

[16] Liyanage PY, Hettiarachchi SD, Zhou Y, et al. Nanoparticle-mediated targeted drug delivery for breast cancer treatment. Biochimica Et Biophysica Acta. Reviews on Cancer. 2019;**1871**(2):419-433. DOI: 10.1016/j.bbcan.2019.04.006

[17] Assali A, Akhavan O, Mottaghitalab F, et al. Cationic graphene oxide nanoplatform mediates miR-101 delivery to promote apoptosis by regulating autophagy and stress. International Journal of Nanomedicine. 2018;**13**:5865-5886. DOI: 10.2147/ijn.s162647

[18] Cheang T-Y, Lei Y-Y, Zhang Z-Q, et al. Graphene oxide–hydroxyapatite nanocomposites effectively deliver HSV-TK suicide gene to inhibit human breast cancer growth. Journal of Biomaterials Applications. 2018;**33**(2):216-226. DOI: 10.1177/0885328218788242

[19] Luo C, Li Y, Guo L, et al. Graphene quantum dots downregulate multiple multidrug-resistant genes via interacting with their C-rich promoters. Advanced Helthcare Materials. 2017;**6**(21):1700328. DOI: 10.1002/adhm.201700328

[20] Liu Y, Zhao C, Sabirsh A, et al. A novel graphene quantum dot-based mrna delivery platform. ChemistryOpen. 2021;**10**(7):666-671. DOI: 10.1002/open.202000200

[21] Dong H, Dai W, Ju H, et al. Multifunctional poly(l-lactide)–polyethylene glycol-grafted graphene quantum dots for intracellular microRNA imaging and combined specific-gene-targeting agents delivery for improved therapeutics. ACS Applied Materials & Interfaces. 2015;7(20):11015-11023. DOI: 10.1021/acsami.5b02803

[22] Felix DM, Rebelo Alencar LM, Duarte de Menezes F, et al. Graphene quantum dots decorated with imatinib for leukemia treatment. Journal of Drug Delivery Science and Technology. 2021;**61**:102117. DOI: 10.1016/j.jddst.2020.102117

[23] Tian Z, Yao X, Ma K, et al. Metal-organic framework/graphene quantum dot nanoparticles used for synergistic chemo- and photothermal therapy. ACS Omega. 2017;**2**(3):1249-1258. DOI: 10.1021/acsomega.6b00385

[24] Bukowski K, Kciuk M, Kontek R. Mechanisms of multidrug resistance in cancer chemotherapy. International Journal of Molecular Sciences. 2020;**21**(9):3233. DOI: 10.3390/ijms21093233

[25] Ruan J, Wang Y, Li F, et al. Graphene quantum dots for radiotherapy. ACS Applied Materials & Interfaces. 2018;**10**(17):14342-14355. DOI: 10.1021/acsami.7b18975

[26] Zhang X, Li H, Yi C, et al. Host immune response triggered by graphene quantum-dot-mediated photodynamic therapy for oral squamous cell carcinoma. International Journal of Nanomedicine. 2020;**15**:9627-9638. DOI: 10.2147/IJN.S276153

[27] Iannazzo D, Pistone A, Salamò M, et al. Graphene quantum dots for cancer targeted drug delivery. International Journal of Pharmaceutics. 2017;**518**(1-2):185-192. DOI: 10.1016/j.ijpharm.2016.12.060

[28] Sinha R, Purkayastha P. Daunomycin delivery by ultrasmall graphene quantum dots to DNA duplexes: Understanding the dynamics by resonance energy transfer. Journal of Materials Chemistry B. 2020;**8**(42):9756-9763. DOI: 10.1039/d0tb01831g

[29] Ko NR, Nafiujjaman M, Lee JS, Lim H-N, Lee Y, Kwon IK. Graphene quantum dot-based theranostic agents for active targeting of breast cancer. RSC Advances. 2017;7(19):11420-11427. DOI: 10.1039/c6ra25949a

[30] Zhu X, Zhang H, Huang H, Zhang Y, Hou L, Zhang Z. Functionalized graphene oxide-based thermosensitive hydrogel for magnetic hyperthermia therapy on tumors. Nanotechnology. 2015;**26**(36):365103. DOI: 10.1088/0957-4484/26/36/365103

[31] Liu X, Yan B, Li Y, et al. Graphene oxide-grafted magnetic nanorings mediated magnetothermodynamic therapy favoring reactive oxygen species-related immune response for enhanced antitumor efficacy. ACS Nano. 2020;**14**(2):1936-1950. DOI: 10.1021/acsnano.9b08320

[32] Gazzi A, Fusco L, Khan A, et al. Photodynamic therapy based on graphene and MXene in cancer theranostics. Frontiers in Bioengineering and Biotechnology. 2019;**7**:295. DOI: 10.3389/fbioe.2019.00295

[33] Wu C, Tian Y, Zhang Y, et al. Acid-triggered charge-convertible graphene-based all-in-one nanocomplex for enhanced genetic phototherapy of triple-negative breast cancer. Advanced Healthcare Materials. 2020;**9**(1):e1901187. DOI: 10.1002/adhm.201901187

[34] De Sanctis A, Mehew J, Craciun M, Russo S. Graphene-based light sensing: Fabrication, characterisation, physical properties and performance. Materials (Basel). 2018;**11**(9):1762. DOI: 10.3390/ma11091762

[35] Mansuriya B, Altintas Z. Applications of graphene quantum dots in biomedical sensors. Sensors. 2020;**20**(4):1072. DOI: 10.3390/s20041072

[36] Speranza G. Carbon nanomaterials: Synthesis, functionalization and sensing applications. Nanomaterials. 2021;**11**(4):967. DOI: 10.3390/nano11040967

[37] Younis MR, He G, Lin J, Huang P. Recent advances on graphene quantum dots for bioimaging applications. Frontiers in Chemistry. 2020;**8**:1-25. DOI: 10.3389/fchem.2020.00424

[38] Suvarnaphaet P, Pechprasarn S. Graphene-based materials for biosensors: A review. Sensors. 2017;**17**(10):2161. DOI: 10.3390/s17102161

[39] Zhao C, Song X, Liu Y, et al. Synthesis of graphene quantum dots and their applications in drug delivery. Journal of Nanobiotechnology. 2020;**18**(1):142. DOI: 10.1186/s12951-020-00698-z

[40] Gore L, DeGregori J, Porter CC. Targeting developmental pathways in children with cancer: What price success? The Lancet Oncology. 2013;**14**(2):e70-e78. DOI: 10.1016/s1470-2045(12)70530-2

[41] Cekanova M, Rathore K. Animal models and therapeutic molecular targets of cancer: Utility and limitations. Drug Design, Development and Therapy. 2014;**8**:1911-1921. DOI: 10.2147/DDDT.S49584

[42] Iannazzo D, Celesti C, Espro C. Recent advances on graphene quantum

dots as multifunctional nanoplatforms for cancer treatment. Biotechnology Journal. 2020;**16**(2):1900422. DOI: 10.1002/biot.201900422

[43] Sang M, Shin J, Kim K, Yu K. Electronic and thermal properties of graphene and recent advances in graphene based electronics applications. Nanomaterials. 2019;**9**(3):374. DOI: 10.3390/nano9030374

[44] Assali A, Akhavan O, Adeli M, et al. Multifunctional core-shell nanoplatforms (gold@graphene oxide) with mediated NIR thermal therapy to promote miRNA delivery. Nanomedicine: Nanotechnology, Biology and Medicine. 2018;**14**(6):1891-1903. DOI: 10.1016/j.nano.2018.05.016

[45] Agostinis P, Berg K, Cengel KA, et al. Photodynamic therapy of cancer: An update. CA: A Cancer Journal for Clinicians. 2011;**61**(4):250-281. DOI: 10.3322/caac.20114

[46] de Melo-Diogo D, Costa EC, Alves CG, et al. POxylated graphene oxide nanomaterials for combination chemo-phototherapy of breast cancer cells. European Journal of Pharmaceutics and Biopharmaceutics. 2018;**131**:162-169. DOI: 10.1016/j.ejpb.2018.08.008

[47] Zhi F, Dong H, Jia X, et al. Functionalized graphene oxide mediated adriamycin delivery and miR-21 gene silencing to overcome tumor multidrug resistance in vitro. PLoS One. 2013;**8**(3):e60034. DOI: 10.1371/journal.pone.0060034

[48] Tran TH, Nguyen HT, Pham TT, et al. Development of a graphene oxide nanocarrier for dual-drug chemo-phototherapy to overcome drug resistance in cancer. ACS Applied Materials & Interfaces. 2015;7(51):28647-28655. DOI: 10.1021/acsami.5b10426

[49] Yong Y, Zhang C, Gu Z, et al. Polyoxometalate-based radiosensitization platform for treating hypoxic tumors by attenuating radioresistance and enhancing radiation response. ACS Nano. 2017;**11**(7):7164-7176. DOI: 10.1021/acsnano.7b03037

[50] Wagner AM, Knipe JM, Orive G, Peppas NA. Quantum dots in biomedical applications. Acta Biomaterialia. 2019;**94**:44-63. DOI: 10.1016/j.actbio.2019.05.022

[51] Gu H, Tang H, Xiong P, Zhou Z. Biomarkers-based biosensing and bioimaging with graphene for cancer diagnosis. Nanomaterials. 2019;**9**(1):130. DOI: 10.3390/nano9010130

[52] Menaa F, Fatemeh Y, Vashist SK, Iqbal H, Sharts ON, Menaa B. Graphene, an interesting nanocarbon allotrope for biosensing applications: Advances, insights, and prospects. Biomedical Engineering and Computational Biology. 2021;**12**:117959722098382. DOI: 10.1177/1179597220983821

[53] Ding H, Zhang F, Zhao C, et al. Beyond a carrier: Graphene quantum dots as a probe for programmatically monitoring anti-cancer drug delivery, release, and response. ACS Applied Materials & Interfaces. 2017;**9**(33):27396-27401. DOI: 10.1021/acsami.7b08824

[54] Wang X, Sun X, He H, et al. A two-component active targeting theranostic agent based on graphene quantum dots. Journal of Materials Chemistry B. 2015;**3**(17):3583-3590. DOI: 10.1039/c5tb00211g

[55] Tandale P, Choudhary N, Singh J, et al. Fluorescent quantum dots: An insight on synthesis and potential biological application as drug carrier in cancer. Biochemistry and Biophysics

Reports. 2021;**26**:100962. DOI: 10.1016/j.bbrep.2021.100962

[56] Ge J, Lan M, Zhou B, et al. A graphene quantum dot photodynamic therapy agent with high singlet oxygen generation. Nature Communications. 2014;**5**:4596. DOI: 10.1038/ncomms5596

[57] Justin R, Tao K, Román S, et al. Photoluminescent and superparamagnetic reduced graphene oxide–iron oxide quantum dots for dual-modality imaging, drug delivery and photothermal therapy. Carbon. 2016;**97**:54-70. DOI: 10.1016/j.carbon.2015.06.070

[58] Cao Y, Dong H, Yang Z, et al. Aptamer-conjugated graphene quantum dots/porphyrin derivative theranostic agent for intracellular cancer-related microRNA detection and fluorescence-guided photothermal/photodynamic synergetic therapy. ACS Applied Materials & Interfaces. 2017;**9**(1):159-166. DOI: 10.1021/acsami.6b13150

[59] Zhou L, Zhou L, Ge X, Zhou J, Wei S, Shen J. Multicolor imaging and the anticancer effect of a bifunctional silica nanosystem based on the complex of graphene quantum dots and hypocrellin A. Chemical Communications (Cambridge). 2015;**51**(2):421-424. DOI: 10.1039/c4cc06968d

[60] Davies AE, Albeck JG. Microenvironmental signals and biochemical information processing: Cooperative determinants of intratumoral plasticity and heterogeneity. Frontiers in Cell and Development Biology. 2018;**6**:44. DOI: 10.3389/fcell.2018.00044

[61] Sun Y, Li Y, Shi S, Dong C. Exploiting a new approach to destroy the barrier of tumor microenvironment: Nano-architecture delivery systems. Molecules. 2021;**26**(9):2703. DOI: 10.3390/molecules26092703

[62] Wang F, Xiao J, Chen S, et al. Polymer vesicles: Modular platforms for cancer theranostics. Advanced Materials. 2018;**30**(17):e1705674. DOI: 10.1002/adma.201705674

[63] Gu Z, Zhu S, Yan L, Zhao F, Zhao Y. Graphene-based smart platforms for combined cancer therapy. Advanced Materials. 2019;**31**(9):e1800662. DOI: 10.1002/adma.201800662

[64] He X, Li J, An S, Jiang C. pH-sensitive drug-delivery systems for tumor targeting. Therapeutic Delivery. 2013;**4**(12):1499-1510. DOI: 10.4155/tde.13.120

[65] Liu J, Huang Y, Kumar A, et al. pH-sensitive nano-systems for drug delivery in cancer therapy. Biotechnology Advances. 2014;**32**(4):693-710. DOI: 10.1016/j.biotechadv.2013.11.009

[66] Tu Z, Achazi K, Schulz A, et al. Combination of surface charge and size controls the cellular uptake of functionalized graphene sheets. Advanced Functional Materials. 2017;**27**(33):1701837. DOI: 10.1002/adfm.201701837

[67] Karimi S, Namazi H. Simple preparation of maltose-functionalized dendrimer/graphene quantum dots as a pH-sensitive biocompatible carrier for targeted delivery of doxorubicin. International Journal of Biological Macromolecules. 2020;**156**:648-659. DOI: 10.1016/j.ijbiomac.2020.04.037

[68] Frieler M, Pho C, Lee BH, Dobrovolny H, Akkaraju GR, Naumov AV. Effects of doxorubicin delivery by nitrogen-doped graphene quantum dots on cancer cell growth: Experimental study and mathematical

modeling. Nanomaterials (Basel). 2021;**11**(1):140. DOI: 10.3390/nano11010140

[69] Mi P. Stimuli-responsive nanocarriers for drug delivery, tumor imaging, therapy and theranostics. Theranostics. 2020;**10**(10):4557-4588. DOI: 10.7150/thno.38069

[70] Karabasz A, Bzowska M, Szczepanowicz K. Biomedical applications of multifunctional polymeric nanocarriers: A review of current literature. International Journal of Nanomedicine. 2020;**15**:8673-8696. DOI: 10.2147/ijn.s231477

[71] Su S, Kang PM. Recent advances in nanocarrier-assisted therapeutics delivery systems. Pharmaceutics. 2020;**12**(9):837. DOI: 10.3390/pharmaceutics12090837

[72] Zeb A, Rana I, Choi H-I, et al. Potential and applications of nanocarriers for efficient delivery of biopharmaceuticals. Pharmaceutics. 2020;**12**(12):1184. DOI: 10.3390/pharmaceutics12121184

[73] Li SD, Huang L. Stealth nanoparticles: High density but sheddable peg is a key for tumor targeting. Journal of Controlled Release. 2010;**145**:178-181. DOI: 10.1016/j.jconrel.2010.03.016

[74] Georgakilas V, Otyepka M, Bourlinos AB, et al. Functionalization of graphene: Covalent and non-covalent approaches, derivatives and applications. Chemical Reviews. 2012;**112**:6156-6214. DOI: 10.1021/cr3000412

[75] Younis MR, He G, Lin J, Huang P. Recent advances on graphene quantum dots for bioimaging applications. Frontiers in Chemistry. 2020;**8**:424. DOI: 10.3389/fchem.2020.00424

[76] Magne TM, de Oliveira VT, Alencar LMR, et al. Graphene and its derivatives: Understanding the main chemical and medicinal chemistry roles for biomedical applications. Journal of Nanostructure in Chemistry. 2021:1-35. DOI: 10.1007/s40097-021-00444-3

[77] Danial WH, Md Bahri NF, Abdul MZ. Preparation, marriage chemistry and applications of graphene quantum dots–nanocellulose composite: A brief review. Molecules. 2021;**26**(20):6158. DOI: 10.3390/molecules26206158

[78] Wang Y, Tang M. Dysfunction of various organelles provokes multiple cell death after quantum dot exposure. International Journal of Nanomedicine. 2018;**13**:2729-2742. DOI: 10.2147/IJN.S157135

[79] Malhotra N, Villaflores OB, Audira G, et al. Toxicity studies on graphene-based nanomaterials in aquatic organisms: Current understanding. Molecules. 2020;**25**(16):3618. DOI: 10.3390/molecules25163618

[80] Fasbender S, Allani S, Wimmenauer C, et al. Uptake dynamics of graphene quantum dots into primary human blood cells following in vitro exposure. RSC Advances. 2017;**7**(20):12208-12216. DOI: 10.1039/c6ra27829a

[81] Nurunnabi M, Khatun Z, Huh KM, et al. In vivo biodistribution and toxicology of carboxylated graphene quantum dots. ACS Nano. 2013;**7**(8):6858-6867. DOI: 10.1021/nn402043c

[82] Qiu J, Li D, Mou X, et al. Effects of graphene quantum dots on the self-renewal and differentiation of mesenchymal stem cells. Advanced Healthcare Materials. 2016;**5**(6):702-710. DOI: 10.1002/adhm.201500770

[83] Xie Y, Wan B, Yang Y, Cui X, Xin Y, Guo L-H. Cytotoxicity and autophagy induction by graphene quantum dots with different functional groups. Journal of Environmental Sciences. 2019;**77**:198-209. DOI: 10.1016/j.jes.2018.07.014

[84] Xiaoli F, Yaqing Z, Ruhui L, et al. Graphene oxide disrupted mitochondrial homeostasis through inducing intracellular redox deviation and autophagy-lysosomal network dysfunction in SH-SY5Y cells. Journal of Hazardous Materials. 2021;**416**:126158. DOI: 10.1016/j.jhazmat.2021.126158

[85] Barrios AC, Wang Y, Gilbertson LM, Perreault F. Structure–property–toxicity relationships of graphene oxide: Role of surface chemistry on the mechanisms of interaction with bacteria. Environmental Science & Technology. 2019;**53**(24):14679-14687. DOI: 10.1021/acs.est.9b05057

[86] Li R, Guiney LM, Chang CH, et al. Surface oxidation of graphene oxide determines membrane damage, lipid peroxidation, and cytotoxicity in macrophages in a pulmonary toxicity model. ACS Nano. 2018;**12**(2):1390-1402. DOI: 10.1021/acsnano.7b07737

[87] Xiaoli F, Qiyue C, Weihong G, et al. Toxicology data of graphene-family nanomaterials: An update. Archives of Toxicology. 2020;**94**(6):1915-1939. DOI: 10.1007/s00204-020-02717-2

[88] Sun Y, Dai H, Chen S, et al. Graphene oxide regulates cox2 in human embryonic kidney 293T cells via epigenetic mechanisms: Dynamic chromosomal interactions. Nanotoxicology. 2018;**12**(2):117-137. DOI: 10.1080/17435390.2018.1425498

[89] Piperno A, Scala A, Mazzaglia A, et al. Cellular signaling pathways activated by functional graphene nanomaterials. International Journal of Molecular Sciences. 2018;**19**(11):3365. DOI: 10.3390/ijms19113365

[90] Ji Y, Li Y-M, Seo JG, et al. Biological potential of polyethylene glycol (PEG)-functionalized graphene quantum dots in in vitro neural stem/progenitor cells. Nanomaterials. 2021;**11**(6):1446. DOI: 10.3390/nano11061446

[91] Jiang D, Chen Y, Li N, et al. Synthesis of luminescent graphene quantum dots with high quantum yield and their toxicity study. PLoS One. 2015;**10**(12):e0144906. DOI: 10.1371/journal.pone.0144906

[92] Chong Y, Ma Y, Shen H, et al. The in vitro and in vivo toxicity of graphene quantum dots. Biomaterials. 2014;**35**(19):5041-5048. DOI: 10.1016/j.biomaterials.2014.03.021

[93] Yuan X, Liu Z, Guo Z, Ji Y, Jin M, Wang X. Cellular distribution and cytotoxicity of graphene quantum dots with different functional groups. Nanoscale Research Letters. 2014;**9**(1):108. DOI: 10.1186/1556-276x-9-108

[94] Mu Q, Su G, Li L, et al. Size-dependent cell uptake of protein-coated graphene oxide nanosheets. ACS Applied Materials & Interfaces. 2012;**4**(4):2259-2266. DOI: 10.1021/am300253c

[95] Wang XY, Lei R, Huang HD, et al. The permeability and transport mechanism of gaphene quantum dots (GQDs) across the biological barrier. Nanoscale. 2015;7(5):2034-2041. DOI: 10.1039/c4nr04136d

[96] Xu L, Dai Y, Wang Z, et al. Graphene quantum dots in alveolar macrophage: Uptake-exocytosis, accumulation in nuclei, nuclear responses and DNA cleavage. Particle and Fibre

Toxicology. 2018;**15**(1):45. DOI: 10.1186/s12989-018-0279-8

[97] Lalwani G, D'Agati M, Khan AM, Sitharaman B. Toxicology of graphene-based nanomaterials. Advanced Drug Delivery Reviews. 2016;**105**(Pt B):109-144. DOI: 10.1016/j.addr.2016.04.028

[98] Zheng W, Wei M, Li S, Le W. Nanomaterial-modulated autophagy: Underlying mechanisms and functional consequences. Nanomedicine (London, England). 2016;**11**(11):1417-1430. DOI: 10.2217/nnm-2016-0040

[99] Ji X, Xu B, Yao M, et al. Graphene oxide quantum dots disrupt autophagic flux by inhibiting lysosome activity in GC-2 and TM4 cell lines. Toxicology. 2016;**374**:10-17. DOI: 10.1016/j.tox.2016.11.009

[100] Tian X, Yang Z, Duan G, et al. Graphene oxide nanosheets retard cellular migration via disruption of actin cytoskeleton. Small. 2017;**13**(3):10-11. DOI: 10.1002/smll.201602133

[101] Wu K, Zhou Q, Ouyang S. Direct and indirect genotoxicity of graphene family nanomaterials on DNA—a review. Nanomaterials. 2021;**11**(11):2889. DOI: 10.3390/nano11112889

[102] Xu H, Wang X, Zhang X, et al. A deep learning analysis reveals nitrogen-doped graphene quantum dots damage neurons of nematode *Caenorhabditis elegans*. Nanomaterials. 2021;**11**(12):3314. DOI: 10.3390/nano11123314

[103] Roy P, Periasamy AP, Lin CY, et al. Photoluminescent graphene quantum dots for in vivo imaging of apoptotic cells. Nanoscale. 2015;7(6):2504-2510. DOI: 10.1039/c4nr07005d

[104] Jeong J, Cho H-J, Choi M, Lee WS, Chung BH, Lee J-S. In vivo toxicity asessment of angiogenesis and the live distribution of nano-graphene oxide and its PEGylated derivatives using the developing zebrafish embryo. Carbon. 2015;**93**:431-440. DOI: 10.1016/j.carbon.2015.05.024

[105] Zhu Z, Qian J, Zhao X, et al. Stable and size-tunable aggregation-induced emission nanoparticles encapsulated with nanographene oxide and applications in three-photon fluorescence bioimaging. ACS Nano. 2016;**10**(1):588-597. DOI: 10.1021/acsnano.5b05606

[106] Wang ZG, Zhou R, Jiang D, et al. Toxicity of graphene quantum dots in zebrafish embryo. Biomedical and Environmental Sciences. 2015;**28**(5):341-351. DOI: 10.3967/bes2015.048

[107] Zhang JH, Sun T, Niu A, et al. Perturbation effect of reduced graphene oxide quantum dots (rGOQDs) on aryl hydrocarbon receptor (AhR) pathway in zebrafish. Biomaterials. 2017;**133**:49-59. DOI: 10.1016/j.biomaterials.2017.04.026

[108] Lu K, Dong S, Petersen EJ, et al. Biological uptake, distribution, and depuration of radio-labeled graphene in adult zebrafish: Effects of graphene size and natural organic matter. ACS Nano. 2017;**11**(3):2872-2885. DOI: 10.1021/acsnano.6b07982

[109] Manjunatha B, Park SH, Kim K, Kundapur RR, Lee SJ. In vivo toxicity evaluation of pristine graphene in developing zebrafish (*Danio rerio*) embryos. Environmental Science and Pollution Research. 2018;**25**(13):12821-12829. DOI: 10.1007/s11356-018-1420-9

[110] Dasmahapatra AK, Dasari TPS, Tchounwou PB. Graphene-based nanomaterials toxicity in fish. Reviews of Environmental Contamination and Toxicology. 2019;**247**:1-58. DOI: 10.1007/398_2018_15

[111] Kurantowicz N, Sawosz E, Halik G, et al. Toxicity studies of six types of carbon nanoparticles in a chicken-embryo model. International Journal of Nanomedicine. 2017;**12**:2887-2898. DOI: 10.2147/ijn.s131960

[112] Jaworski S, Hinzmann M, Sawosz E, et al. Interaction of different forms of graphene with chicken embryo red blood cells. Environmental Science and Pollution Research. 2017;**24**(27):21671-21679. DOI: 10.1007/s11356-017-9788-5

[113] Sawosz E, Jaworski S, Kutwin M, et al. Toxicity of pristine graphene in experiments in a chicken embryo model. International Journal of Nanomedicine. 2014;**9**:3913-3922. DOI: 10.2147/IJN.S65633

[114] Li J, Zhang X, Jiang J, et al. Systematic assessment of the toxicity and potential mechanism of graphene derivatives in vitro and in vivo. Toxicological Sciences. 2019;**167**(1):269-281. DOI: 10.1093/toxsci/kfy235

[115] Tabish TA, Lin L, Ali M, et al. Investigating the bioavailability of graphene quantum dots in lung tissues via Fourier transform infrared spectroscopy. Interface Focus. 2018;**8**(3):20170054. DOI: 10.1098/rsfs.2017.0054

[116] Tabish TA, Scotton CJ, Ferguson DCJ, et al. Biocompatibility and toxicity of graphene quantum dots for potential application in photodynamic therapy. Nanomedicine. 2018;**13**(15):1923-1937. DOI: 10.2217/nnm-2018-0018

[117] Ema M, Gamo M, Honda K. A review of toxicity studies on graphene-based nanomaterials in laboratory animals. Regulatory Toxicology and Pharmacology. 2017;**85**:7-24. DOI: 10.1016/j.yrtph.2017.01.011

[118] Mao L, Hu M, Pan B, Xie Y, Petersen EJ. Biodistribution and toxicity of radio-labeled few layer graphene in mice after intratracheal instillation. Particle and Fibre Toxicology. 2016;**13**:7. DOI: 10.1186/s12989-016-0120-1

[119] Kim JK, Shin JH, Lee JS, et al. 28-Day inhalation toxicity of graphene nanoplatelets in Sprague-Dawley rats. Nanotoxicology. 2016;**10**(7):891-901. DOI: 10.3109/17435390.2015.1133865

[120] Patlolla AK, Randolph J, Kumari SA, Tchounwou PB. Toxicity evaluation of graphene oxide in kidneys of Sprague-Dawley rats. International Journal of Environmental Research and Public Health. 2016;**13**(4):380. DOI: 10.3390/ijerph13040380

[121] Liu Y, Luo Y, Wu J, et al. Graphene oxide can induce in vitro and in vivo mutagenesis. Scientific Reports. 2013;**3**:3469. DOI: 10.1038/srep03469

[122] Kurantowicz N, Strojny B, Sawosz E, et al. Biodistribution of a high dose of diamond, graphite, and graphene oxide nanoparticles after multiple intraperitoneal injections in rats. Nanoscale Research Letters. 2015;**10**(1):398. DOI: 10.1186/s11671-015-1107-9

[123] Xu S, Zhang Z, Chu M. Long-term toxicity of reduced graphene oxide nanosheets: Effects on female mouse reproductive ability and offspring development. Biomaterials. 2015;**54**:188-200. DOI: 10.1016/j.biomaterials.2015.03.015

[124] Pelin M, Sosa S, Prato M, Tubaro A. Occupational exposure to graphene-based nanomaterials: Risk assessment. Nanoscale. 2018;**10**(34):15894-15903. DOI: 10.1039/c8nr04950e

[125] Arvidsson R, Molander S, Sandén B. Review of potential environmental

and health risks of the nanomaterial graphene. Human and Ecological Risk Assessment: An International Journal. 2013;**19**(4):873-887. DOI: 10.1080/10807039.2012.702039

[126] Fadeel B, Bussy C, Merino S, et al. Safety assessment of graphene-based materials: Focus on human health and the environment. ACS Nano. 2018;**12**(11):10582-10620. DOI: 10.1021/acsnano.8b04758

Section 2

Nanocarriers

Chapter 6

A Microfluidic Device as a Drug Carrier

Fikadu Ejeta

Abstract

The development of nanomedicine or medical nanotechnology, has brought important new ways to the development of medicines and biotechnology products. As a result of groundbreaking discoveries in the use of nanoscale materials significant commercialization initiatives have been launched and are at the forefront of the rapidly expanding field of nanotechnology by using smart particles. Microfluidic technologies use nano-and micro-scale manufacturing technologies to develop controlled and reproducible liquid microenvironments. Lead compounds with controlled physicochemical properties can be obtained using microfluidics, characterized by high productivity, and evaluated by biomimetic methods. Microfluidics, for example, can not only produce nanoparticles in a well-controlled, reproducible, and high-throughput manner, but it can also continuously create three-dimensional environments to mimic physiological and/or pathological processes. Materials with smart properties can be manipulated to respond in a controllable and reversible way, modifying some of their properties as a result of external stimuli such as mechanical stress or a certain temperature. All in all, microfluidic technology offers a potential platform for the rapid synthesis of various novel drug delivery systems. Therefore, these smart particles are equally necessary as the drug in drug delivery.

Keywords: smart materials, nanomedicine, microfluidic devices, drug delivery, nanocarriers

1. Introduction

Nanomedicine is a branch of medicine. Its goal is to use nanotechnology—manipulation and manufacturing of materials and devices with diameters of 1–100 nanometers—to prevent diseases and imaging, diagnose, monitor, treat, repair, and regenerate biological systems [1]. The development of nanomedicine or medical nanotechnology, has brought important new ways to the development of medicines and biotechnology products [2]. As a result of groundbreaking discoveries in the use of nanoscale materials significant commercialization, initiatives have been launched and are at the forefront of the rapidly expanding field of nanotechnology [3, 4], and they are expected to overcome the continuing challenges of ineffective drug delivery systems [5].

Materials with smart properties can be manipulated to respond in a controllable and reversible way, modifying some of their properties as a result of external stimuli such as mechanical stress or a certain temperature. Because of their small size, customizable chemical surface qualities, high volume-to-surface ratio, and, fundamentally, the ability to load active medicinal components and imaging agents, nanoparticulate drug delivery has been discovered to successfully affect nanomedicine [6]. In addition, nano-drug delivery media have been proven to improve beneficial results or effects, and reduce the side effects associated with drugs that have already been approved on the market, enabling new treatment methods and inspiring further improvements in the undesirable drug properties of active biological products. Research that was previously considered undeveloped [7].

Microfluidic technologies use nano-and micro-scale manufacturing technologies to develop controlled and reproducible liquid microenvironments [8, 9]. Lead compounds with controlled physicochemical properties can be obtained using microfluidics, characterized by high productivity, and evaluated by the biomimetic method *in vitro* for a human organ on a chip [8, 10]. The microfluidic generation has become an efficient device for the manufacture of microparticles with controlled morphology and preferred properties due to its ability to precisely control the emulsification procedure and generate droplets of monodisperse compounds in microchannels [11]. Microfluidics' ability to produce double emulsions having one, two, three, or more numbers of droplets with remarkable precision displays the degree of control it provides [12]. Since the size of the particles has a substantial influence on carrier release profile [13], it's crucial to place together polymer matrix with appropriate sizes and size distributions to accurately regulate the release of payloads. The loading of medicines onto the polymeric matrix and the release of payloads can both be controlled by changing their interior structures [14]. Multiple medication delivery can be achieved by altering the size and number of interior partitions [14, 15]. Another way to control the release of the payload is to synthesize polymer fragments by using stimulus-responsive substances [16]. After the environmental triggers (including pH, temperature, or ionic strength) are disclosed, the fragments will pass through physicochemical alternatives and then release the payload [17, 18].

Microfluidic technology has advantages in terms of small particle size distribution, lower polydispersity index, higher packaging and loading efficiency, better batch-to-batch uniformity, and the possibility of easy scaling [19]. Interestingly, the preparation of microfluidic chips is simple and easy to implement, thus realizing the economical production of nanocarriers [20]. Various microfluidic chips have been manufactured to synthesize organic, inorganic, polymer, lipid-based vesicular and hybrid nanocarriers [21]. All in all, microfluidic technology offers a potential platform for the rapid synthesis of various novel drug delivery systems [22].

The manufacturing processes for polymer microparticles are becoming increasingly important for applications such as the controlled release of active ingredients, medical-diagnostic tests, the achievement of superhydrophobic surfaces, the optimal design of impact-resistant polymer composites, and food technology [23].

Polymer microparticles are produced using a variety of processes, including suspension or emulsion polymerization, solvent evaporation, spray drying, small-hole spraying of polymer solution and the Shirasu porous glass membrane (SPG) emulsification method. On the other hand, traditional manufacturing processes have several disadvantages, including the fact that they take time, cause particle coalescence, and lead to non-uniform particle sizes and shape irregularities [24]. To work around these limitations, you can use the electrospray method. Furthermore, the electrospray technique offers many benefits over earlier approaches, including minimal residue, the use of very few solvents, low cost, and the use of high molecular weight polymers [25]. The microdevices are made up of two flow-focusing pads that work together in a two-step procedure to make double emulsions. As a result, at low flow rates, the aqueous phase is symmetrically restricted at the initial connection point as a result of which monodisperse aqueous monomer plugs are formed. The oil phase encapsulates liquids 1 and 2 at the second connection point and creates double droplets of aqueous and monomeric phases. The composite droplets then reach a third junction where the channel cross-section is enlarged, whereby they assume spherical shapes. In the large section, conservation of mass forces the droplets to slow down significantly, thereby decreasing the spacing between successive droplets and thus decreasing the spacing between successive droplets, thereby decreasing the spacing between successive droplets [26].

Advances in drug delivery technology can improve pharmacological factors, including efficacy and bioavailability, to discover and develop more effective drugs to improve the treatment effects and quality of life of patients. Manufacturing quality control, fluctuations between product batches, and the inability to obtain physiologically relevant test results in traditional *in vitro* prescreening platforms are all obstacles to nanoparticle drug delivery [10]. Microfluidics has evolved from microliter fluid processing to nanoliter fluid processing, including multidisciplinary methods that can be used in a wide range of applications [27, 28]. Microfluidics (a method of fabrication) provides a mechanism for making highly controllable, reproducible, and scalable methods to produce nanoparticles. When compared to traditional *in vitro* culture methods, the organ-on-chip microfluidic technology provides highly relevant organ-specific testing platforms capable of biologically relevant experimental time scales while employing a fraction of the sample and media volumes [29, 30].

Microfluidic technologies provide low-cost, simple-to-use platforms to control the flow of fluids. Emulsions produced in microfluidic devices have been used in a variety of scientific applications, comprising biomedical field, chemical synthesis, fluid flow, and controlled drugs delivery. T-junctions and flow-focusing nozzles are two types of microfluidic platform devices that are used to make emulsions [31, 32]. Both procedures allow for the production of monodisperse particles as well as a wide range of emulsion sizes. Flow-focusing devices are commonly used to produce monodisperse polymer particles, both spherical and non-spherical. FF devices have been proven to generate photo-curable polymeric particles, ion-cross-linkable thermosensitive gels, polymer-encapsulated cells, and other particles in some situations [33, 34], polymer-encapsulated cells [35, 36], and other particles [21, 37]. Microfluidics can be applied to polylactide particles to make the production of novel drugs easier.

2. Microfluidic devices

There are two main types of microfluidic devices for particle production: microchannels and microcapillaries [38]. Microchannel-based devices are commonly manufactured through processes such as micro-milling, micro-machining, lithography, and shape replication. In such devices, minimizing the interfacial environment causes spontaneous droplet formation, and therefore the droplet size is best dependent on the microchannel geometry while maintaining the oil phase flow rate within an optimal range. Total devices based entirely on microchannels are costly and time-consuming to manufacture, but they enable microsystems to be manufactured with a particle size of only a few tens of micrometers. In addition, the microchannels in such devices can be properly aligned and, in addition to the uniform flow and strong liquefaction of certain droplets or the splitting of droplets to a uniform size, they can serve their equipment, and the systems can be expanded to produce a large number of products. In addition, structures mainly based on capillaries are usually made of low-cost components available on the market and can become microchannels in particle manufacturing. Importantly, these systems can be manufactured in a shorter time and can operate under harsh process conditions [39]. In a complete device based on microchannels, the dispersed phase is very close to the tool wall before being emulsified by the continuous phase, which may cause phase inversion [40]. Although, the affinity of the dispersed relative substance is greater than that of the continuous phase, the dispersed phase preferentially wets the partitions of the tool. This makes the selection of materials produced by the equipment more important than all other materials. However, phase inversion can be avoided by deciding which equipment is suitable for water droplets or organic droplets [41]. On the other hand, capillary-primarily based devices are tremendous for such terms. Here, the droplets are stopped from assembling the device's partitions. Capillary-specific devices allow for the manufacture of oil-in-water or water-in-oil emulsions with a single microsystem [42].

Using a variety of materials and shapes in microfluidic devices to allow future and desirable sort of physical activity and features. Each layer of a laminated microfluidic device is cut separately. The cutting process has a considerable impact on the device's dimensions and functionality. For prototyping and laboratory settings, due to the speed and simplicity each tool offers, cutting is usually done with a knife plotter (i.e., xurography) or laser cutter. A knife plotter works by precisely cutting material with a blade to create the geometry, while a laser cutter uses a focused beam (traditionally, CO_2 lasers are used) [43, 44]. Under these conditions, the droplet diameter can be reduced by increasing the flow rate, density ratio, and viscosity [45]. Bottom-up

***In vitro* culture**	**Advantages**	**Disadvantages**	**Reference**
2D cell culture	Cell cultures are laboratory dishes that are used to grow cells. They are flat and are usually made out of plastic. By sticking cells onto these dishes, scientists are able to study cell behavior using cheap materials. There are several protocols and extensive literature available to analyze data and understand cell behavior.	Limit the simulation of complex cell-cell and cell-matrix interactions to study cell behavior	[48–51]
3D cell culture	Increasing the cell's ability to organize tissue, to express different functions, and improving live imaging.	The cells in the *in vivo* system are in the body, so the *in vitro* system is not exactly like the *in vivo* system when testing cells in a dish.	[10, 52]
(Organ-on-a-chip)	Physiological effects of different tissue types and structures, such as cells and blood vessels, are recreated in a system of fluid and particles to generate forces.	This experiment is very difficult to do and will likely yield inconclusive results, because different humans react differently to the same stimuli.	[29, 53]

Table 1.
Advantages and disadvantages of the methods used in invitro drug screening by microfluidics.

technologies that rely on emulsion or self-assembly on the shape of the equipment used do not always provide fine, pre-designed control over particle geometry (shape, aspect ratio) and composition [46]. A microchannel flow-focusing system (EDCl) was used to study the manufacture of HANP cross-linked with adipic acid hydrazide (ADH) and chlorinated carbodiimide. The focus of this work is to analyze the process parameters of this unique method, which is a continuous nanoprecipitation at the water-organic solvent interface. The influence of the type of organic solvent used, the flow rate of the non-solvent, and the content of hyaluronic acid (HA) on the HANP characteristics of (hyaluronic acid nanoparticles) [47]. Several studies have found that the affinity between water and organic solvents influences the average diameter of nanoparticles (NPs) via water diffusion and the rate of nanoprecipitation. When the non-solvent shows a moderate affinity for water, the polydispersity becomes narrower. In addition, since the process is regulated by convection, lower HA concentrations and higher isopropanol flow rates will produce smaller particles. Regardless of the organic solvent, flow rate, or HA concentration, some stable NPs are formed. The process was found to be simple, repeatable, and fast. This process is expected to be used in the manufacture of oil-free HANP, which is important for medical, pharmacological, and cosmetic applications, as shown in **Table 1** [45, 47].

3. Synthesis of microfluidic nanocarriers

Beyond that, it seems that pharmaceutical formulators have been more interested in using synthetic nanocarriers than natural nanocarriers and colloidal systems, which have not been of much interest. Scientists have recently paid a lot of attention to the production of organic nano-carriers, particularly in pharmaceuticals, as pharmaceutical scientists have begun to recognize the important properties they confer on nano-carriers by microfluidic methods [21, 54]. Nano-carriers are created by spreading premade polymers or inducing polymers to develop through monomer reactions. These nanocarriers can be advanced in a variety of ways, and they are divided into classes based on the processes involved. In the primary group, materials are emulsified, but not necessarily in the other categories. As a result, it gives a straightforward and straightforward synthesis process. When those tactics are applied in typical devices, there is a lack of control over uniform blending, formation, and better impacts on formulation ingredients, and few goods have an excessive particle size dispersion as a result. Microfluidic control structures, on the other hand, can provide control over the aforementioned elements due to their equally sized particles [55]. Lipid polymer hybrid nanoparticles have been merged into high-capacity nanocarriers.

The microfluidic co-flow nanoprecipitation technology has been used to make a large number of LPHNPs. With the help of dissolving poly (lactic-co-glycolic acid) (2 mg/ml) into acetonitrile as a natural phase, the internal fluid changed its ordered state. The outer fluid had a two-to-three mass ratio of lecithin and Distearoyl-sn-glycero-3-phosphoethanolamine-polyethylene glycol 2000 dissolved in 4 percent ethanol and responded in water. These characteristics define a drug's potential to be a good choice for treating breast cancer [21, 22, 55].

Water-to-oil emulsification in a paper-based microfluidic drug carrier results in unique open-channel microfluidics with the capacity to manage the flotation of both adequate and inadequate surface tension liquids. The open channel devices are shown to be effective in limiting a variety of lower surface tension oils at high and low flow rates, allowing for microfluidic emulsification of water in oil in an open channel instrument. The droplets should be formed inside the channel with the aid of an adjustable speed of the continuous phases of the emulsified water and oil. Finally, an instrument has been turned to being used efficiently to synthesize remarkably monodisperse hydrogel microparticles that might contain a drug molecule.

Additional research into the drug delivery properties of manufactured products has yielded promising results. Open channel microfluidic devices have the potential to achieve a high level of fluid manipulation with fast and low-cost production [56]. Dopamine is used as a model drug to quantify electrochemical flow on paper-based devices in a dynamic microfluidic method. Combining electrochemical methods with microfluidic devices to achieve time-resolved detection of neuron-like PC12 cells cultured on filter paper Dopamine [57, 58]. After investigating the attachment of cells to the outside of the paper with a fluorescence microscope; dopamine drug delivery after stimulation with acetylcholine was investigated. As a result, the data collected by the device is consistent with single-cell statistics, demonstrating the effectiveness of the technique for high-throughput quantification of tissues or chemical targets on tissues [59] for higher-throughput quantification of chemical targets on tissues or organs-on-a-chip [58].

In general, microfluidic devices maintain many qualities in pharmaceutical science, consisting of appropriate doses, ideal drug delivery, site-targeted delivery, sustained release and controlled release, reduced repeated doses, and minimal side effects. To do so, these advantages are the key quality of the drug delivery system. Microfluidic technology has been routinely used in many active moiety carriers, direct drug delivery systems, high-throughput screening, and the production of polymers as superior carriers for additives and drugs. Cheaper and easily produced paper-based materials are good substrates that do solve several problems associated with transportation, filtration and storage, concentrators, valves, and multiplexing [59]. Going forward, creating microfluids on paper in controlled drug delivery programs can offer exciting opportunities to broaden the scope of the subject matter and support improved the scientific translation of drug delivery systems. A device for the controlled release of vinblastine (VBL) drug responsive to stimuli from magneto-sensitive chitosan capsules, which is a magnetically sensitive device for controlled drug delivery, was developed by embedding superparamagnetic iron oxide (SPIO) nanoparticles (NPs) into a chitosan matrix and external magnet. Thus, the release rate, time, and dose of VBL released have become controlled by an exterior magnet. The prepared VBL and SPIO NPs-loaded chitosan microparticles were characterized and showed individual and distinctive controlled release patterns. In addition, droplet microfluidics, which is a unique technique for producing polymer spheres, has grown to be used for the manufacturing of monodispersed chitosan microparticles [60]. Because of their distinct physicochemical behavior and synergistic effects in the prevention and inhibition of colorectal cancer progression, atorvastatin and celecoxib were chosen as the version dosage form. For precisely controlled multi-drug delivery, a microfluidic collection of monodisperse multistage pH-responsive polymer/porous silicone composites were developed [61]. Fabrication incorporating hypromerose succinate acetate, which does not dissolve in acidic conditions but incredibly dissolves in basic (alkaline) pH environments, is effective in preventing and suppressing the acceleration of colon and rectal cancers. Microcomposite [62] of Atorvastatin, which benefits from the larger pore volume of porous silicon (PSi), is first loaded into the PSi matrix and then encapsulated via microfluidics into pH-responsive polymer microparticles containing celecoxib, a multidrug obtained Road

Polymer/PSi microcomposite. The manufactured microcomposites were confirmed to have a monodisperse size distribution, multistage pH-response, a particular ratiometric controllable loading extent closer to the concurrently loaded drug molecules, and tailored-made drug release kinetics. This attractive microcomposite technology prevents payloads from being released at low pH values and promotes medicine delivery at higher pH values, and could be used to prevent and treat colon and rectum cancers in the future. Overall, the pH-responsive polymer/PSi-based fully micro composite [63] might be employed as a common platform for combining drug delivery systems for multiple drug compounds [61].

The preparation of monodisperse microparticles of a biodegradable polymer was carried out using an instrument for focusing a microfluidic flow for controlled drug delivery. The manufacture of monodisperse microparticles containing a drug from biodegradable polymers, the use of devices for focusing a microfluidic flow, and the drug delivery properties of these particles have been described [64]. The particle size ranges from 10 to 50 mm. These particles are practically monodispersed with a polydispersity index of 3.9% [65]. Bupivacaine (amphiphilic) is included in a biodegradable debris matrix to characterize the formulation as a model drug [65–67]. The kinetic evaluation suggests that drug release from these monodisperse microparticles is slower than conventional strategies with the same average size, but reveals a larger particle size distribution and, more importantly, a significant reduction in a primary burst than that found with traditional methods, as shown in **Figure 1** [65, 67]. The difference in the preliminary kinetics of drug release is explained by the even distribution of the drug within the particles created using microfluidic strategies. These results demonstrated the application of microfluidic flow-focusing to homogeneous particle system technology for drug delivery [65].

Recently, thermosensitive liposome-controlled release using a disposable microfluidic instrument was developed, with the release of the encapsulated drug from the liposome nanocarrier expected to increase local drug delivery while reducing the toxic effects of increased temperature. High Intensity Focused Ultrasound (HIFU) [68–71], microfluidic devices with micro-HIFU (MHIFU), allow simulation of the bulky HIFU transmission instrument with lower energy consumption and to control of the release of the investigated low-temperature liposomes (LTSL) [52, 72]. In addition, when transitioning to a local temperature of 41–43°C, the structure changes from a gel to a liquid crystal phase, and the encapsulated drug is released by an external hyperthermia source (such as a microwave or infrared radiation laser). The

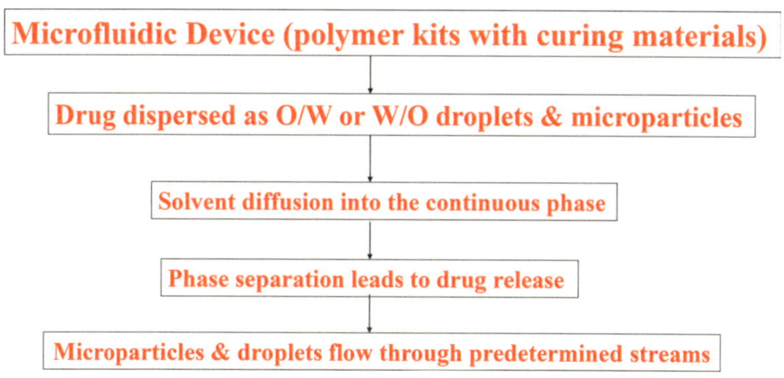

Figure 1.
A strategy for producing dispersed drugs using microfluidic techniques.

lipid membrane structure of low temperature-sensitive liposomes (LTSL) [73]. The era of microfluidics may also provide a promising method for studying ultrasound and the complex dynamics of organisms at the ultramicro level [74]. The main task of improving polymer nanoparticles for many procedures is to specifically engineer preferred physicochemical properties in a repeatable manner [67].

Microfluid self-assembly [9, 75] of polymer nanoparticles with adjustable compactness for controlled drug delivery is predominantly self-assembled hydrophobically modified chitosan (HMC) biopolymer-based nanos. The particle compactness can be determined by adjustable high-speed blending with hydrodynamic flow focusing on microfluidic channels. It has been demonstrated that the self-organizing properties of the chain can be controlled by optimizing the size and compactness of the species, as well as the more restricted particle size distribution, through various flow rates as well as the hydrophobicity of the chitosan chain of nanoparticles [67, 76]. The particle size of the formulation components increased with increasing blending time, while the chitosan produced smaller and more compact nanoparticles with a much smaller variety of aggregated chains and a higher degree of hydrophobicity.

The scientists found that nanoparticles with nearly equal forms of hydrophobic adhesion were formed by blending the two liquids. The scientists found that the lack of affinity for the aqueous medium and the blending times longer than the time of aggregation hindered the formation of nanoparticles with different forms of hydrophobic adhesion.

Moreover, researchers investigating the effectiveness of microfluidics for assembling HMCs and enclosing paclitaxel, a typical anticancer medication, showed that it has a significantly greater encapsulation efficiency and overall quality than the traditional bulk technique. The impact of the components of the synthetic medication on the parameters of the release of paclitaxel from nanoparticles was investigated. [31]. The predicted 50% paclitaxel diffusion coefficient upon drug release meant sustainability in controlling drug release for nanoparticle compactness and superior results compared to traditional bulk blending methods [31, 77]. These results show an excess of microfluidic methods for specific bottom-up control of the physicochemical properties of polymer nanoparticles in many programs [78], including controlled drug delivery [31, 67, 77].

An electrokinetic microfluidic device for rapid, low-power drug delivery in self-sustaining microcontrollers evolved as a low-power, powerful, electrically active

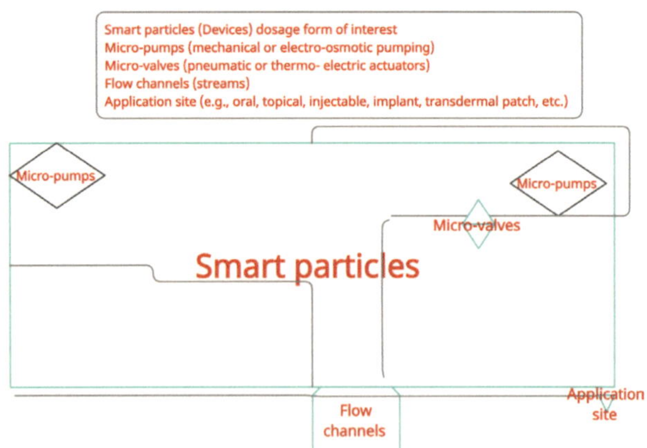

Figure 2.
Fluid-handling systems for the microfabrication of smart materials, including pumps, valves, and flow channels.

microwell intended for use in self-sustaining microcontrollers. The tool features a silicon primary base shape at the top that represents the drug storage location and PDMS (polydimethylsiloxane) that is electrically functionalized as a polymer. The drug release mechanism evolved here utilizes local electrokinetic results of controlled drug release times and compound velocities stored in appropriate, unbiased storage areas [79, 80]. This proves that the dose time can be reduced from hours to seconds over the preceding diffusion, primarily based on the use of low intensities of 20 mJ for the dose. Release techniques are completed in less than 2 minutes or with the use of low energy of 20 mJ. Each of these has an advantage over the state of the artwork subsystem [79]. A version of the electrokinetic delivery involved in the release technique used detailed 3D numerical simulations. The simulated model showed that a large part of the content is released by this technology at an early stage. It also provides a physical view of the delivery process [20, 79]. Such microfabrication is illustrated [81] in **Figure 2**.

4. Conclusions

In conclusion, microfluidic technology allows for incredibly accurate fluid delivery. It could be coupled to an actuator system that delivers drugs on demand or continuously. Microfluidics has revolutionized the design of devices for direct drug delivery in general, as well as the manufacturing of drug carriers. Microfluidic technology is required for the manufacture of drug carriers with a reproducible release profile as well as the controlled release of several substances with varied release characteristics. Materials with smart properties can be manipulated to respond in a controllable and reversible way, modifying some of their properties as a result of external stimuli such as mechanical stress or a certain temperature.

Conflict of interest

The author declares no conflict of interest.

Author details

Fikadu Ejeta
Department of Pharmaceutics and Social Pharmacy, School of Pharmacy, College of Medicine and Health Sciences, Mizan-Tepi University, Ethiopia

*Address all correspondence to: fikaduejeta@gmail.com

References

[1] Viseu A. Nanomedicine. Encyclopedia Britannica. 2020. Available from: https://www.britannica.com/science/nanomedicine. [Accessed: 31 July 2021]

[2] Farokhzad OC, Langer R. Impact of nanotechnology on drug delivery. ACS Nano. 2009;**3**(1):1-7. DOI: 10.1021/nn900002m

[3] Juliano R. Nanomedicine: Is the wave cresting? Nature Reviews. Drug Discovery. 2013;**12**(3):171-172. DOI: 10.1038/nrd3958

[4] Wagner V, Dullaart A, Bock AK, Zweck A. The emerging nanomedicine landscape. Nature Biotechnology. 2006;**24**(10):1211-1217. DOI: 10.1038/nbt1006-1211

[5] Park K. Facing the truth about nanotechnology in drug delivery. ACS Nano. 2013;**7**(9):7442-7447. DOI: 10.1021/nn404501g

[6] Tomeh MA, Zhao X. Recent advances in microfluidics for the preparation of drug and gene delivery systems. Molecular Pharmaceutics. 2020;**17**(12):4421-4434. DOI: 10.1021/acs.molpharmaceut.0c00913

[7] Riahi R, Tamayol A, Shaegh SAM, Ghaemmaghami AM, Dokmeci MR, Khademshosseini A. Microfluidics for advanced drug delivery systems. Current Opinion in Chemical Engineering. 2015;**7**:101-112. DOI: 10.1016/j.coche.2014.12.001

[8] Kwak B, Ozcelikkale A, Shin CS, Park K, Han B. Simulation of complex transport of nanoparticles around a tumor using tumor-microenvironment-on-chip. Journal of Controlled Release. 2014;**194**:157-167. DOI: 10.1016/j.jconrel.2014.08.027

[9] Shamsi M, Zahedi P, Ghourchian H, Minaeian S. Microfluidic-aided fabrication of nanoparticles blend based on chitosan for a transdermal multidrug delivery application. International Journal of Biological Macromolecules. 2017;**99**:433-442. DOI: 10.1016/j.ijbiomac.2017.03.013

[10] Ahn J, Ko J, Lee S, Yu J, Kim YT, Jeon NL. Microfluidics in nanoparticle drug delivery: From synthesis to pre-clinical screening. Advanced Drug Delivery Reviews. 2018;**128**:29-53. DOI: 10.1016/j.addr.2018.04.001

[11] Zhao X et al. Hierarchically porous composite microparticles from microfluidics for controllable drug delivery. Nanoscale. 2018;**10**(26):12595-12604. DOI: 10.1039/c8nr03728k

[12] Liu D, Zhang H, Fontana F, Hirvonen JT, Santos HA. Microfluidic-assisted fabrication of carriers for controlled drug delivery. Lab on a Chip. 2017;**17**(11):1856-1883. DOI: 10.1039/c7lc00242d

[13] Berkland C, King M, Cox A, Kim K, Pack DW. Precise control of PLG microsphere size provides enhanced control of drug release rate. Journal of Controlled Release. 2002;**82**(1):137-147. DOI: 10.1016/S0168-3659(02)00136-0

[14] Duncanson WJ, Lin T, Abate AR, Seiffert S, Shah RK, Weitz DA. Microfluidic synthesis of advanced microparticles for encapsulation and controlled release. Lab on a Chip. 2012;**12**(12):2135-2145. DOI: 10.1039/c2lc21164e

[15] Araújo F et al. Microfluidic assembly of a multifunctional tailorable composite system designed for site specific

combined oral delivery of peptide drugs. ACS Nano. 2015;**9**(8):8291-8302. DOI: 10.1021/acsnano.5b02762

[16] Stuart MAC et al. Emerging applications of stimuli-responsive polymer materials. Nature Materials. 2010;**9**(2):101-113. DOI: 10.1038/nmat2614

[17] Zhao CX. Multiphase flow microfluidics for the production of single or multiple emulsions for drug delivery. Advanced Drug Delivery Reviews. 2013;**65**(11-12):1420-1446. DOI: 10.1016/j.addr.2013.05.009

[18] Mura S, Nicolas J, Couvreur P. Stimuli-responsive nanocarriers for drug delivery. Nature Materials. 2013;**12**(11):991-1003. DOI: 10.1038/nmat3776

[19] Huang X et al. Microfluidic hydrodynamic focusing synthesis of polymer-lipid nanoparticles for siRNA delivery. Oncotarget. 2017;**8**(57):96826-96836. DOI: 10.18632/oncotarget.18281

[20] Lin YS et al. Microfluidic synthesis of microfibers for magnetic-responsive controlled drug release and cell culture. PLoS One. 2012;**7**(3):4-11. DOI: 10.1371/journal.pone.0033184

[21] Karnik R et al. Microfluidic platform for controlled synthesis of polymeric nanoparticles. Nano Letters. 2008;**8**(9):60-75

[22] Tahir N et al. Microfluidic fabrication and characterization of Sorafenib-loaded lipid-polymer hybrid nanoparticles for controlled drug delivery. International Journal of Pharmaceutics. 2020;**581**(March):119275. DOI: 10.1016/j.ijpharm.2020.119275

[23] Tasci ME et al. Production, optimization and characterization of polylactic acid microparticles using electrospray with porous structure. Applied Sciences. 2021;**11**(11):1-13. DOI: 10.3390/app11115090

[24] Fantini D, Zanetti M, Costa L. Polystyrene microspheres and nanospheres produced by electrospray. Macromolecular Rapid Communications. 2006;**27**(23):2038-2042. DOI: 10.1002/marc.200600532

[25] Xu Y, Hanna MA. Electrospray encapsulation of water-soluble protein with polylactide: Effects of formulations on morphology, encapsulation efficiency and release profile of particles. International Journal of Pharmaceutics. 2006;**320**(1):30-36. DOI: 10.1016/j.ijpharm.2006.03.046

[26] Hennequin Y et al. Synthesizing microcapsules with controlled geometrical and mechanical properties with microfluidic double emulsion technology. Langmuir. 2009;**25**(14):7857-7861. DOI: 10.1021/la9004449

[27] Whitesides GM. The origins and the future of microfluidics. Nature. 2006;**442**(7101):368-373. DOI: 10.1038/nature05058

[28] Tokeshi M, Sato K. Micro/nano devices for chemical analysis. Micromachines. 2016;**7**(9):6-8. DOI: 10.3390/mi7090164

[29] Huh D, Matthews BD, Mammoto A, Montoya-Zavala M, Hsin HY, Ingber DE. Reconstituting organ-level lung functions on a chip. Science (80-). 2010;**328**(5986):1662-1668. DOI: 10.1126/science.1188302

[30] Bhise NS et al. Organ-on-a-chip platforms for studying drug delivery systems. Journal of Controlled Release. 2014;**190**:82-93. DOI: 10.1016/j.jconrel.2014.05.004

[31] Thorsen T, Roberts RW, Arnold FH, Quake SR. Dynamic pattern formation in a vesicle-generating microfluidic device. Physical Review Letters. 2001;**86**(18):4163-4166. DOI: 10.1103/PhysRevLett.86.4163

[32] Nisisako T, Torii T, Higuchi T. Droplet formation in a microchannel network. Lab on a Chip. 2002;**2**(1):24-26. DOI: 10.1039/b108740c

[33] Kim JW, Fernández-Nieves A, Dan N, Utada AS, Marquez M, and Weitz DA. "Colloidal assembly route for responsive colloidosomes with tunable permeability," Nano Letters. 2007;7(9):2876-2880. DOI: 10.1021/nl0715948

[34] De Geest BG, Urbanski JP, Thorsen T, Demeester J, and De Smedt SC. "Synthesis of monodisperse biodegradable microgels in microfluidic devices," Langmuir. 2005;**21**(23):10275-10279. DOI: 10.1021/la051527y

[35] Tan WH, Takeuchi S. Monodisperse alginate hydrogel microbeads for cell encapsulation. Advanced Materials. 2007;**19**(18):2696-2701. DOI: 10.1002/adma.200700433

[36] Clausell-Tormos J et al. Droplet-based microfluidic platforms for the encapsulation and screening of mammalian cells and multicellular organisms. Chemistry & Biology. 2008;**15**(5):427-437. DOI: 10.1016/j.chembiol.2008.04.004

[37] Chang J-Y, Yang C-H, Huang K-S. Microfluidic assisted preparation of CdSe/ZnS nanocrystals encapsulated into poly(DL-lactide-co-glycolide) microcapsules. Nanotechnology. 2007;**18**(30):305305. DOI: 10.1088/0957-4484/18/30/305305

[38] Zhao X, Bian F, Sun L, Cai L, Li L, Zhao Y. Microfluidic generation of nanomaterials for biomedical applications. Small. 2020;**16**(9):1-19. DOI: 10.1002/smll.201901943

[39] Herranz-Blanco B, Ginestar E, Zhang H, Hirvonen J, Santos HA. Microfluidics platform for glass capillaries and its application in droplet and nanoparticle fabrication. International Journal of Pharmaceutics. 2017;**516**(1-2):100-105. DOI: 10.1016/j.ijpharm.2016.11.024

[40] J. Pessi, H. A. Santos, I. Miroshnyk, Joukoyliruusi, D. A. Weitz, and S. Mirza, "Microfluidics-assisted engineering of polymeric microcapsules with high encapsulation efficiency for protein drug delivery," International Journal of Pharmaceutics. 2014;**472**(1-2):82-87. DOI: 10.1016/j. ijpharm.2014.06.012

[41] Olanrewaju A, Beaugrand M, Yafia M, Juncker D. Capillary microfluidics in microchannels: From microfluidic networks to capillaric circuits. Lab on a Chip. 2018;**18**(16):2323-2347. DOI: 10.1039/c8lc00458g

[42] Martins JP, Torrieri G, Santos HA. The importance of microfluidics for the preparation of nanoparticles as advanced drug delivery systems. Expert Opinion on Drug Delivery. 2018;**15**(5):469-479. DOI: 10.1080/17425247.2018.1446936

[43] Gale BK et al. A review of current methods in microfluidic device fabrication and future commercialization prospects. Inventions. 2018;**3**(3):60-75. DOI: 10.3390/inventions3030060

[44] Niculescu AG, Chircov C, Bîrcă AC, Grumezescu AM. Fabrication and applications of microfluidic devices: A review. International Journal of

Molecular Sciences. 2021;**22**(4):1-26. DOI: 10.3390/ijms22042011

[45] Chiesa E et al. The microfluidic technique and the manufacturing of polysaccharide nanoparticles. Pharmaceutics. 2018;**10**(4):267-290. DOI: 10.3390/pharmaceutics10040267

[46] Caldorera-Moore M, Guimard N, Shi L, Roy K. Designer nanoparticles: Incorporating size, shape and triggered release into nanoscale drug carriers. Expert Opinion on Drug Delivery. 2010;7(4):479-495. DOI: 10.1517/17425240903579971

[47] R. C. S. Bicudo and M. H. A. Santana, "Production of hyaluronic acid (HA) nanoparticles by a continuous process inside microchannels: Effects of non-solvents, organic phase flow rate, and HA concentration," Chemical Engineering Science. 2012;**84**:134-141.DOI: 10.1016/j.ces.2012.08.010

[48] Arduino I et al. Preparation of cetyl palmitate-based PEGylated solid lipid nanoparticles by microfluidic technique. Acta Biomaterialia. 2021;**121**(xxxx):566-578. DOI: 10.1016/j.actbio.2020.12.024

[49] Damiati S, Kompella UB, Damiati SA, Kodzius R. Microfluidic devices for drug delivery systems and drug screening. Genes (Basel). 2018;**9**(2):103-127. DOI: 10.3390/genes9020103

[50] Laity P, Cassidy A, Skepper J, Jones B, Cameron R. Investigation into the intragranular structures of microcrystalline cellulose and pre-gelatinised starch. European Journal of Pharmaceutics and Biopharmaceutics. 2010;**74**(2):377-387. DOI: 10.1016/j.ejpb.2009.10.006

[51] Coluccio ML et al. Microfluidic platforms for cell cultures and investigations. Microelectronic Engineering. 2019;**208**(January):14-28. DOI: 10.1016/j.mee.2019.01.004

[52] Grüll H, Langereis S. Hyperthermia-triggered drug delivery from temperature-sensitive liposomes using MRI-guided high intensity focused ultrasound. Journal of Controlled Release. 2012;**161**(2):317-327. DOI: 10.1016/j.jconrel.2012.04.041

[53] Kim HJ, Huh D, Hamilton G, Ingber DE. Human gut-on-a-chip inhabited by microbial flora that experiences intestinal peristalsis-like motions and flow. Lab on a Chip. 2012;**12**(12):2165-2174. DOI: 10.1039/c2lc40074j

[54] Le TN, Nguyen VA, Bach GL, Tran LD, Cao HH. Design and fabrication of a PDMS-based manual micro-valve system for microfluidic applications. Advances in Polymer Technology. 2020;**2020**:1-8. DOI: 10.1155/2020/2460212

[55] Khan IU, Serra CA, Anton N, Vandamme TF. Production of nanoparticle drug delivery systems with microfluidics tools. Expert Opinion on Drug Delivery. 2015;**12**(4):547-562. DOI: 10.1517/17425247.2015.974547

[56] Kim DY, Jin SH, Jeong SG, Lee B, Kang KK, Lee CS. Microfluidic preparation of monodisperse polymeric microspheres coated with silica nanoparticles. Scientific Reports. 2018;**8**(1):1-11. DOI: 10.1038/s41598-018-26829-z

[57] Zhou W, Feng M, Valadez A, Li XJ. One-step surface modification to graft dna codes on paper: The method, mechanism, and its application. Analytical Chemistry. 2020;**92**(10):7045-7053. DOI: 10.1021/acs.analchem.0c00317

[58] Trouillon R, Gijs MAM. Dynamic electrochemical quantitation of dopamine release from a cells-on-paper system. RSC Advances. 2016;**6**(37):31069-31073. DOI: 10.1039/c6ra02487d

[59] Mao K et al. Paper-based microfluidics for rapid diagnostics and drug delivery. Journal of Controlled Release. 2020;**322**(March):187-199. DOI: 10.1016/j.jconrel.2020.03.010

[60] Huang KS, Yang CH, Wang YC, Wang WT, Lu YY. Microfluidic synthesis of vinblastine-loaded multifunctional particles for magnetically responsive controlled drug release. Pharmaceutics. 2019;**11**(5);212-226. DOI: 10.3390/pharmaceutics11050212

[61] Liu D et al. Microfluidic assembly of monodisperse multistage pH-responsive polymer/porous silicon composites for precisely controlled multi-drug delivery. Small. 2014;**10**(10):2029-2038. DOI: 10.1002/smll.201303740

[62] Amoyav B, Benny O. Microfluidic based fabrication and characterization of highly porous polymeric microspheres. Polymers (Basel). 2019;**11**:419. DOI: 10.3390/polym11030419

[63] Vasiliauskas R et al. Simple microfluidic approach to fabricate monodisperse hollow microparticles for multidrug delivery. ACS Applied Materials & Interfaces. 2015;7(27):14822-14832. DOI: 10.1021/acsami.5b04824

[64] Zhang L, Chen Q, Ma Y, Sun J. Microfluidic methods for fabrication and engineering of nanoparticle drug delivery systems. ACS Applied Bio Materials. 2019;**3**(1):107-120. DOI: 10.1021/acsabm.9b00853

[65] Xu Q et al. Preparation of monodisperse biodegradable polymer microparticles using a microfluidic flow-focusing device for controlled drug delivery. Small. 2009;**5**(13):1575-1581. DOI: 10.1002/smll.200801855

[66] Maher S et al. Multifunctional microspherical magnetic and pH responsive carriers for combination anticancer therapy engineered by droplet-based microfluidics. Journal of Materials Chemistry B. 2017;**5**(22):4097-4109. DOI: 10.1039/c7tb00588a

[67] Dashtimoghadam E, Mirzadeh H, Taromi FA, Nyström B. Microfluidic self-assembly of polymeric nanoparticles with tunable compactness for controlled drug delivery. Polymer (Guildf). 2013;**54**(18):4972-4979. DOI: 10.1016/j.polymer.2013.07.022

[68] Mu X, Gan S, Wang Y, Li H, Zhou G. Stimulus-responsive vesicular polymer nano-integrators for drug and gene delivery. International Journal of Nanomedicine. 2019;**14**:5415-5434. DOI: 10.2147/IJN.S203555

[69] Chen W, Meng F, Cheng R, Zhong Z. pH-Sensitive degradable polymersomes for triggered release of anticancer drugs: A comparative study with micelles. Journal of Controlled Release. 2010;**142**(1):40-46. DOI: 10.1016/j.jconrel.2009.09.023

[70] Paasonen L, Laaksonen T, Johans C, Yliperttula M, Kontturi K, Urtti A. Gold nanoparticles enable selective light-induced contents release from liposomes. Journal of Controlled Release. 2007;**122**(1):86-93. DOI: 10.1016/j.jconrel.2007.06.009

[71] Ganta S, Devalapally H, Shahiwala A, Amiji M. A review of stimuli-responsive nanocarriers for drug and gene delivery. Journal of Controlled Release. 2008;**126**(3):187-204. DOI: 10.1016/j.jconrel.2007.12.017

[72] Ranjan A et al. Image-guided drug delivery with magnetic resonance guided high intensity focused ultrasound and temperature sensitive liposomes in a rabbit Vx2 tumor model. Journal of Controlled Release. 2012;**158**(3):487-494. DOI: 10.1016/j.jconrel.2011.12.011

[73] Meng L, Deng Z, Niu L, Cai F, Zheng H. Controlled thermal-sensitive liposomes release on a disposable microfluidic device. Proceedings Under Annual International Conference of the IEEE Engineering in Medicine and Biology Society (EMBC). 2015;**2015**(November):5912-5915. DOI: 10.1109/EMBC.2015.7319737

[74] Meng L et al. A disposable microfluidic device for controlled drug release from thermal-sensitive liposomes by high intensity focused ultrasound. Theranostics. 2015;**5**(11):1203-1213. DOI: 10.7150/thno.12295

[75] Liu D et al. "Core/Shell Nanocomposites Produced by Superfast Sequential Microfluidic Nanoprecipitation." Nano Letters. 2017

[76] Morikawa Y, Tagami T, Hoshikawa A, Ozeki T. The use of an efficient microfluidic mixing system for generating stabilized polymeric nanoparticles for controlled drug release. Biological & Pharmaceutical Bulletin. 2018;**41**(6):899-907. DOI: 10.1248/bpb.b17-01036

[77] Wang J et al. A microfluidic tubing method and its application for controlled synthesis of polymeric nanoparticles. Lab on a Chip. 2014;**14**(10):1673-1677. DOI: 10.1039/c4lc00080c

[78] Bazban-Shotorbani S, Dashtimoghadam E, Karkhaneh A, Hasani-Sadrabadi MM, Jacob KI. Microfluidic directed synthesis of alginate nanogels with tunable pore size for efficient protein delivery. Langmuir. 2016;**32**(19):4996-5003. DOI: 10.1021/acs.langmuir.5b04645

[79] Chung AJ, And DK, Erickson D. Electrokinetic microfluidic devices for rapid, low power drug delivery in autonomous microsystems. Lab on a Chip. 2008;**8**(2):330-338. DOI: 10.1039/b713325a

[80] Santini JT, Richards AC, Scheidt R, Cima MJ, Langer R. Microchips as controlled drug-delivery devices. Angewandte Chemie, International Edition. 2000;**39**(14):2396-2407. DOI: 10.1002/1521-3773(20000717)39:14<2396::AID-ANIE2396>3.0.CO;2-U

[81] Ejeta F. Recent advances of microfluidic platforms for controlled drug delivery in nanomedicine. Drug Design, Development and Therapy. 2021;**15**:3881-3891. DOI: 10.2147/DDDT.S324580

Chapter 7

Lipid Nanoparticulate Drug Delivery Systems: Approaches toward Improvement in Therapeutic Efficacy of Bioactive Molecules

Sudarshan Singh, Tanvi R. Dodiya, Rajesh Dodiya, Yogesh V. Ushir and Slamet Widodo

Abstract

Hybrid lipid polymers significantly changed the postulation of low or less bioavailability of conventional drug delivery systems. Several drug delivery systems already exist for the encapsulation and subsequent release of lipophilic drugs with enhanced therapeutic efficacy and are well described in the scientific literature. Among these, lipid polymer-based nanoparticles have specifically come up for dermal, transdermal, mucosal, intramuscular, and ocular drug administration routes in the last 20 years. Moreover, lipid nanoparticles showed potential for active targeting of anticancer therapy, delivery of DNA or RNA materials, and use as a diagnostic imaging agent. Therefore, the multifarious nanostructured lipid carriers can reduce the undesired effects with maximum utilization of active moiety. In this, chapter a brief discussion is presented on the source of synthetic and natural lipid polymers with the use of surfactants. Moreover, a summary on formulation and pharmaceutical characterization of nanostructured lipid carriers considering solid lipid nanoparticles and vesicular drug delivery systems has been taken into consideration. In addition, a light on bioactive fortified with lipid nanoparticles was reviewed for maximizing its therapeutic efficacy. Furthermore, this chapter's focus to bring out the latest applications via recent scientific publications from the Scopus database on nanostructure carriers that showed promising application for the treatments of potentially life-threatening diseases has been summarized.

Keywords: lipid nanostructures, solid lipid nanoparticles, vesicular drug delivery systems, phytomedicine, lipid

1. Introduction

Nanomedicine is still considered an emerging and effective formulations technique due to the fusion of nanotechnology and medicine, which is one of the most promising ways to develop effective targeted therapies. Several active pharmaceuticals fail to demonstrate the therapeutic efficacy when delivered in conventional dosage forms, which is directly or indirectly linked to their biopharmaceutical classification and hydrophobic nature. Moreover, such poor water-soluble active moiety represents several challenges: low or reduced oral bioavailability, topical permeability, therapeutic efficacy, etc. Nanoparticulate drug delivery systems comprise a wide variety of dosage forms including nanospheres, micelles, solid lipid nanoparticles, nanoliposomes, dendrimers, magnetic nanoparticles, and nanocapsules (**Figure 1**). Lipid nanostructure carriers such as solid lipid nanoparticles (SLNs), vesicular drug delivery system (VDDs), and or nano-structure lipid carriers (NLCs) significantly gained attention among the scientific community due to several advantages including low cost of scale-up with prolonged stability [1]. There are several carriers employed in the delivery of available drugs as an alternative to conventional drug delivery systems such as drug-lipid conjugate, lipid nanocapsules, layersomes, and lipid-polymer nanohybrids. Solid lipid nanoparticles were developed to overcome the limitations of other colloidal carriers, such as emulsions, suspensions, and polymeric nanoparticles due to the effective release mechanism and targeted delivery with physical stability [2]. Nano lipid carriers are modified versions of SLNs that improve the stability and drug loading efficacy. In addition, the potential applications of LNs in drug delivery fabrication, research, topical cosmetics, and clinical medicine indicates its efficacy. These carrier systems are mainly composed of physiologically compatible and

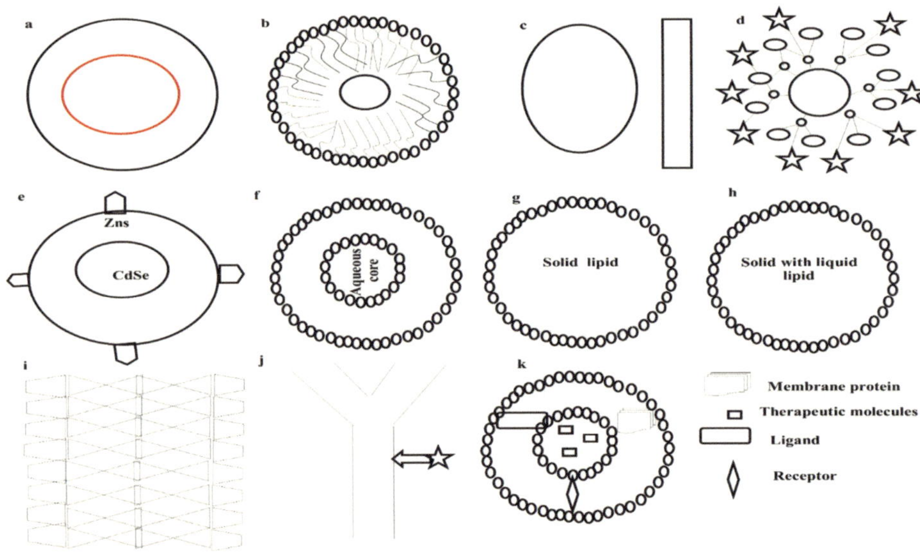

Figure 1.
Various carrier-based polymeric drug delivery systems including polymeric nanoparticle (a), polymeric micelles (b), metallic nanoparticles (c), dendrimer (d), quantum dot (e), liposome (f), solid lipid nanoparticles (g), nanostructure lipid nanoparticle (h), carbon nanotube (i), antibody-drug conjugate (j), exosome (k). Polymeric nanoparticles are particles within the size range from 1 to 1000 nm and can be loaded with active drugs entrapped within or adsorbed on the surface. Polymeric micelles are nanoscopic core or shell structures formed by amphiphilic block copolymers. Metallic nanoparticles are submicron-scale entities fabricated by reduction using synthetic or green materials. Dendrimers are a class of synthetic polymers with a structure of repeatedly branching chains, typically forming spherical macromolecules. A quantum dot is a nanoscale particle of semiconducting materials that can be embedded in cells or organisms for various experimental purposes, such as labeling proteins. A liposome is a spherical vesicle having at least one lipid bilayer that can carry drugs to deliver at the targeted site within the body. Solid lipid nanoparticles or lipid nanostructure carriers are nanoparticles composed of lipids. Carbon nanotubes are tubes made of carbon with diameters typically measured in nanometers. An antibody-drug conjugate is a class of biopharmaceutical drugs designed as a targeted therapy for treating cancer. Whereas, exosomes are a class of cell-derived extracellular vesicles of endosomal origin, and are typically 30–150 nm in diameter.

biodegradable lipid materials, surfactants, and co-surfactants that are generally recognized as safe (GRAS) by food and drug admirations [3].

Vesicles-based drug delivery was the first among the different LNs targeted carrier formulations discovered in 1965 and is still widely accepted in the fabrication of novel pharmaceutical formulations [4]. The word liposome is derived from the Greek words "lipid" which means fat and "soma" which means body. Liposomes are spherical vesicles with a hydrophobic internal sac-like structure enclosed with a lipid bilayer membrane. Moreover, several advantages associated with VDDs include low toxicity, flexibility, cyto-compatibility, biodegradable, protection of active moiety from enzymatic degradation, and non-immunogenicity [5–7]. However, most of the uses in formulations indicate limitations due to specific disadvantages such as low encapsulation efficacy, poor stability, limited shelf-life, and intermembrane transfer [8].

Solid lipid nanoparticles were introduced in the late 90,s as a potential substitute against the carrier-based VDD, emulsion, and polymeric nanoparticles. These carrier-based nanoparticulate offers advantages of spherical size (40–1000 nm), shape, and morphology, composed of single or multiple combined lipids with surfactants, where the dispersed phase is solid lipid fats and surfactant, which act as an emulsifier [9]. The selection and composition of lipid and surfactant affect the physicochemical properties and quality such as drug loading and particle size. The proper combination of lipids and surfactants used in the fabrication of solid lipid nanoparticles demonstrate excellent drug stability and prolonged release compared with VDDs and other polymeric carriers due to the evasion of organic solvent in their fabrication. However, associated disadvantages such as the formation of the crystalline structure of lipids due to inherent low incorporation rates and unpredictable gelation tendency [10, 11].

Nanocapsules have been one of the most widely studied nanosystems for the delivery of functional compounds. Moreover, nanocapsules are also known as nanoparticulate in food science constituted as external polymeric membrane and inner part composed of polymeric matrix containing bioactive compounds. Furthermore, nano-encapsulation involves the incorporation, absorption, or scattering of combinations of bioactive solid, liquid, or gas into small vesicles with nanometer-scale

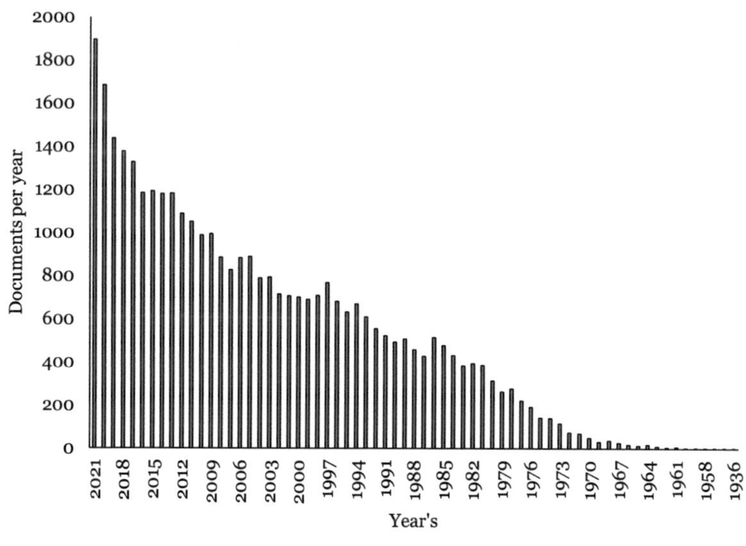

Figure 2.
Total number of publications on LNs from 1936 to 2021 exported from the SCOPUS database on 2 March 2022.

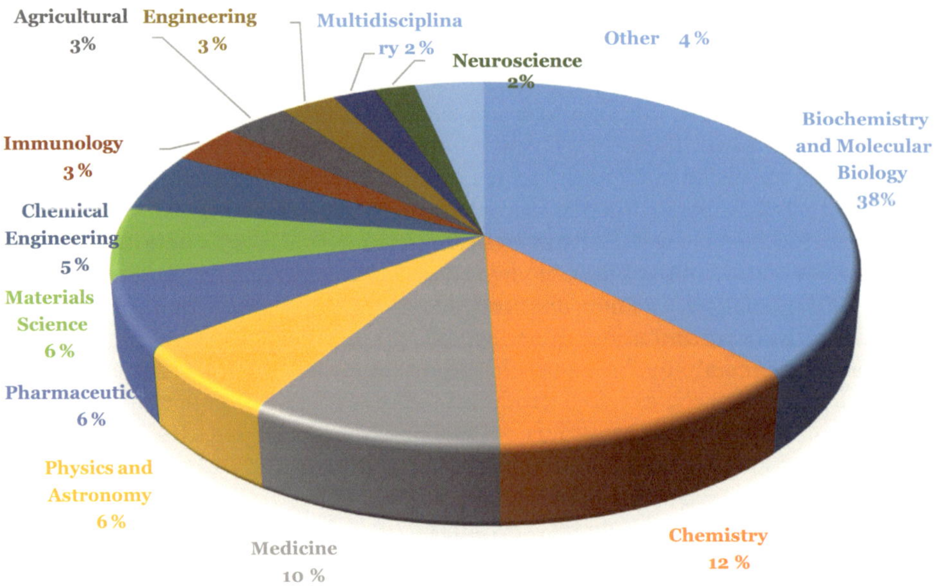

Figure 3.
Total number of publications on lipid nanocarriers subject-wise from 1936 to 2021 exported from the SCOPUS database on 2 March 2022 (for interpretation of the results to color in this figure legend, the reader referred to the web version of this chapter or color print).

diameters. However, lipid nanocapsules are defined as nanovesicular delivery systems with a core-shell structure consisting of polymeric membrane or coating and target active moiety formulation added within the cavity. Moreover, lipid nanocapsules are considered as a sandwich of liposome and nanoemulsion. In addition, nanocapsules have functional properties that are maintained by encapsulation in simple solutions, colloids, emulsions, and biopolymers in food. Lipid nanocapsules are submicron particles with a broader surface area and size below the endothelium fenestration (>100 nm) that present advantages compared to multi-lamellar liposomes, especially with prolonged stability up to 18 months. Thus the lower size of lipid nanocapsules increases the transparency of solution when utilized in clear liquids such as beverages and sauces. Additionally, these lipid carriers can encapsulate efficiently lipophilic drugs, which is a much-needed feature for pharmaceutical colloidal formulations. This chapter presents an overview of the various LNs materials as a potential carrier for the delivery of poorly water-soluble drugs with enhanced therapeutic efficacy. Furthermore, a brief on various fabrication and characterization techniques involved with VDDs and SLNs with their prospect and market challenges concerning the stability. **Figures 2** and **3** indicates the yearly trends of publication for retrieved data from the Scopus database system on keywords "nanocarriers*".

2. Lipids and surfactants

Lipids fulfill various functions in life as membrane constituents, for energy storage, or signaling molecules. Lipids are structurally and functionally diverse organic compounds including fats, oil, and hormones that do not interact appreciably and are insoluble in polar solvents [12]. Lipids are hydrophobic and some of them are amphipathic, which represent a part as hydrophilic and another as hydrophobic. These amphipathic lipids demonstrate

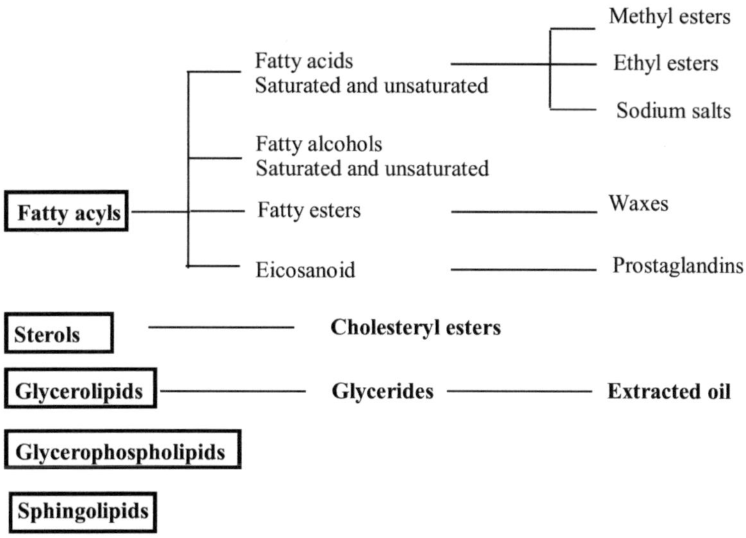

Figure 4.
Fatty acids and their derivatives.

a unique behavior in water that spontaneously form ordered molecular aggregates with their hydrophilic ends on the outside, in contact with the water, and their hydrophobic part on the inside, shielded from the water. Though biological lipids are similar in chemical linking to polymeric materials used for the delivery of active moiety, however they are not large macromolecules. Lipids are classified in several ways and among them, the major groups classified are fatty acids, fatty acid derivatives, cholesterol, and their derivatives, with lipoproteins. The fatty acids are available in abundant in complexed with fats and phospholipids (**Figure 4**). Fatty acids are also known as carboxylic acids composed of a hydrocarbon chain linked with one terminal of the carboxylic group. However, the fragment of a carboxylic acid lacks a hydroxyl group, known as the acyl group. Moreover, fatty acids in the aqueous phase of physiological condition lose a hydrogen ion (H^+) to generate an anionic charged carboxylate group (COO^-) and due to a common biosynthetic pathway within the organism, which involves the linking of the two-carbon unit together produces an even number of carbon atoms within fatty acids [13]. These fatty acid lipids are further classified as saturated, unsaturated, monosaturated (MUFA), and polyunsaturated fatty acids (PUFA). The saturated fatty acids specify the bonding of the maximum possible numbers of hydrogen atoms to each carbon in the molecules. Whereas, unsaturated fatty acids indicate one or more double-bonded carbon–carbon molecules. The number of double bonds attributes to mon or polyunsaturated molecules with one double bond and two or more double bonds, respectively. Common saturated and unsaturated fatty acids are lauric acids, myristic acids, palmitic acids, stearic acid, behenic acid, lignoceric acid and palmitoleic acid, oleic acid, gadoleic acid, erucic acid, and nervonic acid, respectively [14]. Furthermore, frequently polyunsaturated fatty acids used are linoleic acid, linolenic acid, and arachidonic acids. Fatty acids are alternatively also obtained from the hydrolysis of hard animal fats, coconut, palm kernel, soybean oils, and from the fractional distillation of crude tall oil. Other fatty acids are derived from petroleum. Physically, most of these fatty acids are liquid at room temperature. The difference in properties is to a large extent related to the presence of saturation and unsaturation within the molecules. Commonly, solid fats are indicated by the dominance of saturated fatty acids and liquid oils are indications of a high level of unsaturated fatty acids [15]. Cholesterol in the free and combined

Lipoprotein	Density (g/ml)	Size (nm)	Lipoprotein	Density (g/ml)	Size (nm)
Chylomicrons	<0.930	75–1200	LDL	1.019–1.063	18–25
Chylomicron remnants	0.930–1.006	30–80	HDL	1.063–1.210	5–12
VLDL	0.930–1.006	30–80	Lp (a)	1.055–1.085	~30
IDL	1.006–1.019	25–35			

Table 1.
Classification of lipoproteins [17].

state is the most widely occurring sterol in animal tissue. It is an essential compound in the body's production of steroids hormones and bile. It is also an important component for normal skin function. Cholesterol is an important functional excipient used in several pharmaceutical formulations including solid lipid nanoparticles, parenteral mRNA–based drug delivery, vesicular drug delivery, etc. As a part of lipid coating that protects the active drug moiety, and could modulate drug release, enhance the ability of the drug formulation to penetrate cell membranes, and provide a stabilization effect. Recently plant-derived cholesterol including Phytochol®, SyntheChol®, etc., gained significant attention among the researcher due to multifunctional application with lower adverse effects. Lipoproteins are substances made of proteins and fat that carry cholesterol through the bloodstream. Moreover, lipoproteins are complex particles that have a central hydrophobic core of non-polar lipids, primarily cholesterol, ester, and triglycerides [16]. This hydrophobic core is surrounded by a hydrophobic membrane consisting of phospholipids, free cholesterol, and apolipoprotein. Additionally, lipoprotein is a biochemical assembly whose primary function is to transport hydrophobic lipid molecules in water, as in blood plasma or other extracellular fluid. The lipoproteins are broadly classified into several classes, however cholesterol is broadly classified into two categories based on lipoproteins such as high-density lipoprotein (HDL) and low-density lipoprotein (LDL) (**Table 1**). High-density lipoproteins are generally assumed as "good" and low density as "bad" cholesterol [18].

Surfactants have been diligently associated with humans as early as 2800 BC and continue to be a necessity in day-to-day life with great usage in solubility and entrapment efficacy of drugs used within nanocarriers. The earliest record on the usage of surfactant was recorded as sopay traces in clay cylinders at the Babylonian archeological site in Mesopotamia in 2800 BC [19, 20]. The word "Surfactant" is an abbreviation for "surface-active agent", classified as an amphiphilic compound due to the presence of both hydrophilic and hydrophobic groups. Considering hydrophilic group surfactants are broadly classified into four categories such as cationic, anionic, zwitterionic, and non-ionic surfactants. Cationic surfactants contain alkylamine or quaternary ammonium salts that can be absorbed on the negatively charged interface, with the antistatic and disinfectant application. Anionic surfactants contain carboxylic acids salts, sulfonates, sulfate salts, sulfate esters, or phosphate within hydrophobic groups, that offers detergency, foaming, and penetrability use. Zwitterion surfactants contain carboxy betaine, imidazolium betaine, amino ethyl glycine salt, or amine oxide within the hydrophobic structure. They are often used as auxiliary materials to enhance the effectiveness of other surfactants. Non-ionic surfactants have non-dissociable chemical structures in their hydrophilic groups, which are generally used in cosmetics, food emulsifiers, and skin cleaners due to low irritation and toxicity. A wide range of spontaneous, self-assembling surfactants structures in the size range spanning from a few nanometers to tens of micrometers has been reported. Moreover, the role of surfactants in the fabrication of nanocarriers has been proven in various aspects including drug loading, colloidal suspension stability, and

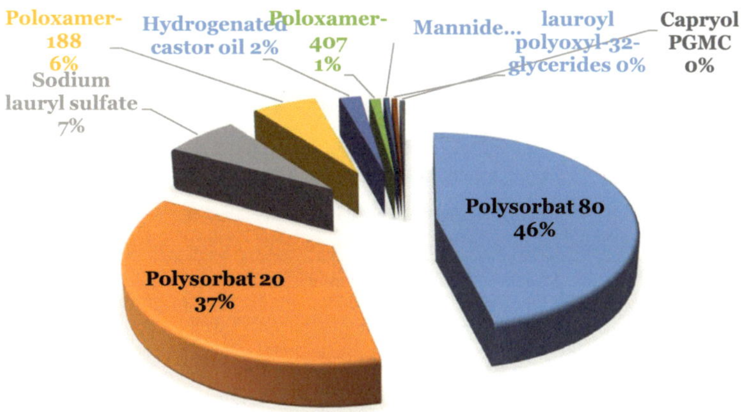

Figure 5.
Percentage of instances for different surfactants found in the composition of the investigational bioactive incorporated dosage form [21].

most important formulation stability on long-term storage. The percentage instances for different surfactants found in the compositions of the investigational bioactive incorporated dosage form are presented in **Figure 5**.

3. Formulation and characterization techniques involved in lipids-based vesicles and nanoparticles

A general method used in the fabrication of VDDs involves the dissolution of the single or mixture of lipids with surfactants, followed by drying the lipid film, and then dispersion of film in an aqueous medium to obtain a multilamellar vesicular system at required hydration temperature. The hydrating temperature used in the formulation of the VDDs should be always above the phase transition temperature of the lipid used. Later developed multilamellar vesicular systems are further processed to obtained small, stable vesicles [22]. The method of

Vesicular drug carriers	Description	Applications
Enzymosomes	Vesicle provide a bio-environment in which covalently enzymes are immobilized or coupled	Targeting tumor cells
Virosomes	Vesicle spiked with virus glycoprotein	Immunological adjuvants
Ufasomes	Long-chain fatty acid incorporated vesicles using a mechanical method	—
Cryptosomes	Vesicle with surface phospholipid coat	Ligand mediated drug delivery
Emulsomes	Microscopic lipid arranged within a polar core	Parenteral administration of hydrophobic drugs
Discomes	Solubilized niosomes within non-ionic surfactant	Ligand mediated drug delivery
Aquasomes	Multi-layered self-assembly composition containing ceramic carbon nano-crystalline particulate	Molecular targeting

Vesicular drug carriers	Description	Applications
Ethosomes	A soft malleable vesicle	Drug delivery to deep skin
Genosomes	Artificial macromolecular complex functionalized gene	Gene transfer
Phytomes	Photolyase encapsulated within liposomes	Photodynamic therapy
Erythrosomes	Chemically crossed linked human erythrocytes	Marco-molecular drug targeting
Hemosomes	Liposome fortified with hemoglobin	Oxygen carrying property
Proteosomes	High molecular weight multi-subunit enzyme complex	Catalytic activity
Vesosome	Embedded bilayer compartment	Multi-compartmental vesicles
Archaeosomes	Archaea glycerolipids composed of vesicles	Serum protectant
Sphingosomes	Consist of an aqueous space sac inside the lipid bilayer to entrap the drug	Improved stability compared to liposomes
Menthosomes	An ultra-deformable vesicles carrier system	Excellent permeability of drug within carrier through the skin
Bilosomes	Bile salt-containing niosomes	Enhance the permeation of the drug by fluidizing the lipoidal bilayer of the vascular system and the stratum corneum.
Invasomes	lipid-based deformable vesicular carriers, enabling the drug to penetrate deeper into the skin or the systemic circulation by non-invasive delivery	Improved dermal delivery due to deformable nature
Niosomes	Made of non-ionic surfactant with neutrally charged compound, compared to the bilayer lipid vesicles	Deliver drug within the dermal layer by perturbation od lipidic membrane
Cubosomes	A cubic-phase lipid-drug delivery system composed of the curved continuous lipid bilayer, which is extending in 3-dimensions and isolating two consistent systems of water channels	Potential delivery of protein, peptides, amino acids, and nucleic acid
Transfersome	An ultra-flexible liposomes composed of bilayer as a backbone and an edge activator	Highly elastic and stress-responsive than the conventional vesicular system
Transethosomes	An advanced VDDs that differs from liposome and niosomes to their fluidic membrane and ethanol concentration with elasticity	Penetrate easily keratinized mammalian skin layer

Table 2.
Market available and various emerging advanced VDDs for therapeutic applications [23, 24].

preparation of vesicular systems is broadly classified into three basic modes of dispersions such as physical dispersion involving handshaking and non-hand shaking technique (i), solvent dispersion including ethanol injection, ether injection, double emulsion, reverse phase evaporation, and stable plurilamellar vesicle

Lipid/surfactant	Applications	Characterization			References
		Zeta potential (mV)	Size (nm)	PDI	
Phospholipid	Solid lipid nanoparticles fortified with Erlotinib indicated a 2.12 fold increase in oral bioavailability with a reduction in pharmacokinetic variabilities, compared with the conventional dosage form	−33	177	—	[27]
Glyceryl mono stearate and Olieac acid	Solid lipid nanoparticles loaded vitamin E within cream indicated good stability at cold temperature with improved and controlled permeability indicated by diffusion study	~ − 24	~210	~ 0.24	[28]
Compritol 888	Rapamycin loaded solid lipid nanoparticles showed promising results for the treatment of lymphagioleiomyomatosis following pulmonary pathway with an appropriate size and necessary charge for controlled aerosol performance	−11.2	237	0.4	[29]
Phospholipid	A two-fold improvement in solubility was demonstrated for BCS class II drug in an entrapped solid lipid nanoparticulate form prepared via lyophilization process.	—	< 1000	—	[30]
Compritol 888 and phospholipid 90 G	Thiopental sodium loaded solid lipid nanoparticles showed cardiac protective effect with altered apoptosis marker, pro-inflammatory cytokines, inflammatory parameters, and reduced p38-MAPK level.	—	~ 68	~0.149	[31]
Glycerin monostearate and soybean lecithin	Paeonol lipid nanoparticulate via high-temperature emulsification-low temperature curing combined with ultrasound indicated improved oral bioavailability compared to alone Paeonol in simulated biological fluid.	~ −10	~ 150	~ 0.22	[32]
Stearic acid	The freeze-dried binary solid lipid nanoparticle of poor oral bioavailable cefixime showed 88% of encapsulation efficacy improvement in bioavailability	- 30.7	206.6	0.271	[33]
Gelucire	Statistically optimized thymoquinone lipid nanoparticles indicated 62.5% of encapsulation efficiency with potential dermal delivery carrier in the treatment of psoriasis	—	84.2	0.26	[34]

Lipid/surfactant	Applications	Characterization			References
		Zeta potential (mV)	Size (nm)	PDI	
Polysorbat 80	Sustained-release carnitine entrapped solid lipid nanoparticles indicated improved bioavailability via oral route of administration	−0.549	68–458.7	—	[35]
Oleic acid	Hydrophobic scaffolds fortified with oleic acid entrapped mRNA lipid nanoparticles showed promising material for curing inflammatory disease	1.5	93	0.08	[36]
Glyceryl monostearate	Nano lipid formulation remarkably improved the bio-efficacy of poorly water-soluble thymoquinone and demonstrated a promising perspective for oral delivery compared with conventional suspension.	- 12.32	188.66	0.319	[37]
Dioleo-yl-*sn*-glycero-phosphatidylcholine	Lipid nanoparticles containing short interfering RNA (siRNA) developed via alcohol dilution-lyophilization with cryoprotectants in a combination of sucrose and polyethylene glycol indicated significant particle stabilization compared to that of conventional ultrafiltration techniques	−1.89	155.0	0.118	[38]
Polyethylene glycol	Glutamic acid derivatives functionalized with non-ionic lipid nanoparticles were exposed as diagnostic tools for diabetic retinopathy.	—	120	0.259	[39]
Phosphatidylcholine	Curcumin loaded lipid vesicular system with surfactant demonstrated entrapment efficacy of 89.6% with Higuchi release kinetic and fickian diffusion	−11	339.3	—	[40]
1-stearoyl-rac-glycerol and L-α-phosphatidylcholine	Artemisone encapsulated nano-vesicular nisomes and solid lipid nanoparticles were evaluated against human melanoma A-375 cells and human keratinocytes cells, the results showed that the formulations have promise for use in cancer chemotherapy	−38 and − 12	211 and 295	—	[41]
Lecithin	Intranasal drug delivery of rizatriptan lipid nanoparticles indicated a significant increase in drug concentration in the brain compared with administered intravenously and could be a promising approach in the treatment of migraine	~ − 20	~ 250	~ 0.35	[42]

DOI: http://dx.doi.org/10.5772/intechopen.104510

Lipid/surfactant	Applications	Characterization			References
		Zeta potential (mV)	Size (nm)	PDI	
Stearic acid	Lopinavir fortified with stearic acid complexed γ-cyclodextrin indicated that inclusion complex can be used in the fabrication of solid lipid nanoparticles	−19.7	212	—	[43]
Coconut and jojoba oil	Lipid nanoparticles prepared using coconut oil indicated high encapsulation efficacy compared with jojoba oil with a regulated release profile	~ − 28	270	—	[44]
Cholesteryl oleate, glyceryl trioleate, cholesterol	Cationic solid lipid nanoparticles, reconstituted from low-density lipoprotein for the delivery of siRNA prepared following solvent-emulsification techniques demonstrated significant uptake by cells.	+ 41.76	117	—	[45]
Sodium taurodeoxycholate, oleic acid, stearic acid	Nanostructured lipid carriers loaded with lopinavir were developed for enhanced drug permeation with significant efficacy for transdermal administration	~ 37.5	179	~ 0.182	[46]
Gelucir and Precirol	Grape seed extract lipid nanoparticles followed melt homogenization an demonstrated increase in antioxidant response in the cells	+ 25.6	139–283	0.44–0.59	[47]
Glyceryl monostearate	Intranasal Repaglinide loaded solid lipid nanoparticles in-situ gel demonstrated maximum therapeutic outcome with dose reduction frequency for diabetes mellitus treatment	—	96.34	—	[48]
Glyceryl monostearate	Flavonoids incorporated solid lipid nanoparticles and nanolipid carrier indicated improved oral bioavailability with sustained therapeutic effect	~ 30	131–189	0.152–0.198	[49]
Lecithin	A temperature-dependent release of doxorubicin from cationic microgels fortified with vesicles indicated retardation at 25°C, compared with temperature between 39 and 41°C	—	—	—	[50]
L-α-phosphatidylcholine	Ethosomal gel fortified with quercetin demonstrated enhanced permeability with effective management of dermatitis on animals study	−26.33 − 39.3	324.1–359	0.241–0.554	[51]

Lipid/surfactant	Applications	Characterization			References
		Zeta potential (mV)	Size (nm)	PDI	
Dioleoylphosphatidylcholine, PEG 2000, cholesteryl hemisuccinate, and cholesteryl	Folate-coated and pH-sensitive liposome drug delivery containing irinotecan showed improved antitumor activity drug alone.	−4.1 – −11.1	159.2–165.2	0.09–0.12	[52]
Hydrogenated phosphatidylcholine, dipalmitoyl-sn-glycero-phosphorylglycerol sodium salt	Isoniazid-hydrogenated phosphatidylcholine induced the formation of ultra-stable quadrupole complexes, characterized by a high temperature showed the effect of isoniazid on the lipid organization that can be possibly employed as anti-TB nano-carries.	−35 – −53	52–57	0.07–0.11	[53]
1,2-dioleoyl-3-dimethylammonium-propane	pH-responsive nanocarrier based on dispersed self-assemblies of 1,2-dioleoyl-3-dimethylammonium-propane with human cathelicidin LL-37 in excess water was characterized and found that the fundamental structure contribute significantly to release of peptide	−4 – +10	269–286	0.16–0.21	[54]
Cholesterol, PEG-2000	Epirubicin is a lysyl oxidase that inhibits the crosslinking of elastin and collagen fibers that were complexed with lipid demonstrated superior inhibition of triple-negative breast cancer with prolonged survival, minimal cytotoxicity, and enhanced biocompatibility compared to free epirubicin.	−21.3 – −30.7	156–231	0.027–0.164	[55]
Kolliphor 188, stearyl amine, oleic acid, tween 80, kolliphor HS 15	pH-responsive multilamellar vesicle loaded vancomycin indicated effective targeting with enhanced antibacterial efficacy	- 5.55	62.5	0.15	[56]
Phosphatidylcholine	Chrysin transfersomes vesicle fortified within chitosan composite showed improvement in the therapeutic performance against doxorubicin-induced cognitive impairment	−26.5 – +46.3	121.5–617.2	0.154–0.66	[57]
Phosphatidylcholine, cholesterol	An attempt for the nose to brain delivery of olanzapine liposome using Design-Expert demonstrated regulated release for 24 h with acceptable physicochemical characterization	−11.46 – −27.53	268.25–325.32	—	[58]

DOI: http://dx.doi.org/10.5772/intechopen.104510

Lipid/surfactant	Applications	Characterization			References
		Zeta potential (mV)	Size (nm)	PDI	
Cholesterol, Dipalmitoyl phosphatidylcholine	Vesicle entrapped amikacin liposome fabricated in aerosol-based drug delivery systems demonstrated efficacious delivery of amikacin after nebulization using lamira nebulizer through inhalation every time with no or low variation	—	269–296	—	[59]
Phospholipon, polysorbate 80	Elastic liposome loaded with desmopressin acetate demonstrated a high permeation flux for therapeutic efficacy on transdermal drug delivery with hemo and biocompatibility	23.6–77.4	111.7–335.6	0.11–0.47	[60]
Amphiphilic block copolymer containing PEG	Synchrotron small-angle x-ray scattering techniques-based synthesis of amphiphilic block copolymer stabilize monoolein nanoparticles containing a range of non-lamellar lyotropic liquid crystal mesophases, demonstrated response towards H2O2, pH, and temperature.	—	140–300	0.38	[61]
Sorbitan monostearate – 60, Tween 80, Brij 97	Carvedilol-loaded nano-spanlastics prepared by ethanol injection techniques demonstrated good deformability index and stability with enhancement in permeability flux after 24 h of release study. Moreover, *in vivo* study indicated superiority in the protection of heart tissue over Carvid®.	—	196.5–512.1	0.21–0.43	[62]
1,2-Dioleoyl-sn-glycero-3-phosphocholine	An integrated quartz crystal microbalance dissipation and localized surface plasmon resonance single sensor were developed to monitor the adsorption and rupture of the liposomes. The results indicated that the device could provide a powerful tool to gain deeper insights into biomolecular interactions, expanding with numerous applications such as monitoring of conformational changes in proteins, oligonucleotides, viruses, bacteria, vesicles, and cells.	—	—	—	[63]
Polyoxyethylenesorbiton monooleate, sodium cholate	Ethosomes and transethosomes loaded cholecalciferol demonstrated rapid intracellular accumulation to support the scientific background for exploring the transdermal and *in vivo* investigation of administration in different experimental and pathological conditions.	—	111.2–276.7	0.085–0.163	[64]

Lipid/surfactant	Applications	Characterization			References
		Zeta potential (mV)	Size (nm)	PDI	
Glycerol	Minoxidil-lo glycerosomesaded demonstrated stable zeta potential, controlled size, and regulated *in vitro* release with excellent stability on storage. Moreover, the presence of high content of glycerol indicated multifaceted application including humectant, emollient, and penetration enhancer.	—	—	—	[65]
Phosphatidylcholine, cholesterol, oleic acid, stearic acid	Amphotericin B-miltefosine nanovesicle prepared using ethanol injection technique showed good compatibility, extended drug release, convenient vesicle size, and high drug entrapment for effective *in vivo* antileishmanial investigations.	−27.3 ± 2.8	169.7–202.6	0.19 ± 0.04	[66]
Dimyristoyl-sn-glycerol3-phosphocholine, dipalmitoyl-sn-glycero-3-phosphocholine	Label-free surface-sensitive quartz crystal microbalance with dissipation monitoring method used to understand the time-dependent phase transition from nano viscosity measurements, the transfer rates, between two vesicle populations consisting of lipids with the same head group and differing alkyl chain length can be estimated.	—	110.0–130.0	0.05–0.12	[67]
Phospholipon®	Topical application across the stratum corneum of unsaturated fatty acid vesicles loaded ammonium gntlycyrrhizinate demonstrated high efficacy compared to its free form.	−42 – −50	146–284	0.17–0.22	[68]
L-α-phosphatidylcholine	The fusion of amphiphilic polypeptides with n-decyl side chains leads to the engulfing of liposomes and multilayered vesicles. Such multilayered vesicle comes with the advantage of reducing the permeability of the cargo in the aqueous core	—	100	—	[69]
Phospholipon 90H	Terbinafine HCl loaded ethosome for enhanced topical application in the management of fungal diseases	−23 – −48	90–199	0.33–0.47	[70]
Hydrogenated soybean lecithin	Black soybean seed coat extract encapsulated nano-dispersion showed improved stability, radical-scavenging capacity with high cellular compatibility	−3.50 – −30.12	27.6–121.1	0.194–0.386	[71]

DOI: http://dx.doi.org/10.5772/intechopen.104510

Lipid/surfactant	Applications	Characterization			References
		Zeta potential (mV)	Size (nm)	PDI	
1,2-Dioleoyl-sn-glycero-3-phosphocholine, cholesterol	Ferulic acid loaded vesicle showed effective membrane surface interaction due to electrostatically zwitterionic polar heads of the lipid, which also depends on the concentration of lipids	−0.4 – 1	117–124	0.06–0.09	[72]
Dipalmitoyl-phosphatidylcholine Hyaluronic acid	Thermosensitive liposomal formulation functionalized with hyaluronic acid encapsulated cisplatin demonstrated a controlled release profile with a possible diffusion rate before reaching 42°C.	20–38	100–130	—	[73]
PEGylated soy lecithin	PEGylated soy lecithin liposome of oxaliplatin showed enhanced activity against human breast cancer cells with reduced cytotoxicity against mouse fibroblast cells.	−39 – −50	180–200	0.2–0.3	[74]
L-α-phosphatidylcholine	*In situ* gel fortified with ketoconazole, trans ethosomes showed no irritation to the cornea with deep penetration to the posterior eye segment without cytotoxicity	12.8–36.8	220.6–1063.3	—	[75]
Pramipexole dihydrochloride, 1,2-Dioleoyl-sn-glycero-3-phosphocholine, 1-Arachidoyl-2Hydroxy-sn-Glycero-3-Phosphocholine, 1–2-didecanoyl-sn-Glycero-3-phosphocholine, cholesterol, sodium cholate, sodium hexadecyl sulfate, cetylpyridinium chloride	Liposomal formulation gel of pramipexole incorporated with edge activators and charge inducer improved the drug permeation, and the extent of penetration depending on phospholipid compared with conventional liposomal gel.	+3.83 – −52.2	117.0–289.7	—	[76]

Table 3.
Recent updates on LNs based drug delivery system considering solid lipid nanoparticles and vesicular drug delivery system.

method (ii), and detergent solubilization (iii). Transferosomes and ethosomes were introduced as VDDs for localized and targeted administration of low or less permeable drugs through the skin, which requires the addition of permeation enhancer, however progression in the research reported that the incorporation of surfactant as edge activator within vesicles can significantly improve the penetration and drug loading capacity. The pharmaceutical characterization involves the determination of size, shape, and size distribution, surface charge, entrapment efficacy, dispersibility, syringeability, lamellarity through freeze-fracture microscopy, phase behaviors, *in vitro – in vivo* drug release, quantitative determination of phospholipid, and cholesterol quantification. Moreover, vesicles fortified in target or localized drug delivery systems are also evaluated for their efficacy including stability, esthetic property, etc. [23]. **Table 2** represents the various types of VDDs with their therapeutic applications.

Solid lipid nanoparticles are generally formulated using high shear homogenization, ultrasonication, microemulsion followed by supercritical liquid innovation, splash drying, dissolvable emulsification/vanishing, dissolvable infusion, and dissolvable emulsification-dissemination techniques [25]. Solid lipid nanoparticles are extensively characterized for size, shape, polydispersity index, zeta potential, entrapment efficacy, crystallization tendency, polymorphic behavior, the viscosity of the solid-state formulation, and *in vitro-in vivo* drug release. Solid lipid nanoparticles are administered via various routes including oral, parenteral, transdermal, pulmonary, rectal, etc. for achieving enhanced therapeutic efficacy of low or less permeable drugs via dermal administration or low water-soluble drugs with improved bioavailability [26]. Recent updates on lipid nanocarriers-based drug delivery systems (solid lipid nanoparticles and vesicle entrapped drug delivery systems) are presented in **Table 3**.

4. Future prospects and challenges with vesicular and solid lipid nanoparticulate drug delivery system

Nanostructured lipid carriers contain an unsaturated solid lipid core that enables the encapsulation of highly lipophilic drugs, protecting them from degradation, and enhancing their stability. Literature indicates that during the past decades, the number of studies elaborating NLCs-based formulations has been drastically increased. Lipid nanostructure carriers such as SLNs, VDDs, and or NLCs have been extensively used and further investigated as carrier systems for drug delivery. Moreover, these nanostructure carrier has demonstrated excellent improvement in the therapeutic efficacy with an increase in targeting specific tissue or organ for low permeable and water-insoluble drugs. The rise in NLCs technology is essentially due to defeated barriers within the technological process of lipid fortified nanoparticles formulation and increased knowledge of the underlying mechanisms of transport of NLCs via varied routes of administration. Although NLCs have shown several advantages, compared with conventional dosage form and promising application in the delivery of various categories of synthetic and bioactive, that presents challenges in their application. The challenges associated with NLCs are as follow: complex manufacturing process, stability during storage, clinical translational barriers, cell-specific delivery, misconceptions, challenges specific to the receptor, ligand, and carriers, etc. [77].

5. Conclusions

Nano lipid structure carriers, composition and formulations techniques have a profound influence on their physicochemical properties and efficacy as drug delivery systems. The lipid carriers have evolved over the years and they have shown promise for treating various clinical diseases and complications including psoriasis, dermatitis, rosacea, vitiligo, acne, fungal infections, several systemic infections, etc. Taking into account the increase in the number of patented NLCs-based formulations and the increase in the availability of data so far, it can be expected that the number of clinical trials pertaining NLCs will substantially increase in near future. Moreover, now NLCs appear to be one step closer to its translation into the market to the clinic.

Author details

Sudarshan Singh[1*], Tanvi R. Dodiya[2], Rajesh Dodiya[3], Yogesh V. Ushir[4] and Slamet Widodo [5]

1 Food Technology and Innovation Center of Excellence, Institute of Research and Innovation, School of Allied Health Sciences, Walailak University, Nakhon Si Thammarat, Thailand

2 Parul Institute of Pharmacy and Research, Parul University, Vadodara, Gujarat, India

3 Laxminarayandev College of Pharmacy, Bharuch, Gujarat, India

4 SMBT Institute of Diploma Pharmacy, Nashik, Maharashtra, India

5 Faculty of Medicine of University of Malahayati, Lampung, Indonesia

*Address all correspondence to: sudarshansingh83@hotmail.com

References

[1] Sainaga Jyothi VGS, Ghouse SM, Khatri DK, Nanduri S, Singh SB, Madan J. Lipid nanoparticles in topical dermal drug delivery: Does chemistry of lipid persuade skin penetration? Journal of Drug Delivery Science and Technology. 2022;**69**:103176

[2] Naseri N, Valizadeh H, Zakeri-Milani P. Solid lipid nanoparticles and nanostructured lipid carriers: Structure, preparation and application. Advanced Pharmaceutical Bulletin. 2015;**5**(3):305-313

[3] Rawal SU, Patel MM. Chapter 2—Lipid nanoparticulate systems: Modern versatile drug carriers. In: Grumezescu AM, editor. Lipid Nanocarriers for Drug Targeting. William Andrew Publishing; 2018. pp. 49-138

[4] Mukherjee S, Ray S, Thakur R. Solid lipid nanoparticles: A modern formulation approach in drug delivery system. Indian Journal of Pharmaceutical Sciences. 2009;**71**(4):349

[5] Sathali A, Ekambaram P, Priyanka K. Solid lipid nanoparticles: A review. Scientific Reviews & Chemical Communications. 2012;**2**(1):80-102

[6] Kamble MS, Vaidya KK, Bhosale AV, Chaudhari PD. Solid lipid nanoparticles and nanostructured lipid carriers—An overview. International Journal of Pharmaceutical, Chemical and Biological Sciences. 2012;**2**(4):681-691

[7] Kumar A, Badde S, Kamble R, Pokharkar VB. Development and characterization of liposomal drug delivery system for nimesulide. International Journal of Pharmacy and Pharmaceutical Sciences. 2010;**2**(4):87-89

[8] Dwivedi C, Sahu R, Tiwari SP, Satapathy T, Roy A. Role of liposome in novel drug delivery system. Journal of Drug Delivery and Therapeutics. 2014;**4**(2):116-129

[9] Attama AA, Momoh MA, Builders PF. Lipid nanoparticulate drug delivery systems: A revolution in dosage form design and development. Recent Advances in Novel Drug Carrier Systems. 2012;**5**:107-140

[10] Das S, Chaudhury A. Recent advances in lipid nanoparticle formulations with solid matrix for oral drug delivery. AAPS PharmSciTech. 2011;**12**(1):62-76

[11] Sinha VR, Srivastava S, Goel H, Jindal V. Solid lipid nanoparticles (SLN'S)-trends and implications in drug targeting. International Journal of Advances in Pharmaceutical Sciences. 2010;**1**(3):212-238

[12] Ashkar A, Sosnik A, Davidovich-Pinhas M. Structured edible lipid-based particle systems for oral drug-delivery. Biotechnology Advances. 2021:107789

[13] Paiva P, Medina FE, Viegas M, Ferreira P, Neves RP, Sousa JoP, et al. Animal fatty acid synthase: A chemical nanofactory. Chemical Reviews. 2021;**121**(15):9502-9553

[14] Liolios V, Tananaki C, Kanelis D, Rodopoulou MA, Argena N. Effect of geographical origin on lipid content and fatty acids composition of bee collected pollen. Journal of Apicultural Research. 2022:1-9

[15] Ramírez Rangel E. Contribution to the Study of Heterogeneous Catalytic Reactions in SCFs: Hydrogenation of Sunflower Oil in Pd Catalysts at Single-Phase Conditions. Catalonia, Spain:

Universitat Politècnica de Catalunya; 2005

[16] Coppens E, Desmaële D, Naret T, Garcia-Argote S, Feuillastre S, Pieters G, et al. Gemcitabine lipid prodrug nanoparticles: Switching the lipid moiety and changing the fate in the bloodstream. International Journal of Pharmaceutics. 2021;**609**:121076

[17] Lewis B. Classification of lipoproteins and lipoprotein disorders. Journal of Clinical Pathology Supplement (Association of Clinical Pathologists). 1973;**5**:26

[18] Madsen CM, Varbo A, Nordestgaard BG. Novel insights from human studies on the role of high-density lipoprotein in mortality and noncardiovascular disease. Arteriosclerosis, Thrombosis, and Vascular Biology. 2021;**41**(1):128-140

[19] Kumar Dutta A. Introductory chapter: Surfactants in household and personal care formulations—An overview. The Journal of Surfactants and Detergents. 2019;**1**:1-10

[20] Hill M, Moaddel T. Soap Structure and Phase Behavior, Soap Manufacturing Technology. London, United Kingdom: Elsevier; 2016. pp. 35-54

[21] Dri DA, Marianecci C, Carafa M, Gaucci E, Gramaglia D. Surfactants, nanomedicines and nanocarriers: A critical evaluation on clinical trials. Pharmaceutics. 2021;**13**(3):381

[22] Saraf S., W. Chunglok, Herbal bioactive: A booster dose for advanced pharmaceutical nanoscience, in: Vivek Dave, Swarnlata Saraf, Ram Kumar Sahu (Ed.), Advanced Pharmaceutical Herbal Nanoscience: Targeted Drug Delivery System, Bentham Science Publishers Pte. Ltd, Singapore, 2022, pp. 53-75.

[23] Biju SS, Talegaonkar S, Mishra PR, Khar RK. Vesicular systems: An overview. The Indian Journal of Pharmaceutical Sciences. 2006;**68**(2):141-153

[24] Chacko IA, Ghate VM, Dsouza L, Lewis SA. Lipid vesicles: A versatile drug delivery platform for dermal and transdermal applications. Colloids and Surfaces. B, Biointerfaces. 2020;**195**:111262

[25] Omray L. Formulation and characterization of solid lipid nanoparticles for transdermal delivery of testosterone. International Journal of Pharmaceutical Sciences and Research. 2014;**5**(7):323-328

[26] Lingayat VJ, Zarekar NS, Shendge RS. Solid lipid nanoparticles: A review. Nanoscience and Nanotechnology Research. 2017;**2**:67-72

[27] Rampaka R, Ommi K, Chella N. Role of solid lipid nanoparticles as drug delivery vehicles on the pharmacokinetic variability of erlotinib HCl. Journal of Drug Delivery Science and Technology. 2021;**66**:102886

[28] Shah F, Sarheed O, Usman S. Development and evaluation of a cream containing solid lipid nanoparticles loaded with vitamin E. Pakistan Journal of Pharmaceutical Sciences. 2021;**34**(6):2109-2119

[29] Landh E, Moir LM, Gomes Dos Reis L, Traini D, Young PM, Ong HX. Inhaled rapamycin solid lipid nano particles for the treatment of lymphangioleiomyomatosis. European Journal of Pharmaceutical Sciences: Official Journal of the European Federation for Pharmaceutical Sciences. 2020;**142**:105098

[30] Karri VVSR, Ananthan S, Mude L. Development, charaterization and solubility enhancement of BCS class

II drug phenytoin by solid dispersion techniques. International Journal of Research In Pharmaceutical Sciences. 2020;**11**(1):403-410

[31] Zhu C, Li W, Wang X, Xue J, Zhao L, Song Y, et al. Thiopental sodium loaded solid lipid nano-particles attenuates obesity-induced cardiac dysfunction and cardiac hypertrophy via inactivation of inflammatory pathway. Drug Delivery. 2020;**27**(1):1188-1200

[32] Sun Y, Li L, Xie H, Wang Y, Gao S, Zhang L, et al. Primary studies on construction and evaluation of ion-sensitive in situ gel loaded with paeonol-solid lipid nanoparticles for intranasal drug delivery. International Journal of Nanomedicine. 2020;**15**:3137-3160

[33] Kamran M, Khan MA, Rehman MU, Shafique M, Khan A, Ahmad S. Binary solid lipid nanosuspension containing cefixime: preparation, characterization and comparative *in-vivo* evaluation. Beilstein Archives. 2019:1-25

[34] Ali A, Ali S, Aqil M, Imam SS, Ahad A, Qadir A. Thymoquinone loaded dermal lipid nano particles: Box Behnken design optimization to preclinical psoriasis assessment. Journal of Drug Delivery Science and Technology. 2019;**52**:713-721

[35] Baskar V, Lakshmi B, Ibrahim K, Shabeer TK, Jawahar Ali A. Modeling of ayurveda ghee based solid lipid nano particles and their comprehensive pharmacokinetics study. Materials Today: Proceedings. 2021;**36**:782-788

[36] Tanaka H, Watanabe A, Konishi M, Nakai Y, Yoshioka H, Ohkawara T, et al. The delivery of mRNA to colon inflammatory lesions by lipid-nano-particles containing environmentally-sensitive lipid-like materials with oleic acid scaffolds. Heliyon. 2018;**4**(12):e00959

[37] Alam M, Najmi AK, Ahmad I, Ahmad FJ, Akhtar MJ, Imam SS, et al. Formulation and evaluation of nano lipid formulation containing CNS acting drug: molecular docking, *in-vitro* assessment and bioactivity detail in rats. Artificial Cells, Nanomedicine, and Biotechnology. 2018;**46**(suppl 2):46-57

[38] Shirane D, Tanaka H, Nakai Y, Yoshioka H, Akita H. Development of an alcohol dilution-lyophilization method for preparing lipid nanoparticles containing encapsulated siRNA. Biological & Pharmaceutical Bulletin. 2018;**41**(8):1291-1294

[39] Ghisaidoobe AB, Yun WS, Chung SJ. Development of stable non-ionic lipid nanoparticles. Journal of Nanoscience and Nanotechnology. 2016;**16**(11):11873-11881

[40] Patel R, Singh S, Singh S, Sheth N, Gendle R. Development and characterization of curcumin loaded transfersome for transdermal delivery. Journal of Pharmaceutical Sciences and Research. 2009;**1**(4):71

[41] Dwivedi A, Mazumder A, du Plessis L, du Preez JL, Haynes RK, du Plessis J. In vitro anti-cancer effects of artemisone nano-vesicular formulations on melanoma cells. Nanomedicine : Nanotechnology, Biology, and Medicine. 2015;**11**(8):2041-2050

[42] Singh A, Ubrane R, Prasad P, Ramteke S. Preparation and characterization of rizatriptan benzoate loaded solid lipid nanoparticles for brain targeting. Materials Today: Proceedings. 2015;**2**(9, Part A):4521-4543

[43] Negi JS, Chattopadhyay P, Sharma AK, Ram V. Preparation of gamma cyclodextrin stabilized solid lipid nanoparticles (SLNS) using stearic acid–γ-cyclodextrin inclusion complex. Journal

of Inclusion Phenomena and Macrocyclic Chemistry. 2014;**80**(3-4):359-368

[44] Kang K-C, Jeong N-H, Lee C-I, Pyo H-B. Preparation and characterization of SLNs (W/O/W type) contained lipoic acid PEG ester by variation lipid. Journal of Industrial and Engineering Chemistry. 2009;**15**(4):529-536

[45] Kim HR, Kim IK, Bae KH, Lee SH, Lee Y, Park TG. Cationic solid lipid nanoparticles reconstituted from low density lipoprotein components for delivery of siRNA. Molecular Pharmaceutics. 2008;**5**(4):622-631

[46] Moura RBP, Andrade LM, Alonso L, Alonso A, Marreto RN, Taveira SF. Combination of lipid nanoparticles and iontophoresis for enhanced lopinavir skin permeation: Impact of electric current on lipid dynamics. European Journal of Pharmaceutical Sciences. 2022;**168**:106048

[47] Trapani A, Esteban MÁ, Curci F, Manno DE, Serra A, Fracchiolla G, et al. Solid lipid nanoparticles administering antioxidant grape seed-derived polyphenol compounds: A potential application in aquaculture. Molecules. 2022;**27**(2):344

[48] Elkarray SM, Farid RM, Abd-Alhaseeb MM, Omran GA, Habib DA. Intranasal repaglinide-solid lipid nanoparticles integrated in situ gel outperform conventional oral route in hypoglycemic activity. Journal of Drug Delivery Science and Technology. 2022;**68**:103086

[49] Ryu S, Jin M, Lee H-K, Wang M-H, Baek J-S, Cho C-W. Effects of lipid nanoparticles on physicochemical properties, cellular uptake, and lymphatic uptake of 6-methoxflavone. Journal of Pharmaceutical Investigation. 2022;**52**:233-241

[50] Panova IG, Sudareva EA, Novoskoltseva OA, Spiridonov VV, Shtilman MI, Richtering W, et al. Temperature-induced unloading of liposomes bound to microgels. Colloids and Surfaces A: Physicochemical and Engineering Aspects. 2021;**630**:127590

[51] Pandey S, Dwivedi D, Asif S, Awasthi V, Kaur G, Nimisha. Investigating the potential of quercetin enthused nano lipoidal system for the management of dermatitis. Research Journal of Pharmacy and Technology. 2021;**14**(12):6516-6526

[52] Nunes SS, Miranda SEM, de Oliveira Silva J, Fernandes RS, de Alcântara Lemos J, de Aguiar Ferreira C, et al. pH-responsive and folate-coated liposomes encapsulating irinotecan as an alternative to improve efficacy of colorectal cancer treatment. Biomedicine & Pharmacotherapy. 2021;**144**:112317

[53] Sciolla F, Truzzolillo D, Chauveau E, Trabalzini S, Di Marzio L, Carafa M, et al. Influence of drug/lipid interaction on the entrapment efficiency of isoniazid in liposomes for antitubercular therapy: A multi-faced investigation. Colloids and Surfaces. B, Biointerfaces. 2021;**208**:112054

[54] Gontsarik M, Mansour AB, Hong L, Guizar-Sicairos M, Salentinig S. pH-responsive aminolipid nanocarriers for antimicrobial peptide delivery. Journal of Colloid and Interface Science. 2021;**603**:398-407

[55] De Vita A, Liverani C, Molinaro R, Martinez JO, Hartman KA, Spadazzi C, et al. Lysyl oxidase engineered lipid nanovesicles for the treatment of triple negative breast cancer. Scientific Reports. 2021;**11**(1):5107

[56] Omolo CA, Hassan D, Devnarain N, Jaglal Y, Mocktar C, Kalhapure RS,

et al. Formulation of pH responsive multilamellar vesicles for targeted delivery of hydrophilic antibiotics. Colloids and Surfaces. B, Biointerfaces. 2021;**207**:112043

[57] Ibrahim SS, Abo Elseoud OG, Mohamedy MH, Amer MM, Mohamed YY, Elmansy SA, et al. Nose-to-brain delivery of chrysin transfersomal and composite vesicles in doxorubicin-induced cognitive impairment in rats: Insights on formulation, oxidative stress and TLR4/NF-kB/NLRP3 pathways. Neuropharmacology. 2021;**197**:108738

[58] Vani GN, Alagusundaram M, Chandrasekar KB. Formulation and optimization and in vitro characterization of olanzapine liposome. International Journal of Applied Pharmaceutics. 2021;**13**(5):109-114

[59] Li Z, Perkins W, Cipolla D. Robustness of aerosol delivery of amikacin liposome inhalation suspension using the eFlow® technology. European Journal of Pharmaceutics and Biopharmaceutics. 2021;**166**:10-18

[60] Altamimi MA, Hussain A, Alshehri S, Imam SS. Experimental design based optimization and *ex vivo* permeation of desmopressin acetate loaded elastic liposomes using rat skin. Pharmaceutics. 2021;**13**(7):1047

[61] Zhai J, Fan B, Thang SH, Drummond CJ. Novel amphiphilic block copolymers for the formation of stimuli-responsive non-lamellar lipid nanoparticles. Molecules. 2021;**26**(12):3648

[62] Sallam NM, Sanad RAB, Ahmed MM, Khafagy ELS, Ghorab M, Gad S. Impact of the mucoadhesive lyophilized wafer loaded with novel carvedilol nano-spanlastics on biochemical markers in the heart of spontaneously hypertensive rat models. Drug Delivery and Translational Research. 2021;**11**(3):1009-1036

[63] Asai N, Matsumoto N, Yamashita I, Shimizu T, Shingubara S, Ito T. Detailed analysis of liposome adsorption and its rupture on the liquid-solid interface monitored by LSPR and QCM-D integrated sensor. Sensing and Bio-Sensing Research. 2021;**32**:100415

[64] Costanzo M, Esposito E, Sguizzato M, Lacavalla MA, Drechsler M, Valacchi G, et al. Formulative study and intracellular fate evaluation of ethosomes and transethosomes for vitamin D3 delivery. International Journal of Molecular Sciences. 2021;**22**(10):5341

[65] Sharma V, Rani D, Manchanda R, Chaurasia H. Formulation, design and optimization of glycerosomes for topical delivery of minoxidil. Research Journal of Pharmacy and Technology. 2021;**14**(5):2367-2374

[66] Bezabeh MF, Werbovetz KA, Murthy KVR. Formulation and evaluation of amphotericin B and miltefosine combination nanovesicles. International Journal of Applied Pharmaceutics. 2021;**13**(3):74-78

[67] Bar L, Cordoyiannis G, Neupane S, Goole J, Grosfils P, Losada-Pérez P. Asymmetric lipid transfer between zwitterionic vesicles by nanoviscosity measurements. Nanomaterials. 2021;**11**(5):1087

[68] Cristiano MC, Mancuso A, Fresta M, Torella D, De Gaetano F, Ventura CA, et al. Topical unsaturated fatty acid vesicles improve antioxidant activity of ammonium glycyrrhizinate. Pharmaceutics. 2021;**13**(4):548

[69] Omarova M, Zhang Y, Mkam Tsengam IK, He J, Yu T, Zhang D, et al.

Hydrophobe containing polypeptoids complex with lipids and induce fusogenesis of lipid vesicles. The Journal of Physical Chemistry B. 2021;**125**(12):3145-3152

[70] Dol HS, Hajare AA. Screening of effective formulation techniques for designing and fabrication of terbinafine hydrochloride ethosomes. Research Journal of Pharmacy and Technology. 2021;**14**(3):1353-1359

[71] Shen P-T, Chiu S-W, Chang J-Y, Chung T-W, Liang C-H, Deng M-J, et al. Formation and characterization of hydrogenated soybean lecithin/ TPGS nano-dispersions as a potential carrier for active herbal agents. Colloids and Surfaces A: Physicochemical and Engineering Aspects. 2021;**611**:125796

[72] Andrade S, Ramalho MJ, Loureiro JA, Pereira MC. The biophysical interaction of ferulic acid with liposomes as biological membrane model: The effect of the lipid bilayer composition. Journal of Molecular Liquids. 2021;**324**:114689

[73] Gomes IP, Malachias Â, Maia ALC, Lages EB, Ferreira FA, Alves RJ, et al. Thermosensitive liposomes containing cisplatin functionalized by hyaluronic acid: Preparation and physicochemical characterization. Journal of Nanoparticle Research. 2022;**24**(2):30

[74] Le NTT, Vu MT, Nguyen NH, Nguyen-Huu A-M, Nguyen DH. Preparation and *in vitro* evaluation of PEGylated liposomes as effective nanocarrier for delivery of oxaliplatin. Journal of Materials Research. 2021;**36**(2):475-486

[75] Ahmed TA, Alzahrani MM, Sirwi A, Alhakamy NA. Study the antifungal and ocular permeation of ketoconazole from ophthalmic formulations containing trans-ethosomes nanoparticles. Pharmaceutics. 2021;**13**(2):151

[76] Trivedi R, Umekar M, Kotagale N, Bonde S, Taksande J. Design, evaluation and *in vivo* pharmacokinetic study of a cationic flexible liposomes for enhanced transdermal delivery of pramipexole. Journal of Drug Delivery Science and Technology. 2021;**61**:102313

[77] Beloqui A, Solinís MÁ, Rodríguez-Gascón A, Almeida AJ, Préat V. Nanostructured lipid carriers: Promising drug delivery systems for future clinics. Nanomedicine: Nanotechnology, Biology and Medicine. 2016;**12**(1):143-161

Chapter 8

Lipid and Polymeric Nanocapsules

Sarai Rochín-Wong and Itziar Vélaz Rivas

Abstract

In recent years, innovative drug nanocarriers have been developed to enhance stability, bioavailability, and provide sustained release. In this chapter, systems based on natural macromolecules, lipids, or polymeric/polyelectrolyte nanocapsules and their principal chemical and functional characteristics are described. Nano-vesicular systems are especially relevant in different fields. Particularly, a promising potential is offered by systems based on colloidal nanocapsules, that exhibit a typical core-shell structure in which the drug can be confined into the cavity or in the polymeric coating that surrounds it. Both the cavity and the active substance can be lipophilic or hydrophilic and in solid or liquid form depending on the materials and methods used, making these nanocapsules attractive carriers for drug delivery. In addition, a compilation of different methods and materials employed in the preparation of these nanosystems and a recent review of applications of lipid and polymeric nanocapsules have been made, focussing on the encapsulation of drugs.

Keywords: drug nanocarriers, core-shell nanocapsules, lipid nanocapsules, colloidal nanocapsules, polymeric nanocapsules, drug delivery

1. Introduction

Nanostructures appear as either nanofibers, nanocompounds, nanomembranes, nanoparticles, or nanotubes, and have applications in different fields, such as medicine, cosmetics, environment, and nutrition. They can be used in biomedicine for diagnosis or the prevention and treatment of different diseases. They are employed as drug, protein, nucleic acid, and peptide carriers, or as biosensors, as well as for medical imaging [1, 2]. The incorporation of active principles in nano- or micrometric scale devices is called encapsulation. The encapsulated material is covered with a different type of material, which can be a polymer, a lipid, or a macromolecule. In general, encapsulation provides an increase in the stability of the encapsulated material, it also preserves its chemical and therapeutic properties, and it enlarges its average life, since it protects it from the effects of pH, heat, light, oxygen, humidity, and even from enzymatic degradation by nucleases and proteases, for instance. Besides, encapsulation offers the possibility to modify the physicochemical properties of the encapsulated material to facilitate manipulation, it reduces the loss of volatile compounds, it can mask unpleasant flavor and odor, improve bioavailability, and help the controlled release of active substances following a certain stimulus (pH, T, P, etc.) [3].

Regarding medical applications, encapsulated systems offer great possibilities of improving the safety and efficiency of countless drugs. They are capable of traveling across biological barriers, such as the skin, the gastrointestinal or respiratory mucous membranes, and even the blood-brain barrier (BBB). They can reach the target organ, tissue, or cell group where the drug has to act; they can even reach intracellular compartments. The distribution of the active principle, and therefore, its concentration in the target, is influenced by the size and the properties of the nanoparticles. This dependence permits minimization of side effects and an increase in the therapeutic power of the released molecule of interest, for example, in cancer treatment. Administration in the form of nanoparticles allows to orally dispense antitumor drugs, as well as biotechnologically originated molecules (peptides, proteins, plasmids, etc.), which are very sensitive to physicochemical and enzymatic degradation and cannot cross the mucous membranes [3].

Organic nanocarriers include nanoparticles such as solid lipid nanocarriers, liposomes, dendrimers, polymeric nanocarriers, micelles, and viral nanocarriers. Nanoparticles are defined as solid vesicles under 1000 nm, usually between 100 and 500 nm, formed by natural macromolecules, lipids, or synthetic polymers. For therapeutic application they must have a size under 200 nm since the width of the microcapillaries of the body is 200 nm [1]. The active principle is incorporated inside the nanoparticle, which can be a nanocapsule or a nanosphere. Nanocapsules are kind of reservoirs, they are vesicular systems, that is to say, traditional hollow shell structures constituted by a polymeric or lipid membrane and an internal core where the molecules of the drug are dissolved or dispersed. As to nanospheres, they are spherical matrixial systems, and the drug is homogeneously dispersed in the solid polymeric matrix [2, 4]. Core-shell nanoparticles offer great versatility and, depending on their composition, permit the encapsulation of a huge variety of molecules in solid, liquid, and semi-solid state. The nanocapsule shells can be prepared from several materials, such as polymers, lipids, phospholipids, and silica [5]. Different methods are used to build the core-shell structure, the polymers and methods employed are chosen according to the properties of the compound to be encapsulated and its application [6].

Some criteria to be considered before nanoencapsulation are clear definition of the desired objective, assurance that the active principle does not degrade during the fabrication process and that it disperses homogeneously inside the nanocapsule, choice of a suitable polymer or macromolecule, and cost/performance optimization. The encapsulating material must be biodegradable/bioerodible and inert with respect to the encapsulated material both in production and storage, offer the highest protection of the active principle, and be processable in suitable solvents for biomedical application. There is a real influence of the nature of the material and the production methodology on the physicochemical properties of the prepared systems. The main characteristics of nanoparticles are their large specific surface area, their homogenous dispersion in fluids, the capacity to encapsulate small molecules, and an adequate release rate [3].

In this chapter, systems based on natural macromolecules, lipids, or polymeric/polyelectrolyte nanocapsules and their principal chemical and functional characteristics are described. In addition, a compilation of different methods and materials employed in the preparation of nanocapsules and a recent review of applications of lipid and polymeric nanocapsules have been made, focussing on the encapsulation of drugs.

2. Common materials

As it has been mentioned above, polymeric nanoparticles and lipid-based systems are included in the research of efficient drug-delivery systems. Lipid polymer hybrid nanoparticles (LPNs) are being explored as well, combining the advantages and properties of polymers and lipids [7]. In this chapter, mainly polymeric and lipid nanocapsules are dealt with.

2.1 Polymeric nanocapsules

Polymeric nanoparticles are colloidal and are prepared from degradable/nondegradable hydrophilic/hydrophobic natural/synthetic polymers. Natural polymers, such as polysaccharides (hyaluronic acid, starch, maltodextrins, chitosan, cyclodextrins, alginate, carrageenan, gums, and agar) or proteins (gliadin, vicilin, legumin, casein, gelatines, and albumin) are not usually used alone due to the variability of their purity. Nanocapsules based on saccharides (glyco nanocapsules) are very interesting for bioapplications. The synthetic polymers usually used are poly(lactic-co-glycolic) acid (PLGA), poly(lactic acid) (PLA), poly(ε-caprolactone) (PCL), polyanionic cellulose (PAC), poly(D,L-glycolide) (PLG), polyethylene glycol (PEG), and poly-cyanoacrylate (PCA) [1, 7–10]. Polymeric nanoparticles made from natural or synthetic polymers are easy to modify superficially and are, in general, stable. Their features can be tuned to achieve better bioavailability and a controlled drug release in specific locations. Biodegradable polymers have been widely used for the preparation of systems to control drug release, which can stabilize certain labile molecules, such as proteins, peptides, or DNA, and can also be used for site-specific drug targeting. The preparation of biodegradable polymeric nanoparticles for application in tissue engineering is also pursued [1]. As they are biodegradable, they can remain for days or even weeks and release the drug in the target during that time. PLA and PLGA have proved to be effective with intracellular drugs. PLGA is usually combined with PEG, as PEGylation increases solubility and stability in water, reduces intramolecular aggregation, decreases immunogenicity, and prolongs the permanence of the drug in the systemic circulation [1, 7]. As an example, a recent review (in press) shows a representation of some modifications on the surface of polymeric nanocapsules (polymer-coating; PEG-coating; layer-by-layer; polymersomes; and inner portion—hollow-core) [5].

Chitosan, alginate, and cellulose are the natural polymers most widely used in medicine due to their geometry, their large specific surface, their mechanic and barrier properties, their low toxicity, and their biodegradability and biocompatibility [11, 12]. Chitosan is a biodegradable cationic polymer that can be obtained from crustaceans, insects, mollusks, and fungi. Usually, it is obtained for industrial use from crustacean exoskeletons, mainly from the waste products of the fishing industry. The properties that make it interesting for use are its molecular weight, deacetylation degree, solubility, biocompatibility, and bioadhesion. It presents antimicrobial activity against fungi, viruses, and bacteria. The application of nanospheres and nanocapsules of chitosan in cartilage and bone regenerative medicine is currently being studied due to the aforementioned properties [13]. The polysaccharide alginate is used in therapeutics because of its biocompatibility, low immunogenicity, and ability to gelation. Moreover, it is a pH-sensitive polymer that can be used to prevent drug release in an acid medium, such as gastric juice, when it is necessary for the active to be released in an alkaline medium (e.g., in oral administration of intestinal targeted drug delivery) [6]. In Ref. [14], nanospheres with alginate and chitosan loaded with the insecticide captan hydrochloride are obtained. Cellulose can be extracted from different natural sources. It is highly abundant, and the development of cellulose-based systems for drug release applicable to cancer therapy has increased enormously in the last decade [11].

Proteins, such as albumin, which are biocompatible and able to be tuned, are also used as polymeric shells for nanocapsules. Albumin is water-soluble and biodegradable. Apart from controlling drug release rate, albumin can reduce the nanosystem immunogenicity, and it can be useful as a drug targeting vector [6].

In Ref. [15] several polymeric systems are described, containing hybrid lecithin/chitosan nanoparticles, PCL nanocapsules stabilized with the non-ionic surfactant polysorbate 80, and polymeric PCL nanocapsules stabilized with a polysaccharide-based surfactant, that is, sodium caproyl hyaluronate. These three systems present interesting physicochemical and structural properties from the biopharmaceutical viewpoint for nasal and nose-to-brain delivery—biocompatibility, drug release, mucoadhesion, and permeation across the nasal mucous membrane. All three systems improved the transport of the hypolipidemic drug simvastatin through the epithelial barrier of the nasal cavity, compared to the traditional formulation.

According to reference [7], polymeric nanoparticles present several disadvantages, such as toxicity, presence of organic solvent residues, inadequate encapsulation of hydrophilic drugs, losses, difficulty of large-scale production, and storage and sterilization issues. Besides, the organism may receive them as strange particles. To avoid this, lipids can be employed. Their instability and the consequent reduction of their average life hinder their clinical applications. Nevertheless, their core-shell structure presents countless advantages, especially for drug delivery. In the case of oily core nanocapsules, the pharmaceutical industry opts for lyophilization, especially if there are thermolabile compounds. Definitely, they result in promising structures as they offer a high capability of drug encapsulation, protection from degradation, and biocompatibility; they hardly irritate tissues and certain polymers have been observed to actively interact with biological fluids [4, 5].

2.2 Lipid-based formulations

Delivery systems with lipid-based formulations are mainly of three types—liquid, solid, and lipid as colloidal carriers (liposomes). The liquid formulations are emulsions or micro-emulsions, self-emulsifying or self-nanoemulsified drug-delivery systems, and solid in oil suspensions. The solid lipid-based systems include solid-state micro-emulsions, solid self-emulsifying drug-delivery systems for dry emulsions, microspheres, nanoparticles, and suppositories. The incorporation of the drug to the matrix or shell-core of the solid lipid nanoparticle relies on the composition and the preparation mode of the formulations [7].

The different types of lipid-based nanocarriers are solid lipid nanoparticles (SLNs), liposomes, lipid-drug conjugates, lipid nanocapsules (LNCs), and nanostructured lipid carriers. Nanocarriers fabricated using lipid biomolecules show low *in vivo* toxicity and are subject to parenteral, oral, transdermal, intranasal, and ocular administration.

SLNs are stable in biological fluids and offer a good therapeutic alternative—their size is between 80 and 100 nm, they are more efficient than polymeric nanoparticles, and have the advantage of being able to be prepared from non-toxic physiological lipids, habitually used as excipients. In Ref. [7] the authors present various advantages compared to other colloidal carriers, such as controlled drug release and targeted therapy; and they protect encapsulated compounds from degradation. Their nature is very versatile and they can be applied in chemotherapy. The solid matrix forms an o/w emulsion, it is formed by well-tolerated lipids, and it allows for the incorporation of hydrophilic and/or hydrophobic drugs. The amount of encapsulated active compounds ranges from 1 to 5% for hydrophilic compounds and reaches 80% for lipophilic ones [16]. The lipids used as the coating can increase bioavailability, they help drug release and protect from water permeability. SLNs are most useful for the oral administration of drugs and vitamins that can solubilize in a lipid medium [17]. They have a lower cost than synthetic polymers, than PLGA for instance, and besides, can bind PEG as ligand [7].

LNCs are hybrid structures between polymeric nanoparticles and liposomes. Their size is small (between 20 and 100 nm), they are very stable, biodegradable and biocompatible, easy to manufacture, they can accommodate one or two drugs together, which can be released in a sustained manner. They show an oily liquid core surrounded by a solid or semisolid hydrophobic shell made of solid lipids and emulsifying agents. They are prepared through micro-emulsification or high-pressure homogenization. The principal components are oils, a lipophilic surfactant, and a non-ionic surfactant. Usually, fatty alcohol or acids; steroids or waxes; mono, di, or triglycerides; and phospholipids are employed [2, 18]. Triglycerides used as excipients, such as caprylic acid (Labrafat®), lauric acid, palmitic acid, oleic acid, and behenic acid, present different chain lengths; mixed glycerides and polar oils like sorbitan trioleate (span 85), and oleic acid, are also used as emulsifying agents. Vegetable oils obtained from castor, soybean, olive, argan, eucalyptus, orange, and sesame are also being tested. Lecithin obtained from egg, soybean, rapeseed, sunflower, and lysolecithin is used as a lipophilic surfactant and is available as Lipoid® and Phospholipon® brands. Phospholipon® is a mixture of nature hydrogenated lecithin and phospholipids. On the other hand, ethanol, glycerol, propylene glycol, and PEG, as well as water-soluble and insoluble (non-ionic) surfactants are used as cosolvents to improve solubility. Water-soluble surfactants have HLB numbers of 12 or more and are, for example, alkyl ether ethoxylate, cremophor RH40 and RH60 (ethoxylated hydrogenated castor oil); and water-insoluble ones have values of HLB from 8 to 12 and can adsorb on the oil-water interface, such as polyoxyethylene and sorbitan trioleate (Tween-85). Finally, anti-oxidants like α-tocopherol, β-carotene, propyl gallate, and butylated hydroxytoluene are added [7, 18]. Among hybrid lipid-polymer nanoparticles (LPNs) are polymer-core lipid shell nanoparticles, formed by a polymer inside the core that is surrounded by one or more membrane-like lipids. The space between the polymer and the lipid is filled with water or aqueous buffer. The core polymer delays drug delivery and favors lipid stability. It is possible to encapsulate lipophilic drugs easily. In the case of highly water-soluble drugs, lipid-polymer complexes can be used [7]. The anti-cancer drug salidroside is incorporated in polymer-core lipid shell NPs formed by PLGA-PEG-PLGA triblock and the lipids lecithin and cholesterol, with high encapsulation efficiency, negative charge, and 150 nm size [19].

There is a type of hollow-core/shell lipid-polymer-lipid hybrid nanoparticles where polymeric NPs and PEGylated lipoplexes are combined. They contain a layer of positively charged lipid, which forms the inner hollow core, a middle layer of PLGA, which is hydrophobic, external to the PEG, and a neuter lipid layer between them. These systems are not simple LPNs, they present the features of PEGylated lipoplexes and PLGA nanoparticles. The positively charged hollow core can accommodate anionic drugs more efficiently than a polymer alone, the polymeric layer of the medium will allow sustained release, and the PEG-lipid layer avoids the particle being recognized by a macrophage, increases stability, and slows down polymer degradation and drug release. The combination of si-RNA and small drug molecules in the hydrophobic layer of PLGA is very useful for the treatment of different diseases, including multidrug-resistant cancers [7, 20].

3. Preparation methods

The production of polymeric nanocapsules has been increasing in the last decade, mainly in relation to the great potential of their applications in the fields of Biology, Medicine, and Pharmaceutics. The characteristics and usability of these nanosystems depend strongly on the production method chosen and the process variables, as well as on the formulation materials used [5]. On these grounds, several methods and processing techniques have been developed in the last two decades to obtain nanocapsules with the desired properties and biological performance according to their purpose. Generally, there are three classical methods for the preparation of polymeric nanocapsules—nanoprecipitation, emulsion template method, and layer-by-layer method [6, 21]. Regardless of the method used, the production of core-shell structures requires a non-solvent/continuous phase (water) and a solvent/dispersed phase (organic solvent that can be removed later), plus one or more polymers and surfactants to contribute to structure and stability, respectively. The nanocapsules are obtained as colloidal dispersions, or in powder if some drying method is added.

3.1 Nanoprecipitation

Nanoprecipitation, also named interfacial deposition method or solvent displacement, was the first method described [22], and it has been widely used in the last two decades, principally because it is fast, and it has extensive applicability, being able to be used with many types of materials, and allowing various drugs to be encapsulated. In addition, it is a low-cost and simple operation technique since it does not require any special equipment [5]. The preparation of nanocapsules using this method involves both an organic and an aqueous phase. Typically, the organic phase, which consists of oil, polymer, and the active compound dissolved in an organic solvent, is added slowly and with moderate stirring to the aqueous phase (in most cases water and a selected surfactant). Hence, the formation of nanocapsules results from a combination of the spontaneous emulsification of oily droplets and the simultaneous precipitation of polymer onto the water-oil interface during the diffusion of phases [23]. Finally, the colloidal aqueous suspension is obtained by eliminating the organic solvent via evaporation or through a drying process [6, 24]. The characteristics of nanocapsules formed by nanoprecipitation are mainly influenced by several process variables, such as nature, concentration, and compatibility of the components [21], volume ratio between organic and aqueous phase, and the selected method for the injection of the organic phase. In fact, there is some evidence that varying the organic phase injection rate, the aqueous phase agitation rate, and adding the organic phase through a thin needle, leads to a significant decrease in the average size of the nanocapsules, compared with the technique consisting in just pouring one phase over the other [25]. This is probably due to the increase of the contact surface between the phases [26].

3.2 Emulsification-based methods

There are different ways to obtain nanocapsules using nanoemulsions as a template, including emulsion-diffusion, emulsion-coacervation, and double emulsification. All of them involve the emulsification of the organic or the aqueous phase in the other using a low or high-energy homogenization technique, causing the surfactant to self-assemble at the interface. The nature of the rest of the materials used in the continuous or in the dispersed phase will depend on the desired characteristics of the nanocapsules to be formulated.

3.2.1 Emulsion-diffusion/evaporation method

Emulsion-diffusion is a technique that involves the emulsification of an organic phase onto an aqueous phase and the subsequent elimination of the organic solvent by diffusion into the external phase or driven by evaporation, which results in the formation of nanocapsules [6, 27]. The formation of a conventional oil-in-water emulsion within a partially water-soluble solvent via diffusion requires a second aqueous phase (also named dilution phase) that promotes the solvent to diffuse into the external phase causing polymer precipitation and interfacial phenomena, forming a core-shell structure. The homogenization of both phases can be attained through low or high-energy shaking (by means of magnetic or mechanical stirring, ultra turrax, ultrasound, high-pressure homogenizers, etc.), being the latter a better option to obtain smaller nanocapsules [5, 28]. The basis of this method, which differentiates it from nanoprecipitation, is mainly the use of an organic phase partially miscible in water and a polymer partially miscible in both phases. Some other factors that can affect the final characteristics of the nanocapsules obtained by this technique are the amount of dilution phase, the surfactant and polymer concentrations, the oil-to-polymer ratio, and the drop size of the primary emulsion [21]. The advantages of this method include better reproducibility, control of particle size, and therefore better scaling response; but enough energy must be spent to remove large amounts of water, and it is a recommended method only for particles with an oily core [5, 23, 29].

3.2.2 Double emulsification method

Multiple emulsion systems are capable of encapsulating both hydrophilic and lipophilic molecules simultaneously and can be obtained through the double emulsification method [20, 30, 31]. Depending on the established phase sequence, double emulsions can be water-in-oil-in-water (w/o/w) or oil-in-water-in-oil (o/w/o). The preparation of nanocapsules using double emulsification involves a two-step emulsification process and the use of two stabilizers or surfactants. In fact, the key to ensuring good interphase stability and improving drug encapsulation and particle size is the correct selection and concentration of surfactants. As an example, based on w/o/w, a low hydrophilic-lipophilic balance (HLB) surfactant is needed to stabilize the w/o interface. In contrast, to stabilize the oil-in-water interface, a high HLB surfactant is required. Finally, particle hardening, or in other words, polymer shell formation, has been reported to be achieved by polymer precipitation, solvent diffusion, coacervation, or a combination of these strategies [5, 32].

3.2.3 Emulsion-coacervation method

Like the methods described in Sections 3.2.1 and 3.2.2, the emulsion-coacervation method uses the emulsion as a template, the difference is that the formation and stabilization of the polymer shell can be achieved by physical coacervation, chemical crosslinking, photopolymerization, sonochemical techniques, *in situ* polymerization, atom transfer radical polymerization (ATRP), and addition-fragmentation chain transfer (RAFT) [5, 33, 34]. Therefore, the materials commonly used for the fabrication of nanocapsules are usually monomers, polymers possessing cross-linking function groups or polyelectrolytes [35]. The general procedure involves the formation of the nanoemulsion firstly, coacervation phase stabilization, and finally, monomer/polymer crosslinking. Thus, some factors that are also necessary for the fabrication of nanocapsules by the emulsion-coacervation method include the addition of coacervation or crosslinking agents and the modification of certain variables, such as pH and temperature [36]. The main advantage of this method is that it permits to obtain a rigid nanocapsule shell structure, which can help to minimize the leakage of the payloads to the external phase. However, the final product may contain monomer residues that did not react [33].

3.3 Layer-by-layer method (LBL)

The layer-by-layer method has a great potential to develop multi-compartmental delivery devices since nanocapsules with multiple polymeric layers around the core are obtained. This method requires a colloidal core, which can be the solid form of the active substance, inorganic particles, biological cells, or an oil-in-water nanoemulsion prepared using any of the methods described in Section 3.2. The mechanism of this nanocapsules formation is the irreversible electrostatic attraction—a sequential adsorption of oppositely charged polyelectrolytes is achieved [5, 37]. The sequential deposition of polycations and polyanions on the inorganic core can be followed by the sacrifice of the template core, resulting in a hollow nanocapsule where the payload can be trapped [6, 38, 39]. The main advantages of the LBL technique are the possibility to simultaneously encapsulate different drugs at different positions, and the possibility to control release properties by modulating the composition and the thickness or number of layers of the polymeric shell [24, 40, 41]. On the other hand, this method bears some difficulties, such as the separation of the polyelectrolyte and the remaining counterions in each deposition cycle. Otherwise, aggregates of these may form. This high number of assembly steps is quite complex and time-consuming. In addition, larger nanocapsules are obtained compared to other methods, due to the number of polymeric layers deposited [21].

3.4 Comparative analysis for the selection of nanocapsules production method

Table 1 summarizes the main advantages and disadvantages of the processing methods described in Section 3 in terms of water volume consumption, additional purification steps, contaminant generation, time consumption, and others. Overall, nanoprecipitation represents a simple, fast, low-cost, and versatile method, but its simplicity can lead to some repeatability and scale-up problems. In contrast, emulsion template methods need agitation and solvent removal equipment and thus the technique becomes more expensive but with better control of particle size and scale response. Finally, the LBL technique offers many possibilities, as several active ingredients of different nature can be encapsulated simultaneously, and the release mechanism can be controlled according to the nature and number of polyelectrolyte layers; however, it becomes a more complex and time-consuming technique and larger particle sizes can be obtained compared to the other methods. The selection of the nanocapsule production method should mainly consider the desired characteristics of the final nanocarrier, the formulation materials, and the availability of laboratory equipment [5].

Method	Advantages	Disadvantages	References
Nanoprecipitation	• Fast and low-cost method • No require any special equipment • Many types of materials and drugs	• Oil core: lipophilic active substance nature • Reproducibility and scale-up problems due to its manual operation	[5, 21, 42]
Emulsion-diffusion	• Better reproducibility, particle size control, and scaling response. • Different ways of homogenization, including low or high-energy shaking	• High water volume consumption (dilution) • Enough energy to remove large amounts of water • Only recommended for particles with an oily core	[5, 23, 28, 29]
Double emulsification	• Encapsulation of hydrophilic and lipophilic molecules simultaneously • Preparation of o/w or w/o emulsions	• Contaminant generation (use of two surfactants) • Additional purification steps	[20, 30, 31]
Emulsion-coacervation	• Rigid nanocapsule shell structure • Good release control and minimization of the "*burst*" effect	• The final product may contain monomer residues	[21, 33]
Layer-by-layer	• Many colloidal core possibilities (solid drug, inorganic particles, biological cells, or an o/w nanoemulsion) • Simultaneous encapsulation of different drugs • Control of the release properties by modulating the composition and the thickness or the number of layers of the polymer shell	• Contaminant generation (remaining polyelectrolyte and counterions in each deposition cycle) • Additional purification steps • Complex and time-consuming technique • Larger nanocapsules compared to other methods	[6, 21, 24, 38–41]

Table 1.
Comparative analysis of the advantages and disadvantages of nanocapsule production methods.

4. Physicochemical characterization of nanocapsules

Next to the technical challenge of fabricating nano-vesicular systems, there is an inevitable need both for monitoring the whole process and characterizing the properties of the nanocapsules produced [43]. A variety of characterization techniques can be found in the literature. Some of them are important techniques required to be done in any colloidal system, while the choice of others depends on the specific area of application of the systems. In this sense, the physicochemical characterization involves techniques to study or determine particle size, morphology, and dynamic stability of the nanocapsule suspension, as well as to know their effectiveness as drug entrapment and release systems.

4.1 Average size and size distribution

The average size and size distribution of submicron particles are usually measured by dynamic light scattering (DLS), which is based on the equivalent sphere principle when an incident beam interacts with the sample particles. Well-prepared nanocapsule systems should be in the nanometer range and with a narrow particle size distribution. Therefore, numerous studies have paid attention to the effect of both the type and the concentration of the constituents, as well as the fabrication process variables, on the size and polydispersity index (PI) of the sample [44]. The disadvantage of DLS is that there are some parameters that may influence data, such as viscosity, pH, and temperature of the suspension medium, as well as concentration, colloidal instability, or the presence of aggregates [23]. On the other hand, microscopic methods are also used to determine nanocapsules' mean size, but they require the imaging of a large number of particles, and the measurement may be affected due to the sample dry state required for the analysis [24]. So, it is generally recommended to use at least two methods to determine the particle size and size distribution [23].

4.2 Morphology

Different microscopy techniques can be used not only to observe the nanocapsule morphology and structure, but also to determine the average size, elemental composition, and state of aggregation. Scanning electron microscopy (SEM) or transmission electron icroscopy (TEM) are the most common techniques, and their choice depends on the size of the studied system and the established purposes [23, 45]. The principle of SEM is to scan the sample with a high-energy electron beam, and image formation is achieved by collecting low-energy secondary electrons or backscattered electrons that are released from the sample surface. For this reason, SEM images present a three-dimensional appearance and are useful to appreciate the structure, shape, and surface defects of the sample [45, 46].

Compared to SEM, TEM needs a higher voltage, resulting in higher resolution (0.2 nm). Since electrons can pass through the sample, the internal structure, whether crystalline or amorphous, can be observed [44]. Both techniques are expensive and require high vacuum, the main difference laying in the preparation of the sample and the information obtained from it. SEM requires sample conductivity, which is usually achieved by coating the sample with a thin layer of gold or platinum. In contrast, for TEM analysis the sample must be thin enough to be electron-transparent [45]. It is worth mentioning that a qualitative or semi-quantitative elemental chemical analysis can be performed by electron microscopy, coupling energy-dispersive X-ray spectroscopy (XEDS) [24]. In addition, the use of scanning transmission electron microscopy (STEM), a technique that combines both principles, has been reported for the characterization of micro- and nanocapsules [47].

Another useful tool for simultaneously determining particle shape, surface structure, and even some mechanical properties is atomic force microscopy (AFM). AFM images are obtained by measuring the displacement of the AFM tip during a raster scanning over the immobilized sample. The result is a high-resolution 3D profile of the surface under study. The principal advantage of AFM over electron microscopy is that it permits the imaging of almost any type of surface and biomolecules under different physicochemical conditions, during biological processes, or even the study of the mechanical properties of delivery systems at the nanoscale [45, 48].

4.3 Stability of nanocapsule suspensions

An important property of colloidal systems is that they remain stable over time and under certain conditions of interest. Some physicochemical instability phenomena of nanocapsules are aggregation, precipitation, creaming, nanocapsule chemical degradation, and consequently, the reduction of drug content within the nanocapsule. All these phenomena can occur during the production process or after storage. Among the main reasons for them are inadequate steric or electrostatic stabilization, and the combination with external agents, such as oxygen, temperature, and ultraviolet radiation. In this way, the stability of nanocapsules is generally evaluated in terms of drug content, variations of zeta potential values, and average particle size as a function of time, pH, or temperature, using DLS or Zeta Potential techniques [23]. In some cases, the visual inspection of the colloidal suspension is also useful. On the other hand, some degradation products can be evaluated by chromatography or spectrometry [49].

4.3.1 Zeta potential

The zeta potential is the electric potential at the interfacial double layer between the dispersed particle and the liquid layer surrounding it, and can be determined by electrophoretic light scattering, where the particle migrates toward the electrode of opposite charge with a velocity that is proportional to the magnitude of the zeta potential [23]. Regarding stability, it is important to ensure that the zeta potential values of the nanosystems are greater than ±30 mV, as this guarantees the strong electrostatic repulsion forces that prevent the occurrence of aggregation phenomena among the particles [50]. In addition to evaluating the stability of nanodevices, zeta potential measurements can also confirm the coating or adsorption of a specific material on the nanocapsules surface, which is useful specifically in the layer-by-layer technique described in Section 3.3 [24].

4.4 Encapsulation efficiency and *in vitro* drug release

Drugs can be loaded onto nanosystems by incorporating them during the nanocapsule production, or either after the formation of the nanocapsules, incubating the carrier with the concentrated drug solution [51]. In both cases, the drug can be physically loaded onto the polymeric matrix or the oily core, or it can be adsorbed on the surface, in the function of the affinity and the physicochemical characteristics of both the drug and the components of the nanocapsules [52]. The total content of a drug in the nanocapsule suspension can be determined after dissolving or extracting the drug from the carrier, or calculated from the difference between the total and free drug concentrations after the separation of nanocapsules by centrifugation or ultrafiltration [23]. The determination of loaded or released drugs can be carried out by means of high-performance liquid chromatography (HPLC), fluorescence spectroscopy, UV-Vis spectroscopy, or another analytical technique.

Nanocapsule erosion or swelling can lead to drug release. *In vitro* drug delivery depends upon the localization of the drug within the particle, the physicochemical properties of both the drug and the nanocapsule constituents, size, morphology, and cross-linking, and also on release conditions, such as pH, temperature, polarity, and the presence of enzymes or an adjuvant. Regarding the release of the active principle, the process is governed by solubility, diffusion, and polymer biodegradation. In the case of nanospheres, where the drug is evenly distributed, drug release occurs through diffusion or matrix erosion. If diffusion is faster than erosion, the release mechanism is said to be controlled by diffusion. If the drug is weakly bound to the surface, a rapid initial release or "*burst*" will take place. If the drug has been incorporated into the polymeric matrix (nanocapsule), it will present a relatively small "*burst*" effect and a sustained release profile instead. In this case, the release will be controlled by drug dissolution and diffusion through the polymeric membrane. To avoid the "*burst*" effect, compounds can be added to the matrix that reduces the drug solubility, or, as in the case of chitosan, ethylene oxide-propylene oxide block copolymer (PEO-PPO) can be added, which increases release rate because it diminishes drug-matrix interaction [1].

Determining the drug release mechanism from the particle system can give valuable information about the interactions between the drug and the nanocapsule. Drug release kinetics from nanocapsules may be obtained using ultracentrifugation, centrifugal ultrafiltration, dialysis techniques, or side-by-side diffusion cells with an artificial or biological membrane [23, 52]. Furthermore, the kinetic data can be fitted to mathematical models to determine the predominant release mechanism, which is very convenient in the design and evaluation of the utility of nanocapsules as drug-delivery systems in pharmaceutical applications [24].

5. Applications of nanocapsules in therapeutics

Nanotechnology has revolutionized cancer diagnosis and therapy. Protein engineering and materials science have contributed to the development of new nanosystems for drug delivery. The major features of nanoparticles for their application in drug delivery are particle size and size distribution. These determine the capacity to reach the target, drug distribution and toxicity, and influence charge and drug release, as well as the stability of nanoparticles. Smaller nanoparticles present a larger surface/volume ratio; in this case, the drug, which is closer to the surface, is expected to be released at a higher speed. Because of their small size, these nanoparticles can cross the sore endothelium, the intestinal epithelium, for example, in tumors, and enter microcapillaries of 5–6 microns diameter, and it also enables them to be selectively captured by cells and cause drug accumulation in certain places. On the other hand, the smaller the particle size, the more the risk of aggregation during the storage, transport, and manipulation. With respect to bigger particles, they allow for a larger drug per particle encapsulation, which derives in a slower release. Therefore, particle size control results in a regulation of the drug release rate. Moreover, size also affects polymeric degradation. In the case of cancer treatment, the aforementioned properties are fundamental; due to their small size, nanoparticles can access tumors and concentrate there through the EPR effect (enhanced permeability and retention). To the moment, many nanotechnological systems have been developed and tested as anticancer drug carriers, however, difficulty arises from the fact that these drugs do not differentiate healthy from tumoral cells. For that reason, it is necessary to investigate strategies that permit systems to reach the tumor specifically [1, 53].

As to the surface properties of nanoparticles, hydrophobicity influences their destiny, as it determines the level of blood components (such as opsonin) that will join them. It is essential to minimize opsonization to prolong the circulation of nanoparticles in blood. With this goal, nanoparticles can be coated with hydrophilic/surfactant and/or biodegradable polymers, such as PEG, polyethylene oxide, poloxamer, poloxamine, and polysorbate 80 (Tween 80) [1]. Targeted delivery can be active or passive. In the first case, the active principle or the nanosystem must conjugate to a specific ligand from the cell or tissue, whereas when the delivery is passive, the drug is released in the target organ. Nanocarriers concentrate preferably in tumors, inflammatory sites, and at antigen sampling sites due to the EPR effect of the vasculature. Anti-neoplastic, anti-viral drugs, and several other drugs are unable to cross the BBB. Nanoparticles with Tween 80 and those formulated with hyper-osmotic mannitol, which breaks the strong unions present, have been proved to be able to cross the BBB and provide a sustained release of drugs for the treatment of brain tumors. Once the target is reached, nanoparticles from biodegradable hydrophobic polymers become like a reservoir and start releasing the active compound in a continuous way. This type of system is usually employed to improve bioavailability and sustained release, and even to solubilize drugs for systemic delivery, and the systems adapt to protect bioactives from enzymatic degradation by nucleases and proteases, for instance [1].

5.1 Drug-delivery systems

Next, some most recent examples are gathered where polymeric and lipid nanocapsules are used to carry a great variety of drugs. In **Table 2** some recent relevant studies are compiled.

5.1.1 Antimicrobial and antibiotics

Several reviews exist about systems developed for the treatment of infections. Specifically, in Ref. [100], the most important works concerning the use of lipid-based formulations from 2000 to 2020 are compiled. Infections caused by bacteria resistant to antimicrobial drugs available for use in humans have increased exponentially. This revision highlights the importance of the development of nanotechnology in lipid systems as an innovative tool for infection treatment. Chitosan nanocapsules, and lecithin-polysorbate 80, containing dapsone, have resulted useful; also, lipid nanocapsules with carvacrol and cinnamaldehyde. Another review about the incorporation of natural substances with antimicrobial activity in polymeric nanoparticles highlights specifically the antifungal activity against *Candida* species of *Glycyrrhiza glabra L.*, which is included in mucoadhesive nanoparticles constituted by PLA, PLGA, and alginate. Nanocapsules were also prepared from polymyxin B cross-linked with sodium alginate and solid lipid nanoparticles with *Ginkgo biloba L.*, and their antimicrobial activity against *Pseudomonas aeruginosa* was studied [101]. For the delivery of fluoxetine, starch nanocapsules with core-shell morphology were prepared and joined to polyurethane. The system presented antibacterial activity against *Staphylococcus aureus* [54]. The incorporation of antimicrobial peptides appears as a promising alternative for infection treatment, as well as carvacrol loaded onto nanocapsules formed by PCL [55]. PCL nanocapsules loaded with amoxicillin trihydrate were prepared to investigate the gastric stability of this drug, as well as its therapeutic activity against *H. pilori* [56]. Eudragit® polymers (polymethacrylate-based copolymers) are easy to handle and are used to prepare formulations for oral administration. Antibiotic florfenicol was encapsulated in Eudragit® nanocapsules [57].

Besides, it was possible to demonstrate the antimicrobial activity of chitosan against *Escherichia coli* through the assembly of bacteria cell membranes. This last finding represents an advance in delivery systems based on chitosan nanocapsules since it can enhance the effects of carried antibiotics [102]. As a strategy to increase the solubility of capsaicin, a major component of chili peppers known for its numerous therapeutic activities, nanocapsules of chitosan in the form of high-payload submicron capsaicin-chitosan colloidal particle complex were prepared. Besides

Pharmacological group	Drug/compound	Type of nanocapsule	References
Antimicrobial and antibiotics	Fluoxetine	Polymeric	[54]
	Carvacrol	Polymeric	[55]
	Amoxicillin	Polymeric	[56]
	Florfenicol	Polymeric	[57]
	Tea tree oil	Polymeric	[58]
	Fusidic acid	Lipid	[59]
	Albendazole	Lipid	[60]
Anticancer drugs	Curcumin	Polymeric	[61–63]
		Hybrid lipid	[64]
		Liquid lipid	[65, 66]
	Docetaxel	Polymeric	[67, 68]
		Lipid	[69]
	Perillyl alcohol	Polymeric	[70]
	Tamoxifen	Polymeric	[71, 72]
	Aprepitant	Polymeric	[73]
	5-fluoroacil	Polymeric	[74, 75]
	Doxorubicin	Polymeric	[76]
	Paclitaxel	Polymeric	[77, 78]
		Lipid	[79]
	Oleic acid	Hybrid	[80]
	Simvastatin	Hybrid	[81]
	Thymoquinone	Polymeric	[82]
	Gemcitabine	Lipid	[83]
	Phloretin	Lipid	[84]
	Itraconazole	Lipid	[85, 86]
	Regorafenib	Lipid	[87]
	Sorafenib	Lipid	[88]
	Imatinib	Lipid	[89]
	Ifosfamide	Lipid	[90]
	Vinorelbine	Lipid	[91]
Anti-leishmaniasis	Glucantime	Polymeric	[92]
Anti-hyperglycaemic	Chrysin	Polimeric	[93]
Inmunological	Imiquimod	Hybrid	[94]
Anti-inflammatory	Diflunisal	Hybrid	[24]
	Celecoxib	Polymeric	[95]
	Nicotine	Lipid	[96]
Antidiabetic	Anthocyanin	Polymeric	[97]
Anesthetics	Prilocaine, Lidocaine	Lipid	[98]
Ophthalmic	Astragaloside	Lipid	[99]

Table 2.
Recent studies based on lipid and polymeric nanocapsules used as drug carriers.

achieving 75% of the loaded compound, capsaicin antimicrobial activity remained intact [103]. Chitosan-PCL core-shell nanocapsules were obtained and loaded with tea tree oil. These nanosystems presented activity against *Cutibacterium acnes*, which makes them useful for topical acne treatment [58]. Also, lipid-core nanocapsules coated with chitosan to test the antimicrobial *in vitro* activity of fusidic acid against Gram-positive bacteria were prepared [59]. The side effects of bedaquiline, a very effective drug against tuberculosis, can be very dangerous. The result of its encapsulation in lipid nanoparticles and chitosan-based nanoparticles suggests that it is possible to achieve a high concentration of the drug in the place of the infection, reducing the dose and therefore, side effects [104]. Encapsulation of the anthelmintic drugs mebendazole, albendazole, and their main metabolite in lipid nanoparticles, showed efficacy for *Cystic echinococcosis* treatment [60]. On the other hand, bacterial biofilms often impede the diffusion and accumulation of antimicrobial compounds, which is why the development of systems able to cross the biofilm is paramount. It has been observed that polymeric nanoparticles can access and change the properties of the biofilm microenvironment due to their size and specific structure. In this way, they interact with bacteria and/or release the encapsulated drugs. Thus, they are systems with a projection in anti-biofilm therapy [105].

5.1.2 Anticancer drugs

Curcumin has been described, among many other applications, to possess anticancer properties against different tumor types, including colorectal cancer. Nevertheless, it presents an inconveniently low bioavailability and a short average life, as well as a limited absorption and quick metabolism. The use of non-toxic nanocapsules prepared from the biodegradable polymer polyallyhydrocarbon proved useful for drugs with low bioavailability, including curcumin. The efficacy of these systems was confirmed with the use of mice as models [61]. In the same way, curcumin was encapsulated in systems prepared from chitosan and carboxymethyl cellulose which presented good stability [62] In Ref. [63], nanocapsules with different polymeric coatings (P80, PEG, chitosan, and Eudragit®) were prepared and compared as curcumin carriers. They evaluated the release of the active, cytotoxicity, and in this case, antimalaria activity was tested instead of antitumoral potential. The highest activity observed was that of nanocapsules prepared from chitosan. On the other hand, a curcumin-loaded nanostructure of hybrid lipid capsules of three different sizes has been shown to present 2.5 times the anti-cancerous efficacy of free curcumin in breast cancer cells and breast cancer stem-like cells [63, 64]. Also, liquid lipid nanocapsules coated with human serum albumin to carry curcumin were proposed. To strengthen the protecting role of the protein layer, this was cross-linked [65]. Moreover, liquid lipid nanocapsules were obtained from olive oil emulsification, where nanocapsules were coated by a protective shell composed of bovine serum albumin and hyaluronic acid [66]. The so-called nanocurcumin was also formulated, consisting of the anti-cancerous compound incorporated into a polymeric nanoparticle, which enhances its solubility. Due precisely to its solubility, its gelifying capacity and its ability to form complexes, pectin has also been widely used for the preparation of diverse nanomaterials, including nanocapsules. It presents medical uses as a coagulant, anti-diarrheic, anti-ulcerous, and anti-cancerous for colon cancer [106].

The anticancer drug docetaxel has been carried in multiple types of nanocapsules. As a novelty, nanocapsules were prepared that consisted of a polymeric shell coating an oily core, targeted to Tn-expressing carcinomas. Chitosan was PEGylated and modified with a monoclonal antibody that recognizes the antigen Tn, which is highly specific for carcinomas. Internalization of nanoparticles and reduction of cellular viability were proved. The release is pH-dependent, being faster in acid pH, which favors intracellular release [67]. Also for docetaxel delivery, nanocapsules were formulated from hyaluronic acid through self-emulsification in absence of organic solvents. They were studied *in vitro* with lung cancer cells and an effective release of the drug was observed [68]. In addition, the system composed of docetaxel and thymoquinone co-encapsulated in PEGylated lipid nanocapsules was explored. Cytotoxicity was improved and enhanced antitumor efficacy and apoptotic effects were observed. Reduced oxidative stress and toxicity to liver and kidney tissues occurred [69]. Chitosan-coated PLC nanocapsules resulted effective for the oral administration of perillyl alcohol, an essential oil with chemo-preventive activity for anticancer therapy. These nanocapsules present the mucoadhesive properties of the oil [70]. Chitosan and gellan gum were combined in the preparation of natural nanocapsules for tamoxifen delivery [71]. Tamoxifen delivery in biocompatible nanocapsules made from a PLA core and a 1,2-dipalmitoyl-sn-glycero-3-phosphoethanolamine-N-[methoxy(polyet hyleneglycol)-2000] shell was studied for breast cancer treatment. Cell proliferation results indicated cytotoxicity of nanocapsules in MCF-7 cells, as compared to free tamoxifen [72].

The drug aprepitant is a selective neurokinin 1 antagonist with low solubility in water, clinically used for the prevention of vomits and sickness provoked by chemotherapy. Chitosan-PEG-coated cyclodextrin nanoparticles and nanocapsules were designed and evaluated *in vitro* and *in vivo* [73]. New topic formulations of the antitumoral drug 5-fluorouracil were studied using sodium alginate and hyaluronic acid-containing AS1411 aptamer-functionalized polymeric nanocapsules. It was proved that nanoencapsulation improves drug permeability, and the nanoparticles prepared showed favorable biosafety and good antitumor effects for skin cancer treatment [74]. To improve the efficiency of the antitumoral treatment, hybrid nanocapsules obtained from the interfacial condensation between chitosan and poly(N-vinyl pyrrolidone-alt-itaconic anhydride), containing both magnetic nanoparticles and 5-fluorouracil, were developed. Their nanometric size and their spherical shape were confirmed by SEM [75].

Polysaccharide-based nanocapsules prepared from furcellaran and chitosan via LBL deposition using electrostatic interaction were studied. To achieve targeted delivery, the surface was modified with a peptide. Doxorubicin was encapsulated with excellent drug loading properties, and release and stability proved to be influenced by pH. This system showed compatibility with eukaryotic organisms and good anticancer effects [76]. Paclitaxel, like most anticancer drugs, is low water-soluble and presents high toxicity at therapeutic doses. Nanoencapsulation seems a good strategy to overcome these difficulties. In Ref. [77] three kinds of nanocapsules using derivates of PEG dimethacrylates as crosslinking agents were obtained. It was possible to prove that the nanocapsule system provides an effective and universal strategy for lung targeting, esterase triggering, and synergy therapy. In another study, paclitaxel was loaded onto chitosan-poly(isobutyl cyanoacrylate) core-shell nanocapsules designed for oral drug delivery. The nanocapsules thus prepared had low polydispersity, spherical shape, and good mucoadhesive properties [78]. Another strategy for the encapsulation of paclitaxel and the reduction of its toxicity is the preparation of lipid and biosurfactant-based core-shell-type nanocapsules. In one such study, Acconon® was the lipid, and stearic-acid-valine conjugate the biosurfactant [79].

Health properties are attributed to the low water-soluble components of garlic oil diallyl disulfide (DADS) and diallyl trisulphide (DATS). Among these is anticancer activity. Both compounds were encapsulated in oil-core nanocapsules of hyaluronic acid. It was proved that encapsulation inhibits the membrane lysis of red blood cells (chiefly provoked by DADS), that the shell acts as a limiting barrier for the sulfur oxidation of the compounds, and that they preserve their biological and anticancer properties after encapsulation. Oleic acid was carried in this same type of nanocapsules and it was concluded that in presence of amphiphilic derivates of hyaluronic acid as a shell of the nanocapsules it is not necessary to include low molecular weight (co)surfactants [80].

Chitosan-coated PCL nanocapsules loaded with simvastatin resulted to be a promising strategy for simvastatin administration within a nose-to-brain approach for brain tumors therapy. Lipid-core nanocapsules coated with chitosan of different molecular weights were prepared by a novel one-pot technique. All formulations presented adequate particle sizes, positive surface charge, narrow droplet size distribution, and high encapsulation efficiency. The nanocapsules allowed for controlled drug release and displayed mucoadhesive properties dependent on the molecular weight of the coating chitosan [81]. Polymeric nanocapsules of Eudragit® were successfully prepared to load thymoquinone. They were conjugated with anisamide as ligand for sigma receptors overexpressed by colon cancer cells [82]. In a bibliographical review, the use of nanocapsules is summarized, among other nanocarriers, for immunotherapy against cancer. As an example, gemcitabine encapsulated in PEGylated lipid nanocapsules is reported. These nanostructures enter macrophages and tumoral cells [107]. Also, lipid nanocapsules (100 nm) loaded with lauroyl-modified gemcitabine efficiently target monocytic myeloid-derived suppressor cells in melanoma patients. The size and charge of nanocapsules can be modulated to reach immunosuppressive cells [83]. The antitumoral effect and the safety of nanocapsules made from a multifunctional component based on Lecigel® phospholipids loaded with the anticancer drug phloretin were tested. This drug is little soluble in an aqueous medium, and therefore, its dermatologic formulations are limited. With the prepared hydrogel, capacity to get through the skin layers was proved, as well as the drug reservoir role in the corneum stratum. Hence, it is presented as an innovative formulation to be applied in melanoma therapy [84]. Itraconazole is an antifungal drug to which are attributed potential anti-cancerous effects with few side effects. Lipid nanocapsules were proposed for the combined therapy with miltefosine and itraconazole, and an increase in the chemotherapeutic efficacy was observed. These nanocapsules were prepared from Labrafil® (oleoyl polyoxyl-6 glycerides), Labrafac® (caprylic-capric acid triglycerides), Transcutol® (diethylene glycol monoethyl ether), and Lipoid® (soybean lecithin, phosphatidylcholine, and phosphatidyl ethanolamine). Lipid systems were also prepared to study their efficacy as topic formulations with fungal and non-fungal effects [85, 86].

In Ref. [87], the possibility to supply intravenously lipid nanocapsules of 50 nm approx. was investigated, and it was checked whether this is viable for the treatment of different cancer types. Six different kinds of drugs were employed; encapsulation efficacy was good and *in vivo* experiments showed that the combination of SN38 and regorafenib in lipid nanocapsules is useful for the treatment of colorectal cancer. Also, sorafenib, a tyrosine kinase inhibitor, was encapsulated in lipid nanocapsules against glioblastoma and the results suggest that they can be used to improve chemotherapy and radiotherapy efficacy [88]. There also exist studies on imatinib, another tyrosine kinase inhibitor, delivered in lipid nanocapsules against melanoma [89]. The therapeutic efficacy against osteosarcoma was increased by ifosfamide-loaded-lipid-core nanocapsules, with significantly higher cytotoxicity of the drug than free ifosfamide at the same concentration. The apoptosis of cancer cells was increased by the prepared system by increasing the expression levels of caspase-3 and caspase-9 in MG63 cells [90]. A hydrophilic antimitotic agent for breast cancer, vinorelbine bitartrate, was incorporated in the lipid aqueous core of nanocapsules protected with a lipid shell. The release mechanism resulted to be Fickian diffusion, and hemocompatibility studies were also carried out to ensure safety in the case of intravenous administration [91].

5.1.3 Genes

The new systems for oncotherapy under development focus on selectivity so that they reach tumor cells without affecting the healthy ones. One strategy is to incorporate genes in non-viral carriers via surface modification to increase selectivity and affinity for the target cell's receptors. Nanocapsules with ter-polymers, to deliver DNA into tumoral cells, were developed. The surface of the nanocapsules was activated with folic acid so as to enable interaction with the folate receptors overexpressed [108]. Folate-decorated reductive-responsive carboxymethylcellulose-based nanocapsules were also prepared for targeted delivery and controlled release of hydrophobic drugs. In this case, the shell was cross-linked by disulfide bonds formed from hydrosulfuryl groups on the thiolated carboxymethylcellulose. These systems could become potential hydrophobic drug carriers for cancer therapy [109]. In addition, the first experiment with DNA-derived nanocapsules designed to reach podocytes, which damage plays a central role in the pathogenesis of idiopathic nephrotic syndrome, as well as in the progression of many chronic glomerular diseases, has been developed. These nanocapsules were composed of chitosan and plasmids, and their size, the number of plasmid layers, and the presence of the solid template were investigated in particular as the main parameters impacting the biological assay [110]. Besides, nanocapsules obtained from chitosan with hyaluronic acid for genes delivery into the lung epithelium were described. The nanocapsules were introduced in mannitol microspheres to facilitate administration in the lungs. This was seen as a good strategy for the delivery of genetic material into the lung [111]. In a different study, spherical nanocapsules were obtained from chitosan and loaded with capsaicin for cystic fibrosis treatment, and wtCFTR-mRNA was linked to the surface. They happened to be highly stable in the cell culture transfection medium [112]. Also, polyarginine was encapsulated in glyceryl-monooleate-based liquid droplets together with the immunomodulator chemokine CCL2 and two RNAi sequences. It was concluded that polymeric shells confer multifunctionality to the nanocapsules due to their versatility, which permits control of the mechanism of the therapeutic action [107]. An analogous of the nucleotide GMP was encapsulated in lipid nanocapsules for the treatment of neurodegenerative retinal degenerations. The nanocapsules were prepared from Labrafac™ lipophile, Kolliphor®, and phospholipids, and remained stable for 6 days in phosphate buffer and in vitreous components, allowing for a sustained release [113].

5.2 Stimuli-responsive systems

Stimuli-responsive drug-delivery systems are of interest because they can restrict drug delivery to the target. Nevertheless, it is difficult for most systems to reach all the cells of the tumoral tissue, due to the natural tumoral barrier. There are nanosystems that can be pre-programmed to alter their structure and release the encapsulated molecule more effectively. In this case, molecular sensors are incorporated which respond to physiological or biological stimuli, such as changes in pH, redox potential, or enzymes. Drug release can occur via passive systemic targeting or active receptor targeting. Plasmids of DNA, si-RNA, and other therapeutic nucleic acids can be carried [1]. The development of pH-sensitive drug-delivery systems for the selective release of anticancer drugs is promising, given that healthy tissue has a pH of 7.4, the average extracellular pH in tumoral tissue is 6.8, and the pH of intracell components such as endosomes and lysosomes varies from 4.5 to 6.5. The cause of this difference is that the high metabolic rate required for tumor growth provokes hypoxia in the tumoral region. Therefore, the specificity of delivery systems for low pH levels is a suitable strategy to improve chemotherapy effectiveness, on one side, and reduce cytotoxicity levels, on the other. Most systems proposed for this kind of strategy are organic, but they still present some inconveniences such as low biocompatibility, complex manufacture, and limited drug release indexes [53]. In the case of melanoma therapy, lipid nanocapsules prepared from N-vinylpyrrolidone and vinyl imidazole showed pH-responsive ability and improved drug entrance into the tumoral cells. The copolymers were inserted into the surface of the nanocapsules, and they particularly changed from neutral charge at physiological pH to positive charge in acid conditions [114]. Besides, polyurea/polyurethane nanocapsules displaying pH-synchronized amphoteric properties were proposed. Such properties facilitate their accumulation and their selectivity for acidic tissues, such as tumoral tissues [115]. Stimuli-responsive multi-layered nanocapsules were also prepared with Eudragit®, chitosan, sodium alginate, and poly-L-arginine. They were loaded with curcumin and delivery was studied under similar pH conditions to those of the gastrointestinal tract. These nanocapsules were observed to shield the compound from being released in the stomach and allow it to be released in the intestine [116]. A LBL nanocapsule was obtained from hyaluronic acid functionalized with anionic azobenzene co-assembled with cationic poly diallyl dimethylammonium chloride. It is a novel UV-induced (365 nm) decomposable nanocapsule. Its size enables it to cross biological barriers, permits a prolonged circulation in the blood, and improves accumulation in the tumor. Later, it can be eliminated after UV-induced dissociation. Similarly, a nanocapsule was prepared with the anionic alginate-azo and cationic chitosan, and the anticancer drug doxorubicin was loaded onto these nanocapsules [117, 118].

5.3 Theragnostics and diagnostics

The field of theragnostics has been rapidly amplified in the last years, thanks to nanotechnology. As it has been commented above, nanomaterials can provide useful action following a great variety of stimuli, be they internal (enzymes, redox potential, pH, and temperature) or external (light, heat, magnetic fields, and ultrasounds-US). In Ref. [119], an interesting review of US-responsive theragnostic nanomaterials under the following categories can be found: microbubbles, micelles, liposomes (conventional and echogenic), niosomes, nanoemulsions, polymeric nanoparticles, chitosan nanocapsules, dendrimers, hydrogels, nanogels, gold nanoparticles, titania nanostructures, carbon nanostructures, mesoporous silica nanoparticles, and fuel-free nano/micro-motors. Theragnostic nanomaterials in service can produce an imaging signal and/or a therapeutic effect, which frequently involves cell death. It is much interesting to combine the ability for theragnostics of the nanocarriers designed with the clinical imaging ultrasound technique. High-intensity-focused ultrasound appears as a promising and minimally invasive therapeutic modality against various solid tumors. Although it has received considerable attention in the biomedical field, both the accuracy and efficacy of this technique are currently unsatisfactory. A nanometer-sized organic/inorganic hybrid enhancement agent for photoacoustic imaging-guided high-intensity-focused ultrasound therapy was designed and fabricated by concurrently encapsulating both Cu2-xS nanodots and perfluorooctyl bromide into a PLGA nanocapsule. These nanocapsules assumed a unique core/satellite/shell sandwich structure and combined the merits of small and uniform particle size, favorable biosafety, and multifunctional theragnostic ability into one system [120]. A biocompatible theragnostic platform consisting of luminescent upconversion nanocapsules encapsulated with cellulose acetate, a biocompatible polymer, was developed. This theragnostic platform is able to simultaneously perform diagnosis and drug delivery. On the one hand, the luminescence properties of the nanocapsules were observed to remain stable even after encapsulation. On the other, the chemotherapeutic drug doxorubicin was successfully loaded onto the nanocapsules [121]. Also, a new theragnostic nanoplatforms based on nanocapsules and PLGA, which were chemically modified so that they could incorporate several imaging moieties was produced. The nanocapsules can be endowed with a magnetic resonance imaging reporter, two fluorescence imaging probes (blue/NIR), and a positron emission tomography (PET) reporter. *In vitro* toxicity was not observed in any of the two different types of human endothelial cells with concentrations up to 100 μg mL^{-1}. Versatile *in vitro/in vivo* multimodal imaging ability was observed, as well as excellent biosafety and over 1% wt protein loading. In the same way, nanocapsules fabricated from biodegradable and photoluminescent polyester with PLGA were reported. Superparamagnetic iron oxide nanoparticles (SPIONs) were incorporated into the polymeric shell so as to transform the system into a magnetic resonance/photoluminescence dual-modal imaging theragnostic platform [122, 123]. Polydopamine is a polymer with adhesive properties; nanoparticles were prepared from it where cisplatin prodrug has been loaded via supramolecular interaction between β-cyclodextrin and adamantyl groups [124]. The nanoparticles exhibited photoacoustic imaging capacity for *in vivo* monitoring of the drug in the tumor site, and the chemo-photothermal therapy of the system showed a powerful anticancer activity against osteosarcoma cells *in vitro*. This is an innovative strategy for the preparation of multifunctional nanotheragnostics for combined anticancer therapy [125]. Polymeric Pluronic-F127-chitosan nanocapsules were obtained and explored as theragnostic agents. IR780 iodide, a near-infrared fluorescent dye that can be applied as a photosensitizer in photodynamic and photothermal therapies, was loaded for single-wavelength NIR laser imaging-assisted dual-modal phototherapy. Besides, the nanocapsules were functionalized with folic acid so as to activate their targeting capacity against folate receptor-expressing ovarian cancer cells [126]. The same compound was encapsulated in PEG-PLA nanocapsules and demonstrated potential as a multifunctional theragnostic agent for breast cancer treatment, with increased cellular uptake and photodynamic activity, and more reliable tracking in cell-image studies [127]. Magnetic lipid nanocapsules that show higher structural stability and better theragnostic properties than traditional lipid-based nanocarriers were reported as therapeutic nanocarriers displaying drug-delivery capacity. These nanocapsules are 16 times more efficient than free drugs and their diagnostic imaging capability was also demonstrated [128]. Increasing attention is being payed to multilayer nanocarriers loaded with optically activated payloads, since they are expected to provide new mechanisms of energy transfer in health-oriented applications, at the same time as they look promising for energy storage and environmental protection. The combination of a careful selection of optical components for efficient Förster resonance energy transfer and surface engineering of the nanocarriers allowed to synthesize and characterize novel theragnostic nanosystems for deep-seated tumors diagnosis and therapy [129]. Recently, a review has been published where the most interesting advances in nanocarriers applications, including polymeric nanocapsules as tools for Alzheimer's diagnosis and treatment, are compiled [130].

5.4 Biosensors

Biosensors measure biological, chemical, and physical signals related to health. They are used to track diseases and thus improve health. A multilayer system via LBL deposition of biopolymers, based on electrostatic interaction and intended to be applied in diabetes detection was developed. They obtained a new glucose-responsive system using poly(lysine) derivatives and alginate as polycation and polyanion, respectively [131]. Also, chitosan-based nanocapsules were demonstrated as *E. coli* bacterial quorum sensing reporter strain [132].

5.5 Others

Next are collected the most recent studies of polymeric and lipid nanocapsules as drug carriers not included in the previous groups:

Regarding polymeric nanocapsules, systems prepared from PLA and PLGA were loaded with glucantime, active against leishmaniasis, and the anti-hyperglycaemic flavonoid chrysin, respectively [92, 93]. Another example is that of the chitosan nanocapsules prepared with the novel excipient Compritol® for transdermal delivery of imiquimod, a modifier of the immunological response [94]. Natural polymers k-carrageenan and chitosan were deposited onto olive oil nanoemulsion droplets via LBL self-assembly. The anti-inflammatory drug diflunisal was used as a lipophilic drug model in the nanocapsules thus prepared and was introduced into the oily core [24]. Also, a new system was developed with optimized hyaluronan nanocapsules for intra-articular delivery of the anti-inflammatory celecoxib [95]. In addition, Eudragit® nanocapsules loaded with nicotine as an adjuvant were studied for the anti-inflammatory therapy of the central nervous system. In this case, some polymer toxicity was observed [96]. An alternative to insulin therapy for diabetes is the use of nanocapsules loaded with anthocyanin. A study explored the potential use of purple sweet potato extract, with high levels of anthocyanin, loaded onto carboxymethyl cellulose and alginate nanocapsules [97].

On the other hand, there are several examples of lipid nanocapsules for the delivery of diverse drugs; lipid spherical nanocapsules with negative zeta potential were prepared with Labrafac® lipophile WL 1349 and Lipoid®, and incorporated in a gel for topical administration. The local anesthetics prilocaine and lidocaine were successfully encapsulated [98]. Phospholipid nanocapsules of three sizes were obtained and loaded with astragaloside to treat age-related macular degeneration. Ocular penetration was corroborated through pharmacokinetic studies [99].

6. Conclusion

The number of publications reporting new strategies for the obtention of nanocapsules for biomedical applications considerably rises every year. New materials are being included for the preparation of nanocapsules, and their applications as stimuli-responsive systems, biosensors, and for theragnostic uses are being explored. The nanocapsule production method depends on the desired characteristics, the formulation materials, and the availability of laboratory equipment. Once the nanocapsules are fabricated, the protocol of characterization of the prepared systems is followed. In general, the nanoparticles described are spherical, with suitable sizes, size distributions, and zeta potentials according to their application, specifically, under 300 nm and with zeta potentials around ±30 mV. On the other hand, the activity of the nanoparticles loaded with the corresponding drug is tested *in vitro* in many of the works, although it is crucial to test that activity *in vivo* so as to access clinical study. For this reason, more and more *in vivo* studies appear, especially in the case of antitumoral therapy, which refers to the activity of the encapsulated drug and the ability of nanocapsules to release it in the desired target, avoiding side effects in healthy cells of the body.

Author details

Sarai Rochín-Wong[1] and Itziar Vélaz Rivas[2*]

1 Department of Chemical and Metallurgical Engineering, University of Sonora, Hermosillo, Mexico

2 Department of Chemistry, University of Navarra, Pamplona, Navarra, Spain

*Address all correspondence to: itzvelaz@unav.es

References

[1] Singh R, Lillard JW. Nanoparticle-based targeted drug delivery. Experimental and Molecular Pathology. 2009;**86**:215-223. DOI: 10.1016/j.yexmp.2008.12.004

[2] Chamundeeswari M, Jeslin J, Verma ML. Nanocarriers for drug delivery applications. Environmental Chemistry Letters. 2019;**17**:849-865. DOI: 10.1007/s10311-018-00841-1

[3] Irache JM. Nanomedicina: Nanopartículas con aplicaciones médicas. Anales del Sistema Sanitario de Navarra. 2008;**31**:7-10. DOI: 10.4321/s1137-66272008000100001

[4] Degobert G, Aydin D. Lyophilization of nanocapsules: Instability sources, formulation and process parameters. Pharmaceutics. 2021;**13**:1112-1137. DOI: 10.3390/pharmaceutics13081112

[5] Lima AL, Gratieri T, Cunha-Filho M, et al. Polymeric nanocapsules: A review on design and production methods for pharmaceutical purpose. Methods. 2022;**199**:54-66. DOI: 10.1016/j.ymeth.2021.07.009

[6] Deng S, Gigliobianco MR, Censi R, et al. Polymeric nanocapsules as nanotechnological alternative for drug delivery system: Current status. Challenges and Opportunities. Nanomaterials. 2020;**10**:847. DOI: 10.3390/nano10050847

[7] Hallan SS, Kaur P, Kaur V, et al. Lipid polymer hybrid as emerging tool in nanocarriers for oral drug delivery. Artificial Cells, Nanomedicine and Biotechnology. 2016;**44**:334-349. DOI: 10.3109/21691401.2014.951721

[8] Urrejola MC, Soto LV, Zumarán CC, et al. Polymeric nanoparticle systems: Structure, elaboration methods, characteristics, properties, biofunctionalization and self-assembly layer by layer technologies. International Journal of Morphology. 2018;**36**:1463-1471. DOI: 10.4067/s0717-95022018000401463

[9] Aguilera-Garrido A, del Castillo-Santaella T, Yang Y, et al. Applications of serum albumins in delivery systems: Differences in interfacial behaviour and interacting abilities with polysaccharides. Advances in Colloid and Interface Science. 2021;**290**:102365. DOI: 10.1016/j.cis.2021.102365

[10] Yan X, Chai L, Fleury E, et al. 'Sweet as a nut': Production and use of nanocapsules made of glycopolymer or polysaccharide shell. Progress in Polymer Science. 2021;**120**:101429. DOI: 10.1016/j.progpolymsci.2021.101429

[11] Montané X, Bajek A, Roszkowski K, et al. Encapsulation for cancer therapy. Molecules. 2020;**25**:1605. DOI: 10.3390/molecules25071605

[12] Murugesan S, Scheibel T. Chitosan-based nanocomposites for medical applications. Journal of Polymer Science. 2021;**59**:1610-1642. DOI: 10.1002/pol.20210251

[13] Shoueir KR, El-Desouky N, Rashad MM, et al. Chitosan based-nanoparticles and nanocapsules: Overview, physicochemical features, applications of a nanofibrous scaffold, and bioprinting. International Journal of Biological Macromolecules. 2021;**167**:1176-1197. DOI: 10.1016/j.ijbiomac.2020.11.072

[14] Kaur I, Agnihotri S, Goyal D. Fabrication of chitosan–alginate nanospheres for controlled release of

cartap hydrochloride. Nanotechnology. 2022;**33**:025701. DOI: 10.1088/1361-6528/ac2d4c

[15] Clementino AR, Pellegrini G, Banella S, et al. Structure and fate of nanoparticles designed for the nasal delivery of poorly soluble drugs. Molecular Pharmaceutics. 2021;**18**:3132-3146. DOI: 10.1021/acs.molpharmaceut.1c00366

[16] Sanna V, Kirschvink N, Gustin P, et al. Preparation and in vivo toxicity study of solid lipid microparticles as carrier for pulmonary administration. AAPS PharmSciTech. 2003;**5**:27

[17] Gutnova TS, Kompantsev DV, Gvozdenko AA, et al. Vitamin D Nanocapsulation. Chemistry & Chemical Technology. 2021;**64**:98-105. DOI: 10.6060/IVKKT.20216405.6399

[18] Dabholkar N, Waghule T, Krishna Rapalli V, et al. Lipid shell lipid nanocapsules as smart generation lipid nanocarriers. Journal of Molecular Liquids. 2021;**339**:117145. DOI: 10.1016/j.molliq.2021.117145

[19] Fang DL, Chen Y, Xu B, et al. Development of lipid-shell and polymer core nanoparticles with water-soluble salidroside for anti-cancer therapy. International Journal of Molecular Sciences. 2014;**15**:3373-3388. DOI: 10.3390/ijms15033373

[20] Hu SH, Chen SY, Gao X. Multifunctional nanocapsules for simultaneous encapsulation of hydrophilic and hydrophobic compounds and on-demand release. ACS Nano. 2012;**6**:2558-2565. DOI: 10.1021/nn205023w

[21] Mora-Huertas CE, Fessi H, Elaissari A. Polymer-based nanocapsules for drug delivery. International Journal of Pharmaceutics. 2010;**385**:113-142. DOI: 10.1016/J.IJPHARM.2009.10.018

[22] Fessi H, Puisieux F, Devissaguet JP, et al. Nanocapsule formation by interfacial polymer deposition following solvent displacement. International Journal of Pharmaceutics. 1989;**55**:1-4. DOI: 10.1016/0378-5173(89)90281-0

[23] Guterres S, Poletto F, Colome L, et al. Polymeric nanocapsules for drug delivery an overview. In: Fanun M, editor. Handbook of Colloids in Drug Delivery. CRC Press-Taylor & Francis Group; 2010. pp. 71-98. DOI: WOS:000285298200004

[24] Rochín-Wong S, Rosas-Durazo A, Zavala-Rivera P, et al. Drug release properties of diflunisal from layer-by-layer self-assembled κ-carrageenan/chitosan nanocapsules: Effect of deposited layers. Polymers. 2018;**10**:760. DOI: 10.3390/polym10070760

[25] Crecente-Campo J, Alonso MJ. Engineering, on-demand manufacturing, and scaling-up of polymeric nanocapsules. Bioengineering & Translational Medicine. 2019;**4**:38-50. DOI: 10.1002/btm2.10118

[26] Jara MO, Catalan-Figueroa J, Landin M, et al. Finding key nanoprecipitation variables for achieving uniform polymeric nanoparticles using neurofuzzy logic technology. Drug Delivery and Translational Research. 2018;**8**:1797-1806. DOI: 10.1007/s13346-017-0446-8

[27] Quintanar-Guerrero D, Ganem-Quintanar A, Allémann E, et al. Influence of the stabilizer coating layer on the purification and freeze-drying of poly(D,L-lactic acid) nanoparticles prepared by an emulsion-diffusion technique. Journal of Microencapsulation. 1998;**15**:107-119. DOI: 10.3109/02652049809006840

[28] Galindo-Pérez MJ, Quintanar-Guerrero D, Cornejo-Villegas MA, et al. Optimization of the emulsification-diffusion method using ultrasound to prepare nanocapsules of different food-core oils. LWT—Food Science and Technology. 2018;**87**:333-341. DOI: 10.1016/j.lwt.2017.09.008

[29] Mora-Huertas CE, Garrigues O, Fessi H, et al. Nanocapsules prepared via nanoprecipitation and emulsification-diffusion methods: Comparative study. European Journal of Pharmaceutics and Biopharmaceutics. 2012;**80**:235-239. DOI: 10.1016/j.ejpb.2011.09.013

[30] Balan V, Dodi G, Tudorachi N, et al. Doxorubicin-loaded magnetic nanocapsules based on N-palmitoyl chitosan and magnetite: Synthesis and characterization. Chemical Engineering Journal. 2015;**279**:188-197. DOI: 10.1016/j.cej.2015.04.152

[31] Chiang CS, Hu SH, Liao BJ, et al. Enhancement of cancer therapy efficacy by trastuzumab-conjugated and pH-sensitive nanocapsules with the simultaneous encapsulation of hydrophilic and hydrophobic compounds. Nanomedicine: Nanotechnology, Biology and Medicine. 2014;**10**:99-107. DOI: 10.1016/j.nano.2013.07.009

[32] Ashjari M, Khoee S, Mahdavian AR. Controlling the morphology and surface property of magnetic/cisplatin-loaded nanocapsules via W/O/W double emulsion method. Colloids and Surfaces A: Physicochemical and Engineering Aspects. 2012;**408**:87-96. DOI: 10.1016/j.colsurfa.2012.05.035

[33] Guimarães TR, Bong YL, Thompson SW, et al. Polymerization-induced self-assembly: Via RAFT in emulsion: Effect of Z-group on the nucleation step. Polymer Chemistry. 2021;**12**:122-133. DOI: 10.1039/d0py01311k

[34] Dubey V, Mohan P, Dangi JS, et al. Brinzolamide loaded chitosan-pectin mucoadhesive nanocapsules for management of glaucoma: Formulation, characterization and pharmacodynamic study. International Journal of Biological Macromolecules. 2020;**152**:1224-1232. DOI: 10.1016/j.ijbiomac.2019.10.219

[35] Xiao Z, Li W, Zhu G, et al. Study of production and the stability of styrallyl acetate nanocapsules using complex coacervation. Flavour and Fragrance Journal. 2016;**31**:283-289. DOI: 10.1002/ffj.3306

[36] Liang X, Ma C, Yan X, et al. Structure, rheology and functionality of whey protein emulsion gels: Effects of double cross-linking with transglutaminase and calcium ions. Food Hydrocolloids. 2020;**102**:105569. DOI: 10.1016/j.foodhyd.2019.105569

[37] Preetz C, Rübe A, Reiche I, et al. Preparation and characterization of biocompatible oil-loaded polyelectrolyte nanocapsules. Nanomedicine: Nanotechnology, Biology and Medicine. 2008;**4**:106-114. DOI: 10.1016/j.nano.2008.03.003

[38] Ji F, Li J, Qin Z, et al. Engineering pectin-based hollow nanocapsules for delivery of anticancer drug. Carbohydrate Polymers. 2017;**177**:86-96. DOI: 10.1016/j.carbpol.2017.08.107

[39] Belbekhouche S, Oniszczuk J, Pawlak A, et al. Cationic poly(cyclodextrin)/alginate nanocapsules: From design to application as efficient delivery vehicle of 4-hydroxy tamoxifen to podocyte in vitro. Colloids Surfaces B Biointerfaces. 2019;**179**:128-135. DOI: 10.1016/j.colsurfb.2019.03.060

[40] Ledo AM, Sasso MS, Bronte V, et al. Co-delivery of RNAi and chemokine by polyarginine nanocapsules enables

the modulation of myeloid-derived suppressor cells. Journal of Controlled Release. 2019;**295**:60-73. DOI: 10.1016/j.jconrel.2018.12.041

[41] Cuomo F, Lopez F, Piludu M, et al. Release of small hydrophilic molecules from polyelectrolyte capsules: Effect of the wall thickness. Journal of Colloid and Interface Science. 2015;**447**:211-216. DOI: 10.1016/j.jcis.2014.10.060

[42] Rietscher R, Thum C, Lehr CM, et al. Semi-automated nanoprecipitation-system—An option for operator independent, scalable and size adjustable nanoparticle synthesis. Pharmaceutical Research. 2015;**32**:1859-1863. DOI: 10.1007/s11095-014-1612-z

[43] Bekas DG, Tsirka K, Baltzis D, et al. Self-healing materials: A review of advances in materials, evaluation, characterization and monitoring techniques. Composites. Part B, Engineering. 2016;**87**:92-119. DOI: 10.1016/j.compositesb.2015.09.057

[44] Peng H, Wang J, Zhang X, et al. A review on synthesis, characterization and application of nanoencapsulated phase change materials for thermal energy storage systems. Applied Thermal Engineering. 2021;**185**:116326. DOI: 10.1016/j.applthermaleng.2020.116326

[45] Luykx DMAM, Peters RJB, Van Ruth SM, et al. A review of analytical methods for the identification and characterization of nano delivery systems in food. Journal of Agricultural and Food Chemistry. 2008;**56**:8231-8247. DOI: 10.1021/jf8013926

[46] Wang Y, Wang J, Nan G, et al. A novel method for the preparation of narrow-disperse nanoencapsulated phase change materials by phase inversion emulsification and suspension polymerization. Industrial and Engineering Chemistry Research. 2015;**54**:9307-9313. DOI: 10.1021/acs.iecr.5b01026

[47] Hodoroaba VD, Akcakayiran D, Grigoriev DO, et al. Characterization of micro- and nanocapsules for self-healing anti-corrosion coatings by high-resolution SEM with coupled transmission mode and EDX. The Analyst. 2014;**139**:2004-2010. DOI: 10.1039/c3an01717f

[48] Uebel F, Thérien-Aubin H, Landfester K. Tailoring the mechanoresponsive release from silica nanocapsules. Nanoscale. 2021;**13**:15415-15421. DOI: 10.1039/d1nr04697g

[49] Müller CR, Haas SE, Bassani VL, et al. Degradação e estabilização do diclofenaco em nanocápsulas poliméricas. Quimica Nova. 2004;**27**:555-560. DOI: 10.1590/S0100-40422004000400008

[50] Liu Y, Yang J, Zhao Z, et al. Formation and characterization of natural polysaccharide hollow nanocapsules via template layer-by-layer self-assembly. Journal of Colloid and Interface Science. 2012;**379**:130-140. DOI: 10.1016/j.jcis.2012.04.058

[51] Yih TC, Al-Fandi M. Engineered nanoparticles as precise drug delivery systems. Journal of Cellular Biochemistry. 2006;**97**:1184-1190. DOI: 10.1002/jcb.20796

[52] Jawahar N, Meyyanathan S. Polymeric nanoparticles for drug delivery and targeting: A comprehensive review. International Journal of Health & Allied Sciences. 2012;**1**:217. DOI: 10.4103/2278-344x.107832

[53] Qian WY, Sun DM, Zhu RR, et al. pH-sensitive strontium carbonate

nanoparticles as new anticancer vehicles for controlled etoposide release. International Journal of Nanomedicine. 2012;7:5781-5792. DOI: 10.2147/IJN.S34773

[54] dos Santos SBF, Pereira SA, Rodrigues FAM, et al. Antibacterial activity of fluoxetine-loaded starch nanocapsules. International Journal of Biological Macromolecules. 2020;**164**:2813-2817. DOI: 10.1016/j.ijbiomac.2020.08.184

[55] Kapustová M, Puškárová A, Bučková M, et al. Biofilm inhibition by biocompatible poly(ε-caprolactone) nanocapsules loaded with essential oils and their cyto/genotoxicity to human keratinocyte cell line. International Journal of Pharmaceutics. 2021;**606**:120846. DOI: 10.1016/j.ijpharm.2021.120846

[56] Abdelghany A, El-Desouky MA, Shemis M. Synthesis and characterization of amoxicillin-loaded polymeric nanocapsules as a drug delivery system targeting *Helicobacter pylori*. Arab Journal of Gastroenterology. 2021;**22**:278-284. DOI: 10.1016/j.ajg.2021.06.002

[57] Castañeda PS, Olvera LG, Bernad MJB, et al. Development of a spectrophotometric method for the determination of florfenicol in eudragit nanocapsules. Pharmaceutical Chemistry Journal. 2021;**54**:1181-1185. DOI: 10.1007/s11094-021-02340-0

[58] da Silva NP, Rapozo EC, Duarte LM, et al. Improved anti-Cutibacterium acnes activity of tea tree oil-loaded chitosan-poly(ε-caprolactone) core-shell nanocapsules. Colloids Surfaces B Biointerfaces. 2020;**196**:111371. DOI: 10.1016/j.colsurfb.2020.111371

[59] Cé R, Pacheco BZ, Ciocheta TM, et al. Antibacterial activity against Gram-positive bacteria using fusidic acid-loaded lipid-core nanocapsules. Reactive and Functional Polymers. 2021;**162**:104876. DOI: 10.1016/j.reactfunctpolym.2021.104876

[60] Ullio Gamboa GV, Pensel PE, Elissondo MC, et al. Albendazole-lipid nanocapsules: Optimization, characterization and chemoprophylactic efficacy in mice infected with Echinococcus granulosus. Experimental Parasitology. 2019;**198**:79-86. DOI: 10.1016/j.exppara.2019.02.002

[61] Al Moubarak A, El Joumaa M, Slika L, et al. Curcumin-Polyallyhydrocarbon nanocapsules potently suppress 1,2-dimethylhydrazine-induced colorectal cancer in mice by inhibiting Wnt/β-catenin pathway. Bionanoscience. 2021;**11**:518-525. DOI: 10.1007/s12668-021-00842-5

[62] Abbas S, Chang D, Riaz N, et al. In-vitro stress stability, digestibility and bioaccessibility of curcumin-loaded polymeric nanocapsules. Journal of Experimental Nanoscience. 2021;**16**:229-245. DOI: 10.1080/17458080.2021.1952185

[63] dos Santos RB, Nakama KA, Pacheco CO, et al. Curcumin-loaded nanocapsules: Influence of surface characteristics on technological parameters and potential antimalarial activity. Materials Science and Engineering: C. 2021;**118**:111356. DOI: 10.1016/j.msec.2020.111356

[64] Yadava SK, Basu SM, Valsalakumari R, et al. Curcumin-loaded nanostructure hybrid lipid capsules for co-eradication of breast cancer and cancer stem cells with enhanced anticancer efficacy. ACS Applied Bio Materials. 2020;**3**:6811-6822. DOI: 10.1021/acsabm.0c00764

[65] Galisteo-González F, Molina-Bolívar JA, Navarro SA, et al.

Albumin-covered lipid nanocapsules exhibit enhanced uptake performance by breast-tumor cells. Colloids Surfaces B Biointerfaces. 2018;**165**:103-110. DOI: 10.1016/j.colsurfb.2018.02.024

[66] Aguilera-Garrido A, del Castillo-Santaella T, Galisteo-González F, et al. Investigating the role of hyaluronic acid in improving curcumin bioaccessibility from nanoemulsions. Food Chemistry. 2021;**351**:129301. DOI: 10.1016/j.foodchem.2021.129301

[67] Castro A, Berois N, Malanga A, et al. Docetaxel in chitosan-based nanocapsules conjugated with an anti-Tn antigen mouse/human chimeric antibody as a promising targeting strategy of lung tumors. International Journal of Biological Macromolecules. 2021;**182**:806-814. DOI: 10.1016/j.ijbiomac.2021.04.054

[68] Cadete A, Olivera A, Besev M, et al. Self-assembled hyaluronan nanocapsules for the intracellular delivery of anticancer drugs. Scientific Reports. 2019;**9**:11565. DOI: 10.1038/s41598-019-47995-8

[69] Zafar S, Akhter S, Garg N, et al. Co-encapsulation of docetaxel and thymoquinone in mPEG-DSPE-vitamin E TPGS-lipid nanocapsules for breast cancer therapy: Formulation optimization and implications on cellular and in vivo toxicity. European Journal of Pharmaceutics and Biopharmaceutics. 2020;**148**:10-26. DOI: 10.1016/j.ejpb.2019.12.016

[70] Penteado L, Lopes VF, Karam TK, et al. Chitosan-coated poly (ε-caprolactone) nanocapsules for mucoadhesive applications of perillyl alcohol. Soft Materials. 2022;**20**:1-11. DOI: 10.1080/1539445X.2021.1906702

[71] Kathle PK, Gautam N, Kesavan K. Tamoxifen citrate loaded chitosan-gellan nanocapsules for breast cancer therapy: Development, characterisation and in-vitro cell viability study. Journal of Microencapsulation. 2018;**35**:292-300. DOI: 10.1080/02652048.2018.1477844

[72] Behdarvand N, Bikhof Torbati M, Shaabanzadeh M. Tamoxifen-loaded PLA/DPPE-PEG lipid-polymeric nanocapsules for inhibiting the growth of estrogen-positive human breast cancer cells through cell cycle arrest. Journal of Nanoparticle Research. 2020;**22**:262. DOI: 10.1007/s11051-020-04990-9

[73] Erdoğar N, Akkın S, Nielsen TT, et al. Development of oral aprepitant-loaded chitosan–polyethylene glycol-coated cyclodextrin nanocapsules: Formulation, characterization, and pharmacokinetic evaluation. Journal of Pharmaceutical Investigation. 2021;**51**:297-310. DOI: 10.1007/s40005-020-00511-x

[74] Rata DM, Cadinoiu AN, Atanase LI, et al. Topical formulations containing aptamer-functionalized nanocapsules loaded with 5-fluorouracil—An innovative concept for the skin cancer therapy. Materials Science and Engineering: C. 2021;**119**:111591. DOI: 10.1016/j.msec.2020.111591

[75] Dellali KZ, Rata DM, Popa M, et al. Antitumoral drug: Loaded hybrid nanocapsules based on chitosan with potential effects in breast cancer therapy. International Journal of Molecular Sciences. 2020;**21**:5659. DOI: 10.3390/ijms21165659

[76] Milosavljevic V, Jamroz E, Gagic M, et al. Encapsulation of doxorubicin in furcellaran/chitosan nanocapsules by layer-by-layer technique for selectively controlled drug delivery. Biomacromolecules. 2020;**21**:418-434. DOI: 10.1021/acs.biomac.9b01175

[77] Zhao D, Jiang K, Wang Y, et al. Out-of-the-box nanocapsules packed with on-demand hydrophobic anticancer drugs for lung targeting, esterase triggering, and synergy therapy. Advanced Healthcare Materials. 2021;**10**:2001803. DOI: 10.1002/adhm.202001803

[78] Xavier-Jr FH, Gueutin C, Chacun H, et al. Mucoadhesive paclitaxel-loaded chitosan-poly (isobutyl cyanoacrylate) core-shell nanocapsules containing copaiba oil designed for oral drug delivery. Journal of Drug Delivery Science and Technology. 2019;**53**:101194. DOI: 10.1016/j.jddst.2019.101194

[79] Katiyar SS, Ghadi R, Kushwah V, et al. Lipid and biosurfactant based core–shell-type nanocapsules having high drug loading of paclitaxel for improved breast cancer therapy. ACS Biomaterials Science & Engineering. 2020;**6**:6760-6769. DOI: 10.1021/acsbiomaterials.0c01290

[80] Janik-Hazuka M, Szafraniec-Szczęsny J, Kamiński K, et al. Uptake and in vitro anticancer activity of oleic acid delivered in nanocapsules stabilized by amphiphilic derivatives of hyaluronic acid and chitosan. International Journal of Biological Macromolecules. 2020;**164**:2000-2009. DOI: 10.1016/j.ijbiomac.2020.07.288

[81] Bruinsmann F, Pigana S, Aguirre T, et al. Chitosan-coated nanoparticles: Effect of chitosan molecular weight on nasal transmucosal delivery. Pharmaceutics. 2019;**11**:86. DOI: 10.3390/pharmaceutics11020086

[82] Ramzy L, Metwally AA, Nasr M, et al. Novel thymoquinone lipidic core nanocapsules with anisamide-polymethacrylate shell for colon cancer cells overexpressing sigma receptors. Scientific Reports. 2020;**10**:10987. DOI: 10.1038/s41598-020-67748-2

[83] Pinton L, Magri S, Masetto E, et al. Targeting of immunosuppressive myeloid cells from glioblastoma patients by modulation of size and surface charge of lipid nanocapsules. Journal of Nanobiotechnology. 2020;**18**:31. DOI: 10.1186/s12951-020-00589-3

[84] Casarini TPA, Frank LA, Benin T, et al. Innovative hydrogel containing polymeric nanocapsules loaded with phloretin: Enhanced skin penetration and adhesion. Materials Science and Engineering: C. 2021;**120**:111681. DOI: 10.1016/j.msec.2020.111681

[85] El-Sheridy NA, Ramadan AA, Eid AA, et al. Itraconazole lipid nanocapsules gel for dermatological applications: In vitro characteristics and treatment of induced cutaneous candidiasis. Colloids Surfaces B Biointerfaces. 2019;**181**:623-631. DOI: 10.1016/j.colsurfb.2019.05.057

[86] El-Sheridy NA, El-Moslemany RM, Ramadan AA, et al. Enhancing the in vitro and in vivo activity of itraconazole against breast cancer using miltefosine-modified lipid nanocapsules. Drug Delivery. 2021;**28**:906-919. DOI: 10.1080/10717544.2021.1917728

[87] Tsakiris N, Papavasileiou M, Bozzato E, et al. Combinational drug-loaded lipid nanocapsules for the treatment of cancer. International Journal of Pharmaceutics. 2019;**569**:118588. DOI: 10.1016/j.ijpharm.2019.118588

[88] Clavreul A, Roger E, Pourbaghi-Masouleh M, et al. Development and characterization of sorafenib-loaded lipid nanocapsules for the treatment of glioblastoma. Drug Delivery. 2018;**25**:1756-1765. DOI: 10.1080/10717544.2018.1507061

[89] Molaahmadi MR, Varshosaz J, Taymouri S, et al. Lipid nanocapsules for imatinib delivery: Design, optimization and evaluation of anticancer activity against melanoma cell line. Iranian Journal of Pharmaceutical Research. 2019;**18**:1676-1693. DOI: 10.22037/ijpr.2019.1100870

[90] Wang S-Q, Zhang Q, Sun C, et al. Ifosfamide-loaded lipid-core-nanocapsules to increase the anticancer efficacy in MG63 osteosarcoma cells. Saudi Journal of Biological Sciences. 2018;**25**:1140-1145. DOI: 10.1016/j.sjbs.2016.12.001

[91] Lakshmi SS, Vijayakumar MR, et al. Lipid based aqueous core nanocapsules (ACNs) for encapsulating hydrophillic vinorelbine bitartrate: Preparation, optimization, characterization and in vitro safety assessment for intravenous administration. Current Drug Delivery. 2018;**15**:1284-1293. DOI: 10.2174/1567201815666180716112457

[92] Cosco D, Bruno F, Castelli G, et al. Meglumine antimoniate-loaded aqueous-core PLA nanocapsules: Old drug, new formulation against Leishmania-related diseases. Macromolecular Bioscience. 2021;**21**:2100046. DOI: 10.1002/mabi.202100046

[93] El-Hussien D, El-Zaafarany GM, Nasr M, et al. Chrysin nanocapsules with dual anti-glycemic and anti-hyperlipidemic effects: Chemometric optimization, physicochemical characterization and pharmacodynamic assessment. International Journal of Pharmaceutics. 2021;**592**:120044. DOI: 10.1016/j.ijpharm.2020.120044

[94] Alvarez-Figueroa MJ, Narváez-Araya D, Armijo-Escalona N, et al. Design of chitosan nanocapsules with compritol 888 ATO® for imiquimod transdermal administration. Evaluation of their skin absorption by Raman microscopy. Pharmaceutical Research. 2020;**37**:195. DOI: 10.1007/s11095-020-02925-6

[95] El-Gogary RI, Khattab MA, Abd-Allah H. Intra-articular multifunctional celecoxib loaded hyaluronan nanocapsules for the suppression of inflammation in an osteoarthritic rat model. International Journal of Pharmaceutics. 2020;**583**:119378. DOI: 10.1016/j.ijpharm.2020.119378

[96] Landau C, Sperling LE, Iglesias D, et al. Characterization, cytotoxicity and anti-inflammatory effect evaluation of nanocapsules containing nicotine. Bioengineering. 2021;**8**:172. DOI: 10.3390/bioengineering8110172

[97] Itishom R, Wafa IA, Budi DS, et al. Oral delivery of purple sweet potato (*Ipomoea batatas* L.) extract-loaded Carboxymethyl chitosan and alginate nanocapsule in streptozotocininduced diabetic mice. Indian Journal of Pharmaceutical Education and Research. 2021;**55**:709-714. DOI: 10.5530/ijper.55.3.143

[98] Cordeiro P, David de Moura L, Freitas de Lima F, et al. Lipid nanocapsules loaded with prilocaine and lidocaine and incorporated in gel for topical application. International Journal of Pharmaceutics. 2021;**602**:120675. DOI: 10.1016/j.ijpharm.2021.120675

[99] Sun R, Zhang A, Ge Y, et al. Ultra-small-size Astragaloside-IV loaded lipid nanocapsules eye drops for the effective management of dry age-related macular degeneration. Expert Opinion on Drug Delivery. 2020;**17**:1305-1320. DOI: 10.1080/17425247.2020.1783236

[100] dos Santos Ramos MA, de Toledo LG, Spósito L, et al. Nanotechnology-based lipid systems

applied to resistant bacterial control: A review of their use in the past two decades. International Journal of Pharmaceutics. 2021;**603**:120706. DOI: 10.1016/j.ijpharm.2021.120706

[101] Stan D, Enciu A-M, Mateescu AL, et al. Natural compounds with antimicrobial and antiviral effect and nanocarriers used for their transportation. Frontiers in Pharmacology. 2021;**12**:723233. DOI: 10.3389/fphar.2021.723233

[102] Gomes LP, Anjo SI, Manadas B, et al. Proteomic analyses reveal new insights on the antimicrobial mechanisms of chitosan biopolymers and their nanosized particles against *Escherichia coli*. International Journal of Molecular Sciences. 2020;**21**:225-240. DOI: 10.3390/ijms21010225

[103] Tran TT, Hadinoto K. A new solubility enhancement strategy of capsaicin in the form of high-payload submicron capsaicin-chitosan colloidal complex. Colloids and Surfaces A: Physicochemical and Engineering Aspects. 2017;**520**:62-71. DOI: 10.1016/j.colsurfa.2017.01.069

[104] De Matteis L, Jary D, Lucía A, et al. New active formulations against M. tuberculosis: Bedaquiline encapsulation in lipid nanoparticles and chitosan nanocapsules. Chemical Engineering Journal. 2018;**340**:181-191. DOI: 10.1016/j.cej.2017.12.110

[105] Li C, Cornel EJ, Du J. Advances and prospects of polymeric particles for the treatment of bacterial biofilms. ACS Applied Polymer Materials. 2021;**3**:2218-2232. DOI: 10.1021/acsapm.1c00003

[106] Induru J. Pectin-based nanomaterials in drug delivery applications. In: Biopolymer-Based Nanomaterials in Drug Delivery and Biomedical Applications. London, United Kingdom: Elsevier; 2021. pp. 87-117. DOI: 10.1016/B978-0-12-820874-8.00011-7

[107] Dai X, Ren L, Liu M, et al. Nanomedicines modulating myeloid-derived suppressor cells for improving cancer immunotherapy. Nano Today. 2021;**39**:101163. DOI: 10.1016/j.nantod.2021.101163

[108] Bellotti E, Cascone MG, Barbani N, et al. Targeting cancer cells overexpressing folate receptors with new terpolymer-based nanocapsules: Toward a novel targeted DNA delivery system for cancer therapy. Biomedicine. 2021;**9**:1275. DOI: 10.3390/biomedicines9091275

[109] He S, Zhong S, Meng Q, et al. Sonochemical preparation of folate-decorated reductive-responsive carboxymethylcellulose-based nanocapsules for targeted drug delivery. Carbohydrate Polymers. 2021;**266**:118174. DOI: 10.1016/j.carbpol.2021.118174

[110] Oniszczuk J, Le Floch F, Mansour O, et al. Kidney–Targeted drug delivery systems based on tailor-made nanocapsules. Chemical Engineering Journal. 2021;**404**:126475. DOI: 10.1016/j.cej.2020.126475

[111] Fernández-Paz E, Feijoo-Siota L, Gaspar MM, et al. Microencapsulated chitosan-based nanocapsules: A new platform for pulmonary gene delivery. Pharmaceutics. 2021;**13**:1-24. DOI: 10.3390/pharmaceutics13091377

[112] Kolonko AK, Efing J, González-Espinosa Y, et al. Capsaicin-loaded chitosan nanocapsules for wtCFTR-mRNA delivery to a cystic fibrosis cell line. Biomedicine. 2020;**8**:364-384. DOI: 10.3390/BIOMEDICINES8090364

[113] Urimi D, Widenbring R, Pérez García RO, et al. Formulation development and upscaling of lipid nanocapsules as a drug delivery system for a novel cyclic GMP analogue intended for retinal drug delivery. International Journal of Pharmaceutics. 2021;**602**:120640. DOI: 10.1016/j.ijpharm.2021.120640

[114] Pautu V, Lepeltier E, Mellinger A, et al. pH-responsive lipid nanocapsules: A promising strategy for improved resistant melanoma cell internalization. Cancers. 2021;**13**:2028-2044. DOI: 10.3390/cancers13092028

[115] Pérez-Hernández M, Cuscó C, Benítez-García C, et al. Multi-smart and scalable bioligands-free nanomedical platform for intratumorally targeted tambjamine delivery, a difficult to administrate highly cytotoxic drug. Biomedicine. 2021;**9**:508-527. DOI: 10.3390/biomedicines9050508

[116] Elbaz NM, Owen A, Rannard S, et al. Controlled synthesis of calcium carbonate nanoparticles and stimuli-responsive multi-layered nanocapsules for oral drug delivery. International Journal of Pharmaceutics. 2020;**574**:118866. DOI: 10.1016/j.ijpharm.2019.118866

[117] Chen Q, Li X, Xie Y, et al. Azo modified hyaluronic acid based nanocapsules: CD44 targeted, UV-responsive decomposition and drug release in liver cancer cells. Carbohydrate Polymers. 2021;**267**:118152. DOI: 10.1016/j.carbpol.2021.118152

[118] Chen Q, Li X, Xie Y, et al. Alginate-azo/chitosan nanocapsules in vitro drug delivery for hepatic carcinoma cells: UV-stimulated decomposition and drug release based on trans-to-cis isomerization. International Journal of Biological Macromolecules. 2021;**187**:214-222. DOI: 10.1016/j.ijbiomac.2021.07.119

[119] Fateh ST, Moradi L, Kohan E, et al. Comprehensive review on ultrasound-responsive theranostic nanomaterials: Mechanisms, structures and medical applications. Beilstein Journal of Nanotechnology. 2021;**12**:808-862. DOI: 10.3762/bjnano.12.64

[120] Yao M, Ma M, Xu H, et al. Small PLGA nanocapsules co-encapsulating copper sulfide nanodots and fluorocarbon compound for photoacoustic imaging-guided HIFU synergistic therapy. RSC Advances. 2018;**8**:4514-4524. DOI: 10.1039/c7ra12074e

[121] Topel SD, Balcioglu S, Ateş B, et al. Cellulose acetate encapsulated upconversion nanoparticles—A novel theranostic platform. Materials Today Communications. 2021;**26**:101829. DOI: 10.1016/j.mtcomm.2020.101829

[122] Zhang Y, García-Gabilondo M, Grayston A, et al. PLGA protein nanocarriers with tailor-made fluorescence/MRI/PET imaging modalities. Nanoscale. 2020;**12**:4988-5002. DOI: 10.1039/c9nr10620k

[123] Zhang Y, García-Gabilondo M, Rosell A, et al. Mri/photoluminescence dual-modal imaging magnetic PLGA nanocapsules for theranostics. Pharmaceutics. 2020;**12**:16-31. DOI: 10.3390/pharmaceutics12010016

[124] González-Gaitano G, Isasi JR, Vélaz I, et al. Drug carrier systems based on cyclodextrin supramolecular assemblies and polymers: Present and perspectives. Current Pharmaceutical Design. 2017;**23**:411-432. DOI: 10.2174/1381612823666161118145309

[125] Du XF, Li Y, Long J, et al. Fabrication of cisplatin-loaded polydopamine nanoparticles via supramolecular self-assembly for photoacoustic imaging guided chemo-photothermal cancer therapy. Applied Materials Today. 2021;**23**:101019. DOI: 10.1016/j.apmt.2021.101019

[126] Potara M, Nagy-Simon T, Focsan M, et al. Folate-targeted Pluronic-chitosan nanocapsules loaded with IR780 for near-infrared fluorescence imaging and photothermal-photodynamic therapy of ovarian cancer. Colloids Surfaces B Biointerfaces. 2021;**203**:111755. DOI: 10.1016/j.colsurfb.2021.111755

[127] Machado MGC, de Oliveira MA, Lanna EG, et al. Photodynamic therapy with the dual-mode association of IR780 to PEG-PLA nanocapsules and the effects on human breast cancer cells. Biomedicine & Pharmacotherapy. 2022;**145**:112464. DOI: 10.1016/j.biopha.2021.112464

[128] Nandwana V, Singh A, You MM, et al. Magnetic lipid nanocapsules (MLNCs): Self-assembled lipid-based nanoconstruct for non-invasive theranostic applications. Journal of Materials Chemistry B. 2018;**6**:1026-1034. DOI: 10.1039/c7tb03160b

[129] Wawrzyńczyk D, Bazylińska U, Lamch Ł, et al. Förster resonance energy transfer-activated processes in smart nanotheranostics fabricated in a sustainable manner. ChemSusChem. 2019;**12**:706-719. DOI: 10.1002/cssc.201801441

[130] Bilal M, Barani M, Sabir F, et al. Nanomaterials for the treatment and diagnosis of Alzheimer's disease: An overview. NanoImpact. 2020;**20**:100251. DOI: 10.1016/j.impact.2020.100251

[131] Mansour O, Peker T, Hamadi S, et al. Glucose-responsive capsules based on (phenylboronic-modified poly(lysine)/alginate) system. European Polymer Journal. 2019;**120**:109248. DOI: 10.1016/j.eurpolymj.2019.109248

[132] Qin X, Engwer C, Desai S, et al. An investigation of the interactions between an *E. coli* bacterial quorum sensing biosensor and chitosan-based nanocapsules. Colloids Surfaces B Biointerfaces. 2017;**149**:358-368. DOI: 10.1016/j.colsurfb.2016.10.031

Chapter 9

Plant Gum Based Drug Carriers

Melika Masoudi, Amirhossein Tashakor and Davood Mansury

Abstract

Recently, there have been various chemical carriers and routines for treatment of infections. Plant gum nanoparticles are being used greatly for this purpose. They have several advantages over chemical drug carriers including being biodegradable, biocompatible, nontoxic, providing better tolerance to the patient, and having fewer side effects. They also do not cause allergies in humans, do not irritate the skin or eyes, and have low production costs. The use of plant gums as drug carriers is limited due to a series of disadvantages. They may have microbial contamination because of the moisture in their content. Also, in storage, their viscosity decreases due to contact with water. By green nanoparticle synthesis of these plant gums as drug carriers, the disadvantages can be limited. There are several studies showing that plant gum drug carriers can have a great combination with various drugs and nanoparticles, thus they could be extremely effective against multi-resistant bacteria and even systemic illness like cancer. These days, the need for green synthesis of medicine and drug carriers has become quite popular and it will be even more essential in the future because of emerging antibiotic-resistant bacteria and climate change.

Keywords: plant gums, drug carriers, nanoparticle synthesis, antibacterial agents, silver nanoparticles

1. Introduction

The use of Synthetic polymers as drug carriers is common nowadays. They do have several advantages, yet there are noticeable disadvantages, including poor adaptation to the patient's body, high cost, and also causing acute and chronic side effects, for example poly-(methyl methacrylate) (PMMA) can cause skin and eye irritation. Other disadvantages of synthetic polymers utilized in tissue engineering include low biocompatibility, the release of acidic products during degradation that may cause systemic and native reactions, and rapid loss of mechanical strength [1].

The use of plant gum nanoparticles as drug carriers is one of the several ways that is employed greatly for the treatment of infections and various illnesses like cancer and this has been stated in various researches [2].

Plant gums are the native gum-producing trees, growing freely within the country's forests, and represent abundantly available materials. Plant-derived gums consist of polysaccharides and a few of them are applied medicinally for several years, including gum Tragacanth which has been used since third century B.C. Various studies have shown the advantage of using Green chemistry-based drug carriers for various purposes compared with using synthetic and chemical substances. Plant gum

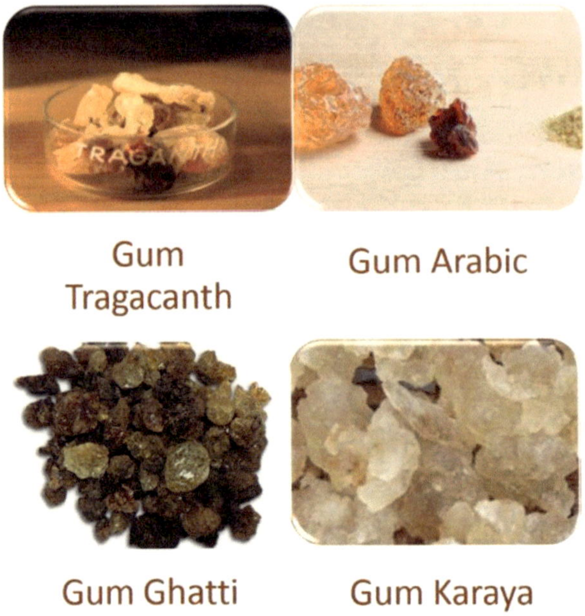

Figure 1.
The images related to the four famous plant gums: gum Tragacanth, gum Arabic, Gum Ghatti, gum Karaya.

drug carriers can have advantages in the pharmaceutical industry including being biodegradable, biocompatible, nontoxic, providing better tolerance to the patient, and having fewer side effects. They also do not cause allergies in humans, do not irritate the skin or eyes, and have low production costs [3]. The extensive use of antibiotics has led to serious issues including resistance toward multiple antibiotics. Now there are articles showing that the use of plant gum nanoparticles loaded with drugs was successful in the treatment of multi-drug resistant bacteria including MRSA,[1] VRE,[2] and MDR-GNB[3] [4, 5].

Natural gums constitute a structurally diverse class of biological macromolecules with a broad range of physicochemical properties, therefore they can be loaded with various drugs and can have a multi-target therapeutic effect. In this case, there will not be the need for consuming several drugs for the treatment of systemic disease.

That being said, the use of plant gums is limited due to a series of disadvantages. They may have microbial contamination because of the moisture in their content. Also, in storage, their viscosity decreases due to contact with water. This situation can be handled by creating nanoparticles from these plant gums and then using them as drug carriers. Green chemistry-based NPs[4] are often applied for designing and manufacturing products by applying sustainable materials which may eliminate or reduce the appliance and formation of unsafe and toxic substances. In this regard, plant gum polysaccharides and their nanostructures are often applied as drug carriers. Natural nanoparticles, improve the stability and bioavailability, as well as the biological distribution of natural products,

[1] Methicillin-resistant *Staphylococcus aureus*.

[2] Vancomycin-Resistant Enterococci.

[3] Multidrug-resistant Gram-negative bacteria.

[4] Nano-particles.

and also significantly reduce the adverse effects of drug uptake. That's why gum-based nano formulations for creating drug carriers have attracted a lot of attention [6].

The important tree exudate gums available on the market are as follows: gum Arabic (GA), gum Karaya (GK), gum Tragacanth (GT), Kondagogu gum (KG), gum Ghatti (GG), and gum Guar. **Figure 1** demonstrates the images related to the four of these famous plant gums. There also are several ways within which plant gum nanoparticles are created including mixing and agitation in a controlled environment, Microwave (MW)-assisted technique, ultrasonic irradiation, etc. The biosynthesis of nanoparticles, nanofibers, and composites for supported tree gums would be very beneficial within the pursuit of relevance to medication for various health issues.

The purpose of this chapter is to review the beneficial medical aspects of these plant gum-based drug carriers. There are several researches that have been done in order to show the advantages of these substances in infection and illness treatment. Various plant gums and routines have been used in order to create nanoparticles with minimum side effects which will be discussed in this chapter.

2. Chemical character and chemical composition of plant gums

Toxic reagents are used in the synthesis and stabilization of commercially generated metal/metal oxide nanoparticles, raising the danger of chemical contamination and acute toxicity, which should be considered in clinical applications. As a result of the rising need for environmentally acceptable technology for the synthesis of antimicrobial fillers, safer approaches with reduced toxicity have gotten a lot of attention. As eco-friendly production of metal/metal oxide nanostructures for purposes like drug delivery, diagnosis, bioengineering, bioremediation, catalysis, antibacterial and antifungal agents, etc. is anticipated in the future. Also, greener strategies for nanomaterials synthesis are still being explored [7].

Green chemistry is related to the practices that promote the development of medicine and processes that decrease or eliminate the usage and creation of hazardous compounds. Biopolymers including cellulose, chitosan, dextran, and tree gums, for example, are frequently utilized as reducing and stabilizing agents in metal NP production. Plant-based ingredients (extracts, stems, gums, seeds, and fruits), among other biological sources, have been shown to be an efficient constituent for synthesizing nanoparticles while maintaining other important factors such as material cost, large-scale production capacity, and potential uses in a variety of applications. The pressure, temperature, solvent, and pH of the medium all play a role in the plant-based biogenic production of nanomaterials [8].

Gum Arabic, gum Karaya, gum Kondagogu, gum Tragacanth, gum Ghatti, Cashew gum, Guar gum, Olibanum gum, and Neem gum, are some examples of greener alternatives with useful chemical properties that have been successfully used for the production and stabilization of NPs.

3. Natural gum characteristics and sources and ways to create green nanofibers

Natural gums, which belong to the polysaccharide family, are often used to increase the viscosity of solutions, even at low concentrations. Natural gums are hydrophobic substances mostly obtained from plants or bacteria. Because the gum molecules are biological, they have a wide range of linear chain lengths, branching features, molecular weight, and other characteristics. Gums are divided into four categories based on their source of origin: (a) plant exudate gum (such as gum Karaya, Salai gum, and gum Arabic), (b) seed gum (such as Guar gum, Locust bean gum, and Tamarind gum), (c) microbial gum (such as Xanthan gum, Gellan gum, and Dextran gum), and (d) marine gums (such as alginic acids) [9].

Various techniques are used in the green synthesis of nanofibers. The plant extracts will be used in: (a) mixing and agitation in a controlled environment, (b) autoclaving, (c) microwave (MW)-assisted technique, (d) ultrasonic irradiation, and (e) UV/visible light irradiation.

3.1 Gum Arabic

3.1.1 Chemical composition

Gum Arabic (GA) is a polysaccharide having branching chains of [1–3] connected β-D-galactopyranosyl units comprising α-L-arabinofuranosy, α-L-rhamnopyranosyl, β-D-glucuronopyranosyl, and 4-O-methyl-β-D-glucuronopyranosyl units. It is a water-soluble dietary fiber. Ca^{2+}, K^{+}, and Mg^{2+} are abundant in GA. GA is made from the dried gummy exudates of *Acacia senegal*'s stems and branches. Microorganisms in the colon break down GA into short-chain fatty acids [10].

3.1.2 Manufacturing and application

GA is one of the safest dietary fibers, according to the US Food and Drug Administration. GA is used to treat individuals with chronic kidney disease and end-stage renal disease in Middle Eastern nations [10].

Using a simple and practical approach for making Au nano-architectures with branching forms of GA is considered critical for the intriguing anisotropic. Au structures are beneficial in a variety of research domains. Using gold nanoparticles, reducing agents, and assembling them on gum Arabic under sonication for around 20 minutes at room temperature is described as a natural drug delivery agent [11].

Through a chemical reduction, with the help of gum Arabic, Au particles with a variety of morphologies (e.g., flower-shaped and confieto-shaped) are effectively created. Au nano-flower shapes can have high biocompatibility with human bladder cancer cells (T-24), which might be used in biomedical applications. Sonicating a combination of gum Arabic solution with $KAuBr_4$ and ascorbic acid for around five seconds at room temperature can result in a well-organized approach for manufacturing gold nano-flowers [12].

Gum Arabic can also be used as a drug carrier in order to increase the solubility and stability of curcumin under physiological pH conditions. The compound may demonstrate anticancer activity in human hepatocellular carcinoma (Hep G2) cells, which is claimed to be higher than in human breast carcinoma (MCF-7) cells. Hep G2 cells show a faster accumulation of gum Arabic/curcumin NPs due to the high effectiveness of targeting the galactose groups present in gum Arabic, bypassing the prior hurdles and making it appropriate for drug delivery systems [13].

Biocompatible gold NPs can be created by continuously mixing an aqueous gum Arabic solution (0.2 percent), phosphine amino acid, and $NaAuCl_4$ together. The produced NPs can be used as molecular imaging contrast agents and can exhibit in vitro and in vivo endurance for months in aqueous, salt, and buffered solutions using an X-ray computed tomography scan [14].

In a study, using gum Arabic as a bio-template, a cost-effective and simple one-step technique for the manufacture of extremely stable molybdenum trioxide (MoO_3) nanoparticles was devised. The cytotoxic effects of the NP were measured using 2,3-bis-(2-methoxy-4-nitro-5-sulfophenyl)-2H-tetrazolium-5-carboxanilide assays in Hep G2 (human liver cancer) and HEK293 (human embryonic kidney) cell lines. MoO_3 nanoparticles are benign to Hep G2 cell lines and have low toxicity even at extremely high concentrations (1000 ppm), but have significant toxicity to HEK293 cells, according to the findings of this study [15].

Antibacterial activities of gum Arabic as drug carriers are stated in **Table 2**.

3.2 Gum Karaya

3.2.1 Chemical composition

Natural polysaccharide gum Karaya (GK, Sterculiaurens) is a plant exudates widely available and relatively cheap biomaterial, which is used in food and medical industry. However, GK is insoluble in water and it limits subsequent processing and broader utilization in medicine. That's why it's necessary to use nanoparticles in order to limit this situation [16].

One of the key challenges with inorganic nanoparticles as a medicine delivery technology is their biocompatibility. Sugars, hydrocolloids, and plant extracts have all been proven to have the potential to be used in the green production of biocompatible gold nanoparticles.

3.2.2 Manufacturing and application

The manufacture of gum Karaya (GK) stabilized gold nanoparticles (GKNP)[5] and their application in the delivery of anticancer medicines is described in Ref. [17]. GKNP showed great biocompatibility toward CHO,[6] normal ovary cells, and A549 human non-small cell lung cancer cells. The anti-cancer medication gemcitabine hydrochloride (GEM) was loaded on the surface of gum Karaya with a drug loading efficiency of 19.2%. In anti-proliferation and various experiments, GEM-loaded nanoparticles (GEM-GNP) inhibited cancer cell growth more than regular GEM. This impact was linked to GEM-GNP producing more reactive oxygen species in A549 cells than GEM alone. In conclusion, GK offers tremendous promise for the manufacture of biocompatible gold nanoparticles that might be exploited as a possible anticancer drug delivery carrier. This study also stated that gum Karaya loaded with gold nanoparticles has a longer shelf life and is extremely resistant to factors such as pH and salt. The GK-Au NP combination demonstrated effectiveness as a drug carrier and improved colloidal stability for Au NPs in human lung cancer cells, outperforming the drug gemcitabine hydrochloride in anticancer activity, colony formation suppression, and ROS generation.

Gum Karaya can also be used as a drug carrier for copper oxide (CuO) nanoparticles which have gained a lot of interest because of their catalytic, electric, optical, photonic, textile, Nanofluid, and antibacterial properties, which

[5] Gum Karaya stabilized gold nanoparticles.
[6] Chinese hamster ovary cells.

is based on their size, shape, and surrounding medium. Green technology can be used to make CuO nanoparticles put on the surface of the gum Karaya, which is a harmless natural hydrocolloid. In a study, a colloid-thermal synthesis technique was used to make the CuO nanoparticles. The mixture was kept at 75°C at 250 rpm for 1 h in an orbital shaker with varied concentrations of $CuCl_2 \cdot 2H_2O$ (1 mM, 2 mM, and 3 mM) and gum Karaya (10 mg/mL). CuO nanoparticles of various sizes were obtained by purifying and drying the CuO nanoparticles that had been produced [18].

3.3 Kondagogu gum

3.3.1 Chemical composition

Gum Kondagogu (Cochlospermumgossypium) maybe a tree exudate gum that belongs to the family Bixaceae. Compositional analysis of the gum by HPLC and LC-MS revealed uronic acids to be the key component of the polymer (~26 mol%). Furthermore, analysis of the gum by GC-MS indicated the presence of sugars like arabinose (2.52 mol%), mannose (8.30 mol%), α-D-glucose (2.48 mol%), β-D-glucose (2.52 mol%), rhamnose (12.85 mol%), galactose (18.95 mol%), D-glucuronic acid (19.26 mol%), β-D-galactouronic acid (13.22 mol%), and α-D-galacturonic acid (11.22 mol%). The viscoelastic behavior of gum Kondagogu solutions (1 and 2%) in aqueous as well as in 100 mM NaCl solution shows a unique gel-like system, making it suitable for being used as a drug carrier [19].

3.3.2 Manufacturing and application

Gum Kondagogu (GK) has been used to reduce and cap gold nanoparticle constructions in recent investigations [20].

Antibacterial activity of Kondagogu gum loaded with AuNPs against *Escherichia coli* and *Bacillus subtilis* is reported to be excellent [21].

Using gum Kondagogu, a natural biopolymer, as a reducing and stabilizing agent, for delivering silver nanoparticles has shown to be beneficial. The effect of several factors on the production of nanoparticles was investigated, including gum particle size, gum concentration, silver nitrate concentration, and reaction time. The silver nanoparticles are easily incorporated for diverse applications since they have the best functional properties [22].

A study used sodium borohydride as a reductant and gum Kondagogu as a stabilizer to create selenium nanoparticles (Se NPs). Plant gum is a biopolymer-based feedstock that is sustainable, non-toxic, and non-immunogenic. Using ultraviolet-visible spectroscopy and dynamic light scattering, the role of gum on synthesis and mean particle size was investigated. In comparison to ionic Se, the current work shows that tree gum stabilized Se NPs may be used as a strong antioxidant nutrition supplement at a significantly lower dose [23].

Another study employed a two-stage chemical reduction approach to make copper nanoparticles (CuNPs), with a distinct reducing agent Hydrazine Hydrate (HH), and a separate stabilizing agent Gum Kondagogu extract. The anti-biofilm impact of gum Kondagogu extract stabilized copper NPs against clinical isolate *Klebsiella pneumoniae* was investigated, and the results revealed that the copper NPs film had an efficient anti-biofilm effect [24].

3.4 Gum Ghatti

3.4.1 Chemical composition

Gum Ghatti is a proteinaceous exudate tree gum. It is utilized in traditional medicine. The exudate gum has a glass-like appearance and the color is from dark red to white based on the shape of it which can be either a nodule or spiro [25].

3.4.2 Manufacturing and application

A simple and environmentally acceptable green approach for producing silver nanoparticles from silver nitrate has been devised, utilizing gum Ghatti (Anogeissuslatifolia) as a reducing and stabilizing agent. This approach can have various benefits including better treatment of bacterial illnesses.

The non-toxic, renewable plant polymer gum Ghatti was used as both the reducing and stabilizing agent in a simple and green way to make palladium nanoparticles from palladium chloride. The development of deep brown color and wide continuous absorption spectra in the UV-visible range verified the synthesis of palladium nanoparticles. At a considerably lower nanoparticle dosage, the nanoparticles demonstrated improved antioxidant activity. To evaluate the homogeneous catalytic activity of palladium nanoparticles, dyes such as coomassie brilliant blue G-250, methyl orange, methylene blue, and a nitro compound, 4-nitrophenol, were reduced using sodium borohydride. The nanoparticles showed high catalytic activity in dye degradation, and the findings suggest that biogenic palladium nanoparticles might be used as a nanocatalyst in environmental remediation [26].

Because of the unique intrinsic catalytic properties of diverse size, shape, and surface-functionalized gold nanoparticles, their prospective applications in disciplines such as drug transport, diagnostics and biosensor are being investigated. However, the traditional method of production of these metallic nanoparticles employs hazardous chemicals as reducing agents, an extra capping agent for stability, and surface functionalization for drug delivery objectives. Gum Ghatti can be a great drug delivery option for stabilizing this nanoparticle [27].

3.5 Gum tragacanth

3.5.1 Chemical composition, manufacturing and application

The aqueous extract of gum Tragacanth (Astragalusgummifer), a renewable, nontoxic natural phyto-exudate, can be used to develop a simple and environmentally acceptable technique for the green production of silver nanoparticles. Reductants and stabilizers are provided by the gum's water-soluble components. The probable functional groups involved in nanoparticle reduction and capping have also been identified [28].

The sol-gel technique can be used to make $Ni_{0.35}Cu_{0.25}Zn_{0.4}Fe_2O_4$ nanoparticles utilizing Tragacanth gum as a bio-template and Metals nitrate as a metal supply. The advantages of this approach include a simple set-up, moderate reaction conditions, quick reaction periods, the use of a cost-effective catalyst, and good product yields. The catalyst may be easily recycled and reused several times without losing its catalytic activity [29].

Plant gums	NPs
Gum Arabic	Magnetite, Cu, Ag, Se, Au, Zn, Zein-curcumin, Chitosan/GA, Fe_3O_4
Gum Karaya	Ag, Cu, Au, Magnetite, Pt, Fe_3O_4
Gum Kondagogu	Ag, Au, Cu, Pd, Pt, Ti, Fe_3O_4, Ag_2S
Gum Tragacanth	Ag, ZnO, TiO_2, Carbon dots, Au
Gum Ghatti	Pd, Magnetite, Ag, Au
Guar gum	Ag, Au, Pd, Pt Magnetite, Zn, Palmshell extract/chitosan
Cashew gum	Ag, ZnO
Gellan gum	TiO_2, Ag
Xanthan gum	Au
Gum Olibanum	Ag

Table 1.
Greener synthesis of NPs using plant gums.

Nano-particles that can be loaded on plant gums are stated briefly in **Table 1**.

4. Using plant gums loaded with NPs as antibacterial agents

Different studies have illustrated the benefits of using Plant gums loaded with NPs as antibacterial agents. Metallic NPs and other components can have various antibacterial effects based on the type of plant gum drug carriers and their way of production.

4.1 Silver nanoparticles

These NPs can be loaded on different plant gum drug carriers for various anti-bacterial purposes. AgNPs have a strong bactericidal and catalytic effect according to various studies and they are extremely beneficial for preventing drug-resistant bacteria.

In a study, Gum acacia was loaded with silver NPs mixed with structures of HDN (fruit flavonoid). In this essay, after the preparation of GA-AgNPs (Gum acacia silver NPs loaded with NP structures of HDN), a Bactericidal assay was performed by incubating 108 colony-forming units per mL of MRSA and *E. coli* K1 with various concentrations of GA-AgNPs-HDN and respective controls in 1.5 mL centrifuge tubes at 37°C for 2 h. For negative controls, untreated bacterial cultures were incubated with PBS,[7] while 100 μg/mL gentamicin-treated bacteria were used as positive control. The result for this essay is stated in **Table 2**.

In another study, gum Tragacanth was used as a drug carrier for Ag NPs. The well-diffusion method was used to study the antibacterial activity of the synthesized silver nanoparticles. Bacterial suspension was prepared by growing a single colony of Gram-positive bacterial strain *S. aureus* and Gram-negative bacterial strains *E. coli* and *P. aeruginosa* overnight in nutrient broth and by adjusting the turbidity to 0.5 McFarland standard. Mueller Hinton agar plates were inoculated with this bacterial suspension,

[7] Phosphate buffer saline.

Plant gums loaded with NPs	Result	Antibacterial activity against	Reference
GA-AgNPs	Bactericidal effect of this nanoparticle was more significant on *E. coli* K1 infections than MRSA infections, indicating that this component is more effective on Gram-negative bacteria than Gram-positive but overall these NPs have more bactericidal effects than chemicals	MRSA and *E. coli* K1	[30]
Gum Tragacanth loaded with Silver Nanoparticles	The inhibition zone of about 1 1. 5 ± 0 mm was observed around the Gram-positive bacteria. For Gram-negative bacterial strains *E. coli* and *P. aeruginosa* the inhibition zone was reported 9. 5 ± 0. 4 and 1 0. 5 ± 0, respectively. In the case of positive control plates loaded with erythromycin discs, growth inhibition was noted much less than the loaded NPs	Gram-positive bacterial strain *S. aureus* and Gram-negative bacterial strains *E. coli* and *P. aeruginosa*	[28]
P. domestica gum loaded Silver NPs	*P. domestica* gum-loaded silver nanoparticles can have a potential antibacterial effect against *S. aureus* (19.7 ± 0.4 mm) and *E. coli* (14.4 ± 0.7 mm), and *P. aeruginosa* (13.1 ± 0.2 mm). although this study suggests that streptomycin has an antibacterial effect of higher magnitude as compared to *P. domestica* gum-loaded silver nanoparticles against the tested bacterial strains (23.6 ± 0.8 mm, 21.8 ± 0.2 mm, and 18.6 ± 0.3 mm)	Gram-positive (*Staphylococcus aureus*), Gram-negative (*E. coli*), and *P. aeruginosa*	[2]
P. domestica gum loaded Gold NPs	Gum-loaded gold nanoparticles had the least effect on foregoing bacteria (*S. aureus* (10.5 ± 0.6 mm), *E. coli* (10 ± 0.4) mm, and *P. aeruginosa* (8.2 ± 0.3 mm)) compared to *P. domestica* gum loaded silver NPs and streptomycin	Gram-positive (*S. aureus*), Gram-negative (*Escherichia coli*), and *P. aeruginosa*	[2]
CS/PVA/GG	SEM results showed that surface morphology was more affected by mixing and bonding ratios. Also, The FTIR and XRD confirmed the strong intermolecular bonding between polymers. The study suggests that these blends have great potential to be used against *Pasteurella multocida*, *S. aureus*, *E. coli*, and *B. subtilis* bacterial agents since they managed to have a great bactericidal effect on these organisms	*P. multocida*, *S. aureus*, *E. coli*, and *B. subtilis*	[31]
Gum Karaya loaded with Copper oxide (CuO)	Bactericidal effect on both Gram-negative and positive cultures, especially, smaller NPs (4.8 ± 1.6 nm), which are highly stable and have maximum zone of inhibition compared to the larger size of synthesized CuO nanoparticles (7.8 ± 2.3 nm)	Gram-negative and positive cultures	[18]
Kondagogu gum loaded with Gold nanoparticles	The AuNPs showed good antibacterial activity against *E. coli* and *Bacillus subtilis.*	*E. coli* and *B. subtilis*	[21]

Plant gums loaded with NPs	Result	Antibacterial activity against	Reference
Kondagogu gum loaded with Silver nanoparticles	The minimum inhibitory concentration values were lower by 3.2- and 16-folds for Gram-positive *S. aureus* and Gram-negative *E. coli* strains, respectively. The minimum bactericidal concentration values were lower by 4 and 50-folds. Thus, the biogenic silver nanoparticles were found to be more potent bactericidal agents in terms of concentration. The study implies that this NP has strong effects on biofilms, indicating that it can have great effect on drug-resistant bacterial infections caused by biofilms. Also, the growth curve stated a faster inhibition in Gram-negative bacteria as compared to Gram-positive	Gram-positive *S. aureus* and Gram-negative *E. coli*	[32]
Gum Kondagogu loaded with Selenium nanoparticles	In this study, NPs exhibited growth inhibition activity against Gram-positive bacteria only. *B. subtilis* and *Micrococcus luteus* showed respective inhibition zones of 6.3 and 8.6 mm at 12 μg. This study implies that the tree gum stabilized Se NPs have more applicability as a potent antioxidant nutrition supplement at a much lower dose, in comparison with ionic Se.	*B. subtilis* and *M. luteus*	[23]
Gum Kondagogu loaded with Copper nanoparticles	Anti-biofilm effect of gum Kondagogu extract stabilized copper NPs against clinical isolate *Klebsiella Pneumoniae* was demonstrated in this study	*Klebsiella Pneumoniae*	[24]

Table 2.
Plant gums loaded with NPs as antibacterial agents.

and 5 μg of Gum Tragacanth loaded with silver nanoparticles were added to the center well with a diameter of 6 mm. Culture plates loaded with discs of antibiotic, erythromycin (15 μg/disc) were included as positive controls. The result of this research is stated in **Table 2**.

Silver NPs can also be loaded on *P. domestica* plant gum according to research performed in 2017, which showed an antibacterial effect on both Gram-positive (*Staphylococcus aureus*) and Gram-negative (*E. coli* and *P. aeruginosa*) bacteria. Disc diffusion method was used for Antibacterial assay using Gram-positive (*S. aureus*), Gram-negative (*Escherichia coli*), and *Pseudomonas aeruginosa*, three independent experiments were carried out for each bacterial strain with streptomycin as the positive control. Au/Ag-NPs (5 μg) were dissolved in DMSO[8] and incubated at 30°C for 24 h. the result and reference for this article are stated in the table down below.

Kondagogu gum loaded with silver nanoparticles also demonstrated antibacterial effect against Gram-positive *S. aureus* and Gram-negative *E. coli*. Variety of susceptibility assays was done in this study in order to demonstrate the antibacterial effects including micro-broth dilution, anti-biofilm activity, growth kinetics, cytoplasmic content leakage, membrane permeabilization, etc. The production of reactive oxygen

[8] D-methyl-sulfoxide.

species (ROS) and cell surface damage during bacterial nanoparticle interaction were also demonstrated using dichlorodihydrofluorescein diacetate, N-acetylcysteine; and scanning electron microscopy and energy-dispersive X-ray spectra.

4.2 Gold nanoparticles

Gold nanoparticles (AuNPs) can also be loaded on various plant gum drug carriers and be used as antibacterial agents. Gold nanoparticles (AuNPs) have exceptional stability against oxidation and therefore may play a significant role in the advancement of clinically useful diagnostic and therapeutic Nanomedicines. That being said, conventional process for synthesis of these metallic nanoparticles utilizes toxic reagents as reducing agents, additional capping agents for stability as well as surface functionalization for drug delivery purposes.

Just like silver NPs, *P. domestica* gum can also be loaded with AuNPs. Preparation and assessment in this study were performed like *P. domestica* gum-loaded silver NPs and the antibacterial effect was studied on Gram-positive (*S. aureus*), Gram-negative (*E. coli* and *P. aeruginosa*) bacteria.

Kondagogu gum is also one of the drug carriers that was used in a study for AuNPs in order to demonstrate their effects on *E. coli* and *Bacillus subtilis*. After the preparation of these NPs, their concentration, and reaction time on the synthesis of AuNPs were investigated by using techniques like UV-visible spectroscopy, FTIR, and XRD.

4.3 Copper nanoparticles

These nanoparticles may have great antibacterial effects if they are loaded on suitable plant gum drug carriers.

In a study, copper oxide (CuO) was used as a NP and was loaded on gum Karaya. The CuO nanoparticles were synthesized by a colloid-thermal synthesis process. The synthesized CuO was purified and dried to obtain different sizes of CuO nanoparticles. The well diffusion method was used to study the antibacterial activity of the synthesized CuO nanoparticles on gram-negative and positive cultures. The zone of inhibition, minimum inhibitory concentration, and minimum bactericidal concentration were determined by the broth microdilution method.

Gum Kondagogu loaded with Copper is another example of using plant gums as drug carriers for copper nanoparticles. The synthesized CuNPs were characterized by using Transmission Electron Microscopy (TEM), SEM, UV-visible spectroscopy, XRD, and FTIR experimental methods and then were tested on *Klebsiella Pneumoniae.*

4.4 Other nanoparticles

Various chemicals and drugs can be loaded on plant gums which can have a great antibacterial effects. For instance, in a study, chitosan and polyvinyl alcohol were loaded on Guar gum (CS/PVA/GG), then their effects were studied on *Pasteurella multocida*, *S. aureus*, *E. coli*, and *B. subtilis.* After the preparation of a mixture of chitosan/poly (vinyl alcohol)/guar gum (CS/PVA/GG), the ratio of swelling, together with antimicrobial properties, was studied. These components were characterized by scanning electron microscopy (SEM), Fourier Transform Infra-red (FTIR), and X-ray powder diffraction (XRD).

In another stud, selenium nanoparticles (Se NPs) were loaded on Gum Kondagogu. Role of gum on synthesis and mean particle size was studied using ultraviolet-visible spectroscopy and dynamic light scattering. Size of the NPs was determined (from 44.4 to 200 nm) and mean particle size was 105.6 nm. Antibacterial potential of these NPs on *B. subtilis* and *Micrococcus luteus* were checked with well diffusion assay.

It should be stated that the results for these studies and their related references are stated in the table down below.

5. Conclusion

Plant-based synthesis and stabilization of metal/metal oxide NPs have been successfully implemented by many researchers worldwide. These techniques have various advantages including being more affordable physically and financially, having better drug distribution, and having easier production. The major drawbacks of this method include the use of imprecise evaluation tools for the stability, aggregation behavior, size, shape of the NPs, and the subsequent systematic description of the application of the NPs as a result of their physical and chemical characteristics.

Based on these articles, using plant gums alone is less effective than being loaded with NPs substances and on some occasions, they even may have side effects on human body. For an instant, guar gum can lead to infection because of its high moisture if it's not loaded with NPs.

Various metallic or non-metallic NPs can be created and added to these plant gums. Most frequent of them in these studies are AgNPs and AuNPs. Gold nanoparticles (AuNPs) have exceptional stability against oxidation, and therefore, may play a significant role in the advancement of clinically useful diagnostic and therapeutic Nanomedicines. That being said, conventional process for synthesis of these metallic nanoparticles utilizes toxic reagents as reducing agents, additional capping agents for stability as well as surface functionalization for drug delivery purposes. Also, according to various studies, they are less effective against microorganisms than AgNPs. AgNPs have a strong bactericidal and catalytic effect according to various studies. They are extremely beneficial for preventing drug-resistant bacteria which will be a huge issue in the future.

The influence of different parameters such as gum particle size, concentration of gum, concentration of silver nitrate, and reaction time on the synthesis of nanoparticles is quite significant in various studies. For instants, smaller NPs can have more bactericidal effects compared to their bigger counterparts. Thus, using the right concentration and technique for making these NPs are very important and should be considered.

The future use of tree gums also relies on the development of ultralightweight, high, strength, bio-based, biodegradable, porous, and tunable, two-dimensional (2D) membranes, and three-dimensional (3D) sponges with facile and easy to implement synthetic schemes. Each year scientists are getting more keen on researching about these green NPs because of various reasons including the significant growth in the number of antibiotic-resistant bacteria or climate change. Also, these NPs can be afforded and produced easily.

Acknowledgements

This study was supported by Isfahan University of Medical Sciences, Isfahan, Iran.

DM: designed the study. Supervised, conceptualized the paper, and edited the manuscript, **MM** and **AT** Conducted research and performed writing the manuscript.

Abbreviations

PMMA	poly-methyl methacrylate
MDR-GNB	multidrug-resistant Gram-negative bacteria
VRE	Vancomycin-Resistant Enterococci
MRSA	methicillin-resistant *S. aureus*
NPs	Nano-particles
GA	gum Arabic
GK	gum Karaya
GT	gum Tragacanth
KG	Kondagogu gum
GG	gum Ghatti
Hep G2	hepatocellular carcinoma cells
MCF-7	human breast carcinoma cells
GKNP	gum Karaya stabilized gold nanoparticles
CHO	chinese hamster ovary cells
GEM	gemcitabine hydrochloride
GEM-GNP	gemcitabine hydrochloride loaded nanoparticles
HH	hydrazine hydrate
CuNPs	copper nanoparticles
SGG	selenium-infused guar gum nanoparticles
PBS	phosphate buffer saline
DMSO	D-methyl-sulfoxide
CS/PVA/GG	chitosan/poly(vinyl alcohol)/guar gum
GA-AgNPs	gum acacia silver NPs
HDN	fruit flavonoid
SEM	scanning electron microscopy
FTIR	Fourier Transform Infra-red
XRD	X-ray powder diffraction
AuNPs	gold nanoparticles
AgNPs	silver nanoparticles
CuNPs	copper nanoparticles
Se NPs	selenium nanoparticles
ROS	reactive oxygen species

Author details

Melika Masoudi[1], Amirhossein Tashakor[2] and Davood Mansury[2]*

1 Department of Veterinary Surgery, Tehran University, Tehran, Iran

2 Department of Microbiology, School of Medicine, Isfahan University of Medical Sciences, Isfahan, Iran

*Address all correspondence to: mansuryd@med.mui.ac.ir

References

[1] Khan I, Saeed K, Khan I. Nanoparticles: Properties, applications and toxicities. Arabian Journal of Chemistry. 2019;**12**(7):908-931

[2] Islam NU, Amin R, Shahid M, Amin M, Zaib S, Iqbal J. A multi-target therapeutic potential of Prunusdomestica gum stabilized nanoparticles exhibited prospective anticancer, antibacterial, urease-inhibition, anti-inflammatory and analgesic properties. BMC Complementary and Alternative Medicine. 2017;**17**(1):1-17

[3] Abulafatih H. Medicinal plants in southwestern Saudi Arabia. Economic Botany. 1987;**41**(3):354-360

[4] Siddiqui AH, Koirala J. *Methicillin Resistant Staphylococcus aureus*. Europe: StatPearls; 2020

[5] Levitus M, Rewane A, Perera TB. Vancomycin-Resistant Enterococci (VRE). Europe: StatPearls; 2020

[6] Patra JK, Das G, Fraceto LF, Campos EVR, del Pilar R-TM, Acosta-Torres LS, et al. Nano based drug delivery systems: Recent developments and future prospects. Journal of Nanobiotechnology. 2018;**16**(1):1-33

[7] Padil VV, Zare EN, Makvandi P, Černík M. Nanoparticles and nanofibres based on tree gums: Biosynthesis and applications. Comprehensive Analytical Chemistry. 2021;**94**:223-265

[8] Nguyen NH, Padil VVT, Slaveykova VI, Černík M, Ševců A. Green synthesis of metal and metal oxide nanoparticles and their effect on the unicellular alga Chlamydomonasreinhardtii. Nanoscale Research Letters. 2018;**13**(1):1-13

[9] Sharma G, Sharma S, Kumar A, Ala'a H, Naushad M, Ghfar AA, et al. Guar gum and its composites as potential materials for diverse applications: A review. Carbohydrate Polymers. 2018;**199**:534-545

[10] Nasir O. Renal and extrarenal effects of gum arabic (*Acacia senegal*)-what can be learned from animal experiments? Kidney and Blood Pressure Research. 2013;**37**(4-5):269-279

[11] Wang L, Imura M, Yamauchi Y. Tailored synthesis of various Au nanoarchitectures with branched shapes. CrystEngComm. 2012;**14**(22):7594-7599

[12] Wang L, Liu C-H, Nemoto Y, Fukata N, Wu KC-W, Yamauchi Y. Rapid synthesis of biocompatible gold nanoflowers with tailored surface textures with the assistance of amino acid molecules. RSC Advances. 2012;**2**(11):4608-4611

[13] Sivan SK, Padinjareveetil AK, Padil VV, Pilankatta R, George B, Senan C, et al. Greener assembling of MoO 3 nanoparticles supported on gum arabic: Cytotoxic effects and catalytic efficacy towards reduction of p-nitrophenol. Clean Technologies and Environmental Policy. 2019;**21**(8):1549-1561

[14] Kattumuri V, Katti K, Bhaskaran S, Boote EJ, Casteel SW, Fent GM, et al. Gum arabic as a phytochemical construct for the stabilization of gold nanoparticles: In vivo pharmacokinetics and X-ray-contrast-imaging studies. Small. 2007;**3**(2):333-341

[15] Kothaplamoottil Sivan S, Padinjareveetil AK, Padil VV,

Pilankatta R, George B, Senan C, et al. Greener assembling of MoO3 nanoparticles supported on gum arabic: Cytotoxic effects and catalytic efficacy towards reduction of p-nitrophenol. Clean Technologies and Environmental Policy. 2019;**21**(8):1549-1561

[16] Postulkova H, Chamradova I, Pavlinak D, Humpa O, Jancar J, Vojtova L. Study of effects and conditions on the solubility of natural polysaccharide gum karaya. Food Hydrocolloids. 2017;**67**:148-156

[17] Pooja D, Panyaram S, Kulhari H, Reddy B, Rachamalla SS, Sistla R. Natural polysaccharide functionalized gold nanoparticles as biocompatible drug delivery carrier. International Journal of Biological Macromolecules (India). 2015;**80**:48-56

[18] Padil VVT, Černík M. Green synthesis of copper oxide nanoparticles using gum karaya as a biotemplate and their antibacterial application. International Journal of Nanomedicine. 2013;**8**:889

[19] Vinod V, Sashidhar R, Sarma V, VijayaSaradhi U. Compositional analysis and rheological properties of gum kondagogu (Cochlospermumgossypium): A tree gum from India. Journal of Agricultural and Food Chemistry. 2008;**56**(6):2199-2207

[20] Selvi SK, Kumar JM, Sashidhar R. Anti-proliferative activity of Gum kondagogu (Cochlospermumgossypium)-gold nanoparticle constructs on B16F10 melanoma cells: An in vitro model. Bioactive Carbohydrates and Dietary Fibre. 2017;**11**:38-47

[21] Seku K, Gangapuram BR, Pejjai B, Hussain M, Hussaini SS, Golla N, et al. Eco-friendly synthesis of gold nanoparticles using carboxymethylated gum Cochlospermumgossypium (CMGK) and their catalytic and antibacterial applications. Chemical Papers. 2019;**73**(7):1695-1704

[22] Rastogi L, Sashidhar R, Karunasagar D, Arunachalam J. Gum kondagogu reduced/stabilized silver nanoparticles as direct colorimetric sensor for the sensitive detection of Hg2+ in aqueous system. Talanta. 2014;**118**:111-117

[23] Kora AJ. Tree gum stabilised selenium nanoparticles: Characterisation and antioxidant activity. IET Nanobiotechnology. 2018;**12**(5):658-662

[24] Suresh Y, Annapurna S, Singh A, Chetana A, Pasha C, Bhikshamaiah G. Characterization and evaluation of anti-biofilm effect of green synthesized copper nanoparticles. Materials Today: Proceedings. 2016;**3**(6):1678-1685

[25] Al-Assaf S, Phillips GO, Amar V. Gum ghatti: Handbook of hydrocolloids. Elsevier; 2021. pp. 653-672

[26] Kora AJ. Multifaceted activities of plant gum synthesised platinum nanoparticles: Catalytic, peroxidase, PCR enhancing and antioxidant activities. IET Nanobiotechnology. 2019;**13**(6):602-608

[27] Alam MS, Garg A, Pottoo FH, Saifullah MK, Tareq AI, Manzoor O, et al. Gum ghatti mediated, one pot green synthesis of optimized gold nanoparticles: Investigation of process-variables impact using Box-Behnken based statistical design. International Journal of Biological Macromolecules. 2017;**104**:758-767

[28] Kora AJ, Arunachalam J. Green fabrication of silver nanoparticles by gum tragacanth (Astragalusgummifer): A dual functional reductant and

stabilizer. Journal of Nanomaterials. 2012;**2012**

[29] TaghaviFardood S, Ramazani A, Golfar Z, Joo SW. Green synthesis of Ni-Cu-Zn ferrite nanoparticles using tragacanth gum and their use as an efficient catalyst for the synthesis of polyhydroquinoline derivatives. Applied Organometallic Chemistry. 2017;**31**(12):e3823

[30] Anwar A, Masri A, Rao K, Rajendran K, Khan NA, Shah MR, et al. Antimicrobial activities of green synthesized gums-stabilized nanoparticles loaded with flavonoids. Scientific Reports. 2019;**9**(1):1-12

[31] Iqbal DN, Shafiq S, Khan SM, Ibrahim SM, Abubshait SA, Nazir A, et al. Novel chitosan/guar gum/PVA hydrogel: Preparation, characterization and antimicrobial activity evaluation. International Journal of Biological Macromolecules. 2020;**164**:499-509

[32] Kora AJ, Sashidhar R. Biogenic silver nanoparticles synthesized with rhamnogalacturonan gum: Antibacterial activity, cytotoxicity and its mode of action. Arabian Journal of Chemistry. 2018;**11**(3):313-323